Biosimilarity

The FDA Perspective

Biosimilarity

The FDA Perspective

Sarfaraz K. Niazi, PhD, SI, FRSB, FPAMS, FACB
Adjunct Professor, Biopharmaceutical Sciences, University of Illinois (U.S.), University of Houston (U.S.), HEJ Research Institute (PK), and National University of Science and Technology (PK), Founder, Karyo Biologics, LLC (U.S.), Adello Biologics (U.S.), and Pharmaceutical Scientist, INC (U.S.)

CRC Press
Taylor & Francis Group
Boca Raton London New York

CRC Press is an imprint of the
Taylor & Francis Group, an **informa** business

CRC Press
Taylor & Francis Group
6000 Broken Sound Parkway NW, Suite 300
Boca Raton, FL 33487-2742

Printed on acid-free paper
Version Date: 20151116

International Standard Book Number-13: 978-1-4987-5039-4 (Hardback)

Library of Congress Cataloging-in-Publication Data

Names: Niazi, Sarfaraz, 1949- , author.
Title: Biosimilarity : the FDA perspective / Sarfaraz K. Niazi.
Description: Boca Raton : Taylor & Francis, 2016. | Includes bibliographical references and index.
Identifiers: LCCN 2015043743 | ISBN 9781498750394 (hardcover : alk. paper)
Subjects: | MESH: United States. Food and Drug Administration. | Biosimilar Pharmaceuticals--United States. | Drug Approval--United States. | Government Regulation--United States. | United States Government Agencies--United States.
Classification: LCC RS67.U6 | NLM QV 241 | DDC 615.10973--dc23
LC record available at http://lccn.loc.gov/2015043743

Visit the Taylor & Francis Web site at
http://www.taylorandfrancis.com

and the CRC Press Web site at
http://www.crcpress.com

To Dr. Janet Woodcock, Director, CDER, FDA, whose passion for making biosimilars accessible is only superseded by her determination to assure their safety.

Contents

About the author

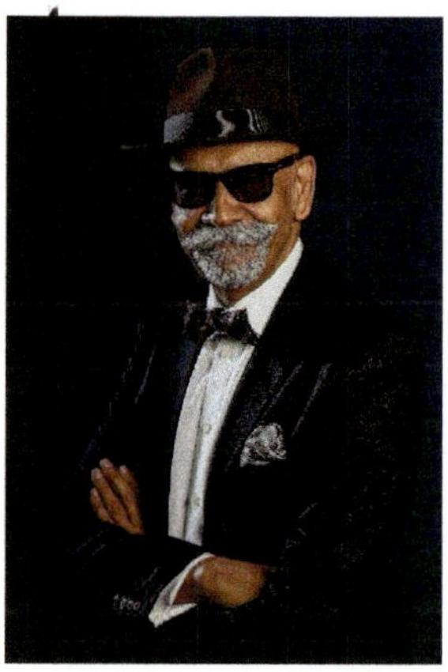

Sarfaraz K. Niazi, PhD, is a lifetime educator of biopharmaceutical sciences, serving at several academic institutions worldwide, who has written the largest number of books on the subject of biosimilars. He is also a founder of two U.S. biosimilar companies that have taken several biosimilar products to Food and Drug Administration. He is the largest solo inventor of bioprocessing inventions that have revolutionized the development and manufacturing of biosimilars. He is recognized as the "most interesting man revolutionizing healthcare," by the *Forbes Magazine*, inducted into the Entrepreneur Hall of Fame, conferred with the highest civil award, Star of Distinction (Pakistan), and honored by prestigious learned academies. He has authored 50+ major books, more than 100 research papers, and hundreds of blogs. He is a US patent law practitioner, a radio broadcaster, a published photographer, a classical guitarist, and a lyricist. Dr. Niazi holds graduate degrees in pharmacy from the Washington State University and the University of Illinois. He lives in Illinois and Wisconsin. He can be reached at niazi@niazi.com. (www.niazi.com) (www.karybio.com) (www.pharmsci.com)

Professional website: http://www.karyobio.com
Author website: http://www.niazi.com
LinkedIn: https://www.linkedin.com/pub/sarfaraz-k-niazi/18/24/592
Wikipedia: http://en.wikipedia.org/wiki/Sarfaraz_K._Niazi
Twitter: @moustaches

Other selected books by the author

- *Textbook of Biopharmaceutics and Clinical Pharmacokinetics*, John Wiley & Sons, New York, NY, 1979; ISBN-13: 9789381075043
- *The Omega Connection*, Esquire Press, Illinois, 1982; ISBN-13: 9780961784102
- *Adsorption and Chelation Therapy*, Esquire Press, Illinois, 1987. ISBN-9780961784140
- *Attacking the Sacred Cows: The Health Hazards of Milk*, Esquire Press, Illinois, 1988; ISBN-13: 9780961784119
- *Endorphins: The Body Opium*, Esquire Press, Illinois, 1988; ISBN 9780961784126
- *Nutritional Myths: The Story No One Wants to Talk About*, Esquire Press, Illinois; ISBN 9780961784133
- *Wellness Guide*, Ferozsons Publishers, Pakistan, 2002; ISBN 9789690017932
- *Love Sonnets of Ghalib: Translations, Explication and Lexicon*, Ferozsons Publishers, Lahore, Pakistan, 2002; and Rupa Publications, New Delhi, India, 2002; ISBN-13: 9788171675968
- *Filing Patents Online*, CRC Press, Boca Raton, Florida, 2003; ISBN-13: 9780849316241
- Pharmacokinetic and Pharmacodynamic Modeling in Early Drug Development, in Charles G. Smith and James T. O'Donnell (eds.), *The Process of New Drug Discovery and Development*, Second Edition, CRC Press, New York, 2004; ISBN-13: 978-0849327797.
- *Handbook of Biogeneric Therapeutic Proteins: Manufacturing, Regulatory, Testing and Patent Issues*, CRC Press, Boca Raton, Florida, 2005; ISBN-13: 9780971474611
- *Handbook of Preformulation: Chemical, Biological and Botanical Drugs*, Informa Healthcare, New York, New York, 2006; ISBN-13: 9780849371936
- *Handbook of Bioequivalence Testing*, Informa Healthcare, New York, 2007; ISBN-13: 978-0849303951
- *Handbook of Pharmaceutical Manufacturing Formulations*, Volume 6, Second Edition: Sterile Products, Informa Healthcare, New York, New York, 2009; ISBN-13: 9781420081305

- *Handbook of Pharmaceutical Manufacturing Formulations*, Volume 1, Second Edition: Compressed Solids, Informa Healthcare, New York, New York, 2009; ISBN-13: 9781420081169
- *Handbook of Pharmaceutical Manufacturing Formulations*, Volume 2, Second Edition: Uncompressed Solids, Informa Healthcare, New York, New York, 2009; ISBN-13: 9781420081183
- *Handbook of Pharmaceutical Manufacturing Formulations*, Volume 3, Second Edition: Liquid Products, Informa Healthcare, New York, New York, 2009; ISBN-13: 9780849317484
- *Handbook of Pharmaceutical Manufacturing Formulations*, Volume 4, Second Edition: Semisolid Products, Informa Healthcare, New York, New York, 2009; ISBN-13: 9781420081268
- *Handbook of Pharmaceutical Manufacturing Formulations*, Volume 5, Second Edition: Over the Counter Products, Informa Healthcare, New York, New York, 2009; ISBN-13: 978-1420081282
- *Textbook of Biopharmaceutics and Clinical Pharmacokinetics*, The Book Syndicate, Hyderabad, India, 2010; ISBN: 978-93-8107-504-3
- *Wine of Passion: Love Poems of Ghalib*, Ferozsons (Pvt) Ltd., Lahore, Pakistan, 2010; ISBN-13: 9780971474611
- *Disposable Bioprocessing Systems*, CRC Press, Boca Raton, Florida, 2012; ISBN-13: 9781439866702
- *Handbook of Bioequivalence Testing*, Second Edition, Informa Healthcare, New York, New York, 2014; ISBN-13: 9781482226379
- *There Is No Wisdom: Selected Love Poems of Bedil*, Translations from Darri Farsi, Sarfaraz K. Niazi, and Maryam Tawoosi, Ferozsons Private (Ltd), Lahore, Pakistan, 2015; ISBN: 978969025036
- *Biosimilars and Interchangeable Biologicals: Strategic Elements*, CRC Press, Boca Raton, Florida, 2015; ISBN: 9781482298918
- *Biosimilars and Interchangeable Biologics: Tactical Elements*, CRC Press, Boca Raton, Florida, 2015; ISBN: 9781482298918
- *Fundamentals of Modern Bioprocessing*, Sarfaraz K. Niazi and Justin L. Brown, CRC Press, Boca Raton, Florida, 2015; ISBN: 9781466585737

Preface

> Efforts to undermine trust in these [biosimilar] products are worrisome and represent a disservice to patients who could benefit from these lower-cost treatments.
>
> **Margaret Hamburg**
> *Former the FDA Commissioner*

1. The motivation

In 2005, when I wrote my first book (*Handbook of Biogeneric Therapeutic Proteins*) about biosimilar drugs, I predicted, with confidence, that within a decade, the United States will have full acceptance of biosimilars. Many reviewers of my book questioned my wisdom, most called it wishful thinking, and some responded by suggesting an Armageddon scene if my predictions were to come true. In 2015, exactly 10 years later, the FDA approved its first biosimilar product, and several 351(k) applications are pending for approval, including applications for licensing of monoclonal antibodies. To commemorate this event, I revised my first book as a two-volume series—*Biosimilars and Interchangeable Biological Products: Strategic Elements* and *Biosimilars and Interchangeable Products: Tactical Elements*, both of which were recently published. However, as I began my own effort to secure approval of the FDA for biosimilar and interchangeable products, I realized that there is a need to share this expertise as it pertains to the mindset of the FDA alone as the largest world market of biosimilars has just opened wide to all. There is no doubt in my mind that by sharing this knowledge, I am inviting my competitors to become stronger, but that is what I want—more companies entering the biosimilar markets. The markets of biosimilar products are enormous and more competitors mean that we may be able to reach the goal of reducing the cost of biological drugs sooner. There is so much suffering in this world, we cannot be selfish.

The scope of this book is clearly defined to elaborate on the mindset of the U.S. FDA in approving biosimilar products under the 351(k) category. The key to this approval lies in understanding the meaning of biosimilarity, a term that is ill-understood, not fully well appreciated, and frequently quoted inaccurately in the literature. A clear understanding of "biosimilarity" as viewed by the FDA, which can be very different from how other regulatory agencies interpret, is the goal of this book.

2. The vocabulary

The FDA defines biosimilarity as a stage of evaluation when it is determined:

> "that the biological product is highly similar to the reference product notwithstanding minor differences in clinically inactive components" and that "there are no clinically meaningful differences between the biological product and the reference product in terms of the safety, purity, and potency of the product" (see section 351(i)(2) of the PHS Act).

This statement needs a description of the following terms.

Reference Product

Under section 351(i)(4), a "reference product" is the single biological product licensed by the FDA under section 351(a) of the PHS Act against which a proposed biological product is evaluated in an application submitted under section 351(k).

Reference Listed Drug

Biosimilars filed under section 505 (b)(2) use information on biologics approved as Listed Drugs, not as biologics, for example, insulin products till 2020.

Biosimilar or Biosimilarity

Under section 351(i)(2), "biosimilar" or "biosimilarity" means that the biological product is highly similar to the reference product notwithstanding minor differences in clinically inactive components, and there are no clinically meaningful differences between the biological product and the reference product in terms of safety, purity, and potency of the product.

Interchangeable Biological Product

Under 351(k)(4), an "interchangeable" biological product is a product that has been shown to be biosimilar to the reference product, and can be expected to produce the same clinical result as the reference product in any given patient. In addition, to be determined to be an interchangeable biological product, it must be shown that for a biological product that is administered more than once to an individual, the risk in terms of safety or diminished efficacy of alternating or switching between use of the biological product and the reference product is not greater than the risk of using the reference product without such alternation or switch.

Reference Product Exclusivity

Section 351(k)(7) of the PHS Act describes reference product exclusivity as the period of time from the date of first licensure of a reference product, the single biological product licensed under section 351(a) of the PHS Act against which a biological product is evaluated in a 351(k) application, during which a 351(k) sponsor is not permitted to submit and the FDA is not permitted to license a 351(k) application that references the reference product. Specifically, if the reference product has reference product exclusivity under this section, approval of a 351(k) application may not be made effective until the date that is 12 years after the date of first licensure of the reference product, and a 351(k) application may not be submitted for review to the FDA until the date that is 4 years after the date of first licensure. See 351(k)(7). For additional information on how the FDA determines the date of first licensure and reference product exclusivity, please see the draft guidance for industry, "Reference Product Exclusivity for Biological Products Filed under Section 351(a) of the PHS Act (PDF—99 kB)."

Reference Product Exclusivity Expiry Date

The reference product exclusivity expiry date indicates (1) the date that is 12 years from the date of first licensure as described in 351(k)(7); plus (2) any pediatric exclusivity granted pursuant to section 505(A) of the FD&C Act, if applicable. The reference product exclusivity expiry date is the date on which a 351(k)-application referencing the reference product may be licensed, assuming it is not blocked by orphan exclusivity and otherwise meets the requirements for licensure under 351(k). To determine whether there is unexpired orphan exclusivity for an indication for which the reference product is licensed, please refer to the searchable database for Orphan Designated and/or Approved Products.

Date of First Licensure

Although the FDA has not decided of the date of first licensure for all 351(a) biological products included on the lists, it does not mean that the biological products on the list are not, or were not, eligible for exclusivity. A determination of the date of first licensure and of when any remaining reference product exclusivity will expire for a biological product submitted under section 351(a) of the PHS Act will generally be made for reasons of regulatory necessity and/or at the request of the 351(a)-application license holder.

The FDA has introduced a new vocabulary in describing the process of establishing biosimilarity; this needs to be understood, as described in various guidance documents, the Q&A reporting, as well as the face-to-face meetings with the FDA, where the FDA goes into greater details how they would like to see the data collected and presented. A lot of discussions provided in this book are based on a firsthand experience in developing biosimilars, discussing the development protocols with regulatory agencies worldwide, and conducting the necessary exercises to complete the 351(k) filing dossiers.

- "Highly similar."
  - This is the third tier of the level of similarity: not similar, similar, highly similar, and finger-print like similar; this is the minimum level of entry to the club.
- "Minor differences in clinically inactive components."
  - "Minor" is debatable; the first biosimilar product approved by the FDA had a different buffer system, a different pH, and likely minor impact on PK profile; however, none of these was considered major.
- "No clinically meaningful difference."
  - Differences are expected as long as these do not affect clinical response (effectiveness) or the adverse events.
- "Safety, purity, and potency."
  - The FDA does not use "efficacy" in the final evaluation; safety is related to immunogenicity, purity refers to analytical similarity, and potency refers to an assessment from in vitro or in vivo methods, and where necessary in human trials.
- "Phase 1 and phase 3."
  - The FDA does not describe the studies as phase 1 or phase 3 studies in its guidance because the clinical studies in developing biosimilar serve a difference purpose and also require a different clinical product and study design.

3. About first biosimilar originators

It is important to recognize that a few decades ago when biological products like therapeutic proteins and monoclonal antibodies were developed, they represented, in many instances, copies of the endogenous molecules like insulin, erythropoietin, filgrastim, etc. In reality, these first waves of products were actually the first biosimilar product to what the body was already producing. It will be, therefore, proper to call them originator products, not an innovator's product. They originated, not invented, and thus I have decided to call them as such and not the innovator. Now we are at a stage where biosimilar companies are emulating the originator's products. Whether the first originators of biological drugs would succeed in developing, a biosimilar program will depend to a considerable degree on whether they can think and act differently from their pedigree. Several large companies like Amgen, Sanofi, Pfizer, and Merck are developing biosimilar products because the markets of these products are so large and fit well within their ROI calculations. However, it remains to be seen if the mindset of large first originators can adopt to biosimilar paradigm.

One of the emerging discussions in the field of biosimilars is the role of creative play companies established exclusively to produce cost-effective biosimilars. In financial management, a create-pure-play company utilizes creative partnerships to develop and supply biosimilars, instead of conducting all work in-house that leads to inevitable capacity constraints as well as high cost and long time to bring biosimilars to the market. I will dwell on it in a later chapter.

4. Purple book

The "Purple Book" lists biological products, including any biosimilar and interchangeable biological products, licensed by the FDA under the Public Health Service Act (the PHS Act). The Purple Book includes the date a biological product was licensed under 351(a) of the PHS Act and whether the FDA evaluated the biological product for reference product exclusivity under section 351(k)(7) of the PHS Act.
The Purple Book, in addition to the date licensed, also includes whether a biological product licensed under section 351(k) of the PHS Act has been determined by the FDA to be biosimilar to or interchangeable with a reference biological product (an already-licensed FDA biological product). The Patient Protection and Affordable Care Act (Affordable Care Act), signed into law by President Barrack Obama on March 23, 2010, amends the PHS Act to create an abbreviated licensure pathway for biological products that are demonstrated to be "biosimilar" to or "interchangeable" with an FDA-licensed biological product. This pathway is provided in the part of the Affordable Care Act known as the Biologics Price Competition and Innovation Act of 2009 (BPCI Act). Biosimilar and interchangeable biological products licensed under section 351(k) of the PHS Act will be listed under the reference product to which biosimilarity or interchangeability was demonstrated.

Healthcare providers can prescribe biosimilar and interchangeable biological products just as they would prescribe other medications. The BPCI Act describes an interchangeable product as a product that may be substituted for the reference product without the intervention of the healthcare provider who prescribed the reference product. In contrast, the FDA expects that a biosimilar product will be specifically prescribed by the healthcare provider and cannot be substituted for a reference product at the pharmacy level.

5. Biosimilar markets

As of 2020, biological drugs are expected to claim a market of over $200 billion (Figure 1), and eventually all of these drugs would be a biosimilar target.

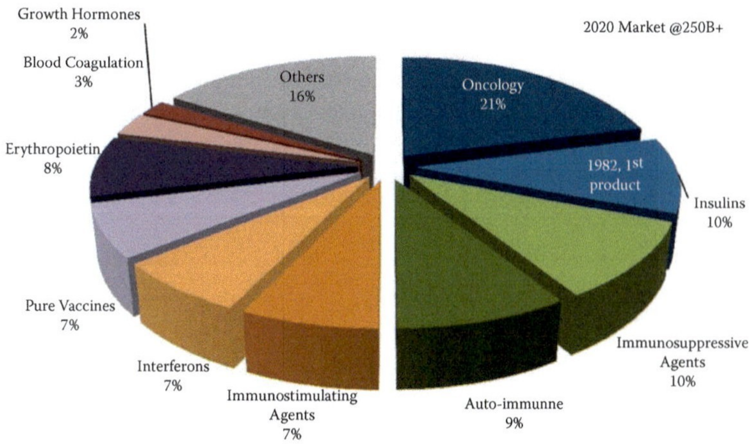

Figure 1 Biological drugs projected to define the 2020 markets.

Table 1 Biological Drugs that are Off-Patent for Main Gene Sequence Patent as of 2017

Activase®: alteplase; Avonex®: interferon beta-1a; BeneFIX®: nonacog alfa; Betaseron®: interferon beta-1b; Bexxar®: tositumomab; Cerezyme®: imiglucerase; Epogen®: epoetin alfa; Fabrazyme®: agalsidase beta; Genotropin®: somatropin; Gonal-F®: follitropin alfa/beta; Helixate®: octocog alfa; Humalog®: insulin lispro; Humatrope®: somatropin; Humira®: adalimumab; Humulin R®: insulin (human); Increlex®: mecasermin [rDNA origin]; insulin analogs: insulin; Kogenate®: octocog alfa; Lantus®: insulin glargine ; Lemtrada®: alemtuzumab; Luveris®: lutropin alfa; Macugen®: pegaptanib sodium; Natrecor®: nesiritide; Neulasta®: pegfilgrastim; Neumega®: oprelvekin; Neupogen®: filgrastim; Norditropin SimpleXx®: somatropin; NovoMix 30®: insulin aspart; NovoRapid®: insulin aspart; NovoSeven®: eptacog alfa; Nutropin®: somatropin; Oncaspar®: pegaspargase; Ontak®: denileukin diftitox; Orgalutran/Antagon®: ganirelix acetate; Orthoclone OKT-3®: muromonab-CD3; Ovidrel®: choriogonadotropin alfa; Pediarix®: DTP, hepatitis B, and polio vaccine; PEGIntron®: peginterferon alfa-2b; Prevnar®: pneumococcal vaccine; Procrit®: epoetin alfa; Proleukin®: aldesleukin; Provenge®: sipuleucel-T; Puregon/Follistim®: follitropin beta; Rebif®: interferon beta-1a; Recothrom®: thrombin alfa; ReFacto AF /Xyntha®: moroctocog alfa; ReoPro®: abciximab; Replagal®: agalsidase alfa; Serostim®: somatropin; Somavert®: pegvisomant; Synagis®: palivizumab; Thyrogen®: thyrotropin alfa

Table 1 lists the biological drugs whose patents have expired, and Table 2 lists the drugs coming off patent from 2018 to 2024.

In terms of the patent expiry and the market of these products, it is a multibillion dollar business (Figure 2).

It should be noted that biological drugs are allowed a 12-year exclusivity period on the market, regardless of the patent expiry, so it is likely that some of the listed drugs may not be available for development as biosimilars, despite their patent expiry. As described below, biosimilar

Table 2 Biological Drugs Coming Off Patent from 2018 to 2024

Advate®: factor VIII (procoagulant); Afrezza®: insulin (human); Aldurazyme®: laronidase; Apidra®: insulin glulisine; Aranesp®: darbepoetin alfa; Arcalyst®: rilonacept; Avastin®: bevacizumab; Benlysta®: belimumab; Blincyto®: blinatumomab; Botox®: onabotulinumtoxinA; Cervarix®: human papillomavirus (HPV) vaccine; ChondroCelect®: autologous cultured hondrocytes; Cimzia®: certolizumab pegol; Cyramza®: ramucirumab; Elaprase®: idursulfase; Elelyso®: taliglucerase alfa; Elonva®: corifollitropin alfa; Entyvio®: vedolizumab; Erbitux®: cetuximab; Forteo®: teriparatide; Herceptin®: trastuzumab; Ilaris®: canakinumab; Imvamune®: smallpox vaccine; Intron A®: interferon alfa-2b; Ixiaro®: japanese encephalitis vaccine; Jetrea®: ocriplasmin; Kadcyla®: ado-trastuzumab emtansine; Kalbitor®: ecallantide; Kepivance®: palifermin; Kineret®: anakinra; Levemir®: insulin detemir; Lucentis®: ranibizumab; Mircera®: methoxy polyethylene glycol-epoetin beta; Myalept®: metreleptin; Myozyme®: alglucosidase alfa; Natpara®: parathyroid hormone; NovoThirteen®: catridecacog; Nplate®: romiplostim; Nulojix®: belatacept; Obizur®: susoctocog alfa; Orencia SC®: abatacept; Orencia®: abatacept; Pegasys®: peginterferon alfa-2a; Prochymal®: remestemcel-L; Prolia®: denosumab; Recombivax HB®: hepatitis B vaccine; Remicade®: infliximab; Rituxan®: rituximab; RotaTeq®: rotavirus vaccine; Saxenda®: liraglutide [rDNA origin]; Simponi®: golimumab; Simulect®: basiliximab; Soliris®: eculizumab; Stelara®: ustekinumab; Tanzeum®: albiglutide; Trulicity®: dulaglutide; Tysabri®: natalizumab; V419®: DTP, hepatitis B, Hib, and polio vaccine; Vectibix®: panitumumab; Victoza®: liraglutide [rDNA origin]; Voraxaze®: glucarpidase; Vpriv®: velaglucerase alfa; Xgeva®: denosumab; Xolair®: omalizumab; Yervoy®: ipilimumab; Zaltrap®: ziv-aflibercept; Zevalin®: ibritumomab tiuxetan

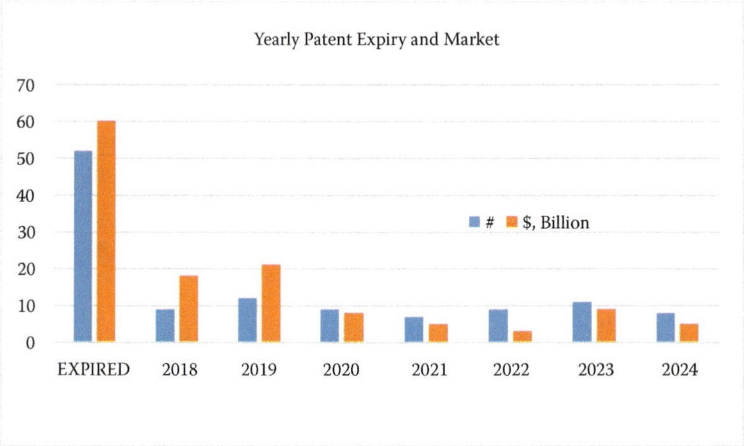

Figure 2 Patent expiry of biological drugs and the current market.

drugs are further subject to patent challenges based on the process used for manufacturing, indications, formulations, and many other attributes that can also delay entry of biosimilars to the market. Still, given that it may take several years to develop a biosimilar product, both lists represent opportunities for biosimilars, making them one of the most lucrative categories of drugs in the history.

While biological drugs have provided a new lease on life to many, the cost of these drugs remains high, even in the markets like the United States. For example, antibodies and fusion proteins used for the treatment of symptoms of rheumatoid arthritis may cost $10,000–$30,000 per year with very high copays making their penetration and availability limited. The same holds true for cytokines like pegylated filgrastim and most of the anticancer drugs. The cost of biological drugs used in the treatment of cancer can run much higher. The high cost of these drugs is justified by the originators based on the complexity and difficulties of their manufacture and a much lower success rate in new discoveries. However, it is abundantly clear now that the price of these drugs is driven mainly by economic incentives supported by complex intellectual property laws that have allowed some of these drugs to have an exclusivity of over 30 years such as in the case of interferon alpha, etanercept, and several others.

One of the hotly debated topics in the healthcare industry today is the cost of these drugs and their affordability. In many instances, the greatest burden lies on the governments that pay for these drugs. For example, the Center for Medicare and Medicaid (CMC) services spend billions of dollars for biological drugs, mandating faster approval and adoption of biosimilars.

5.1 Biosimilars misconceptions

The misconceptions about biosimilar product were, at first, aimed at the regulatory agencies; now it is public at large as seen recently in the legislative actions taken by several states in making the interchangeability of biosimilar product more onerous and often cumbersome with an aim to prevent it.

The most common misconceptions currently spread today about biosimilar product include the following:

- Biosimilar products are inferior because they are not identical.
- Biosimilar products are unsafe.
- Only way to establish safety and efficacy is to demonstrate it in patients.
- There is only one approval pathway for biosimilars.
- There is only one correct way to manufacture biosimilars.
- INN naming will create safety hazards.
- Savings will be minimal due to high development costs.

Given the large and complex molecular structure, the biological drugs will always have structural variability that will be questioned even if it does not impact their safety and efficacy. Lot-to-lot variation in the originator product is common and so is the variability in the product manufactured by our body; variability is part of the structure, not a flaw.

The misconception that biosimilar products are unsafe is routinely aimed at their immunogenicity, but the fact is that biological drugs are one of the safest categories of drugs; most biological products do not have any significant immunogenicity, and where immunogenicity is significant, it is part of their mechanism of action, and not an adverse effect. In an almost a decade of the use of biosimilars, the adverse events reported are far less than what was feared. The reported incidences for erythropoietin, which itself has little immunogenicity, were a result of improper changes made to the packaging that should have been prevented and have nothing to do with any inherent hazard in the use of these products. This incidence has damaged the reputation of the biosimilar product drug industry.

The misconception that unless you show safety and efficacy in patients, the product cannot be declared safe and effective is based on lack of understanding of statistics and the pharmacological aspects of drug action. The originator product is evaluated in several conditions in large patient populations but against a placebo; a biosimilar product would have to demonstrate non-inferiority against the originator product. Often, the number of patients required to prove this will be higher than the studies of the originator; besides, requiring clinical trials in limited indications in a small number of patients would not provide extrapolation possibilities if demonstrated clinical effects are made the ultimate measure. In approving Levonox (small molecular weight heparin) without any clinical trials in patients, the FDA has clearly explained the relative importance of structural and functional similarity.

Whereas most biosimilar product developers will follow the same manufacturing process as that of the originator, there remain many aspects of manufacturing, such as in-process controls, that need to be developed by the biosimilar product developers. The originators take the position that unless the product is made using the same in-process controlled method exactly the same way as they do it, it is not possible to manufacture a safe and effective product. Ironically, when the originators developed a process, it was always "a" process and never "the" process. There are so many changes that can improve the process, and definitely any change or difference is readily justified in the ultimate comparison with the originator product.

The issue of naming has been resolved by the FDA by using a four-letter code as a suffix to the generic name of the drug, even for the originator products, to differentiate any two biological products. This naming structure is to help prevent inadvertent substitution (which could lead to medication errors) of biological products that are not determined to be interchangeable by the FDA and to support safety monitoring of all biological products after they are on the market, by making it easier to track accurate usage of biological products in all settings of care, such as outpatient, hospital, and pharmacy settings. In my opinion, this naming convention does not help in both situations and is a mere bureaucratic intervention that will continue to give originator companies a reason to question the safety and efficacy of biosimilars.

6. About this book

Biosimilarity: The FDA Perspective that you hold in your hand is specific to the topic of biosimilarity; other topics of manufacturing, legality, marketing, cost containment, etc., have been fully covered in the two-volume series published earlier, *Biosimilar and Interchangeable Products: From Cell Lines to Commercial Launch—Strategic Elements* and *Biosimilar and Interchangeable Products: From Cell Lines to Commercial Launch—Tactical Elements* (CRC Press, 2016). In limiting the discussion to a specific topic, it became possible for me to provide an exhaustive discussion dwelling on the current thinking of the FDA and provide advice to the sponsors of biosimilars on avoiding making costly mistakes. One specific goal of this book is to allow biosimilar developers to take the products fast to market. The current cost of $150–200 million and a filing period of five to eight years are untenable; this book anticipates providing advice to break this constraint based on my first-hand experience in developing biosimilar products globally.

It is expected that those consulting this book will have an interest in the regulatory aspect of biosimilar development; as a developer, they would have already produced a product that they consider to be biosimilar and are ready to package it for the FDA review. As a result, a lot of details of manufacturing variability and process selection attributes are left out of this book. These are available in detail in other works by the author.

There are nine chapters in this book, each dealing with a specific subtopic, and the final chapter provides a seamless integration of the process described.

1. Preface. This preamble sets the stages of understanding biosimilarity by providing first the reason why I chose to write this book and then a political view of the field of biosimilars that encompasses the mindset and tactics of the originator companies, the nature of expanding markets for biosimilars, and the gross misconceptions about biosimilars, mostly created by the originator companies and some as a result of ignorance.
2. Chapter 1: Understanding Proteins. Understanding the mindset of the FDA first requires a clearer understanding of the science of protein chemistry, especially the recent advances made

in both analyzing and characterizing the molecular structures at all levels. This chapter is a primer to protein chemistry emphasizing the biosimilar protein studies where structural variability, posttranslational modification, and association and aggregation are investigated.

3. Chapter 2: The Biosimilar Landscape. This chapter begins with a historical perspective on the rise of biosimilars with intention to show how the science of biosimilars has evolved globally; the terminology used by the FDA in its guidance plays a very significant role in understanding the mindset of the FDA—there is a detailed deconstruction of these designations. Further, the chapter delves into global markets and the scientific basis of their approval, keeping in mind that biosimilar developers are likely to take a broader view of their regulatory submissions, given the high cost of development. The chapter also provides an extensive list of the identification of the biosimilar products on the horizon for the next few decades; the global mindset about biosimilars is also important to understand, as this chapter suggests.
4. Chapter 3: The FDA Regulatory Guidance. A comprehensive discussion of every document issued by the US FDA on the biosimilar products, current as of this book going to press (December 2017). Extensive details of the explanation of the expectations of the US FDA in the submissions on a progressive basis, from the Initial Advisory Meeting (IAM) to type II, type II and type IV meeting, and the final submission, are provided. The FDA has yet to issue the guidance on one topic—statistical evaluation—yet the FDA has provided sufficient guidance directly to the author, as well as in its many publications that I consider the guidance to be complete, if not totally clear. I have provided clarity on the guidance relating to scientific aspects as well as clinical pharmacology, all leading to the determination of biosimilarity. Topics like regulatory exclusivities and various choices like 505 (b)(2), 351(a), and 351 (k) are also discussed. A brief discussion of EMA and the FDA comparative mindset as well as topics of pharmacovigilance, the Purple Book, etc., make this perhaps the most pivotal reading.
5. Chapter 4: Understanding Biosimilarity. Introducing a novel approach to understanding the mindset of the US FDA, this chapter is the heart of the book. The concept presented here delineates the progressive understanding of the US FDA. Every definition and expectation of the FDA in the preparation of a 351(k) filing is deconstructed to make it most relevant on a molecule-by-molecule basis. A progressive development plan is provided that includes detailed discussions on the analytical methodologies as well as design study protocols for clinical pharmacology studies, interchangeability studies, as well as

nonclinical studies. This is the longest chapter of the book and prepares a developer to create a formal development program.

6. Chapter 5: Biopharmaceutical Tools. Since the analytical and functional similarity forms the basis of the determination of biosimilarity, this chapter provides details of the tools available to the sponsors, along with their relative importance. Also referred to in this chapter are the novel tools. This chapter heavily emphasizes the need for a very high level of analytical capability development if the FDA expectations are to be met.
7. Chapter 6: Critical Quality Attributes. Prior to any studies to demonstrate analytical and functional similarity, the FDA expects the sponsor to create a list of critical quality attributes based on risk factors as described in various ICH guidelines and the FDA guidance; this chapter takes a significant place in this book because of the paucity of published data on the risk management of biosimilar products vis-à-vis the standalone biological products; a substantially different approach is needed to avoid getting in costly studies that may not be relevant. This chapter provides a step-by-step method to identify the CQAs and create a testing plan to satisfy the FDA expectations of similar identity, safety, potency, and purity.
8. Chapter 7: Safety Similarity. The FDA evaluates biosimilarity not on the basis of efficacy (which is called effectiveness) but primarily on safety, which will include immunogenicity potential as well. This chapter provides extensive details of how protein drugs become immunogenic, and how this potential can be tested side-by-side with the originator product in both humans and animals; the difficulties in these testing for products that do not have a PD model are also described along with plausible solutions.
9. Chapter 8: Formulation Similarity. While most injectable product formulations are fully disclosed, the biosimilar developer faces a unique challenge when the originator formulation is protected by IP, as it has come to front as a measure by the originators to keep the biosimilars out of market; protein formulation science is complex, and the biosimilar developers are apprised of the need to develop a strong scientific basis to allow optimization of formulation stability and to develop tools that will satisfy the FDA needs of biosimilarity; the FDA allows differences in the formulation.
10. Chapter 9: Statistical Approach to Analytical Similarity. This chapter specifically elaborates the FDA expectations of how to analyze and present the analytical similarity data as well as clinical pharmacology studies; this approach of the FDA is distinctly different from what is anticipated in regulatory submissions to other agencies—the FDA is more focused, quantitative, and elaborate in its expectations; while the guidance for

this data treatment is still anticipated, enough has been made public to allow complete understanding of this expectation of the FDA. This chapter includes specific examples of testing, answers dozens of questions that were never elaborated on any publications, and prepares the biosimilar product developer with the ability to develop a good package for the FDA review. This chapter also provides clarification of some basic statistical concepts applied to the tier-based testing expected by the FDA. Also included are specific topics about stability and process-related impurities.

11. Chapter 10: Biosimilarity: The Final Frontier. The closing chapter summarizes in a highly focused manner the expectations of the FDA, the FDA perspective, and a critical analysis of the FDA mindset.

A book of this scope and emphasis could not be produced without the recognition and the arduous support of the publisher. The great folks at CRC Press have been more than kind to me for decades, and I could not thank enough Laurie Oknowsky, without whose untiring encouragement this book could not have been completed.

Last, but not the least, I am thankful for scores of my scientific and professional colleagues and particularly those whom I came to know through the landmark literature in the field but have never met. I may have quoted their work thinking that this is all in the public domain subconsciously; I hope they would excuse me for taking this liberty as it would be impossible to recognize them well. An elaborate bibliography does not necessarily replace this obligation that I have of properly acknowledging their work.

I am dedicating this book to the leadership of the FDA that has been responsive to my many requests and challenges I have made to the FDA guidance; in one stance, Dr. Janet Woodcock approved my citizen's petition to allow discussion of reducing testing in healthy subjects to establish bioequivalence, both for chemical drugs and biologics.

Finally, I would like to admit my mistakes, and I couldn't find a better statement that appeared in the first edition of *Encyclopedia Britannica* (1786):

> "WITH regard to errors, in general, whether falling under the denomination of mental, typographical or accidental, we are conscious of being able to point out a greater number than any critic whatever. Men who are acquainted with the innumerable difficulties attending the execution of a work of such an extensive nature will make proper allowances. To these, I (we) appeal and shall rest satisfied with the judgment they pronounce."

I will just add: please send me an email at niazi@niazi.com to correct my mistakes.

Bibliography

FDA: http://www.fda.gov/downloads/Drugs/GuidanceComplianceRegulatoryInformation/Guidances/UCM459987.pdf

Federal Register: https://www.federalregister.gov/articles/2015/08/28/2015-21383/nonproprietary-naming-of-biological-products-draft-guidance-for-industry-availability

Disclaimer

The author does not accept responsibility for any technical or legal suggestions or advice provided in this book; all views expressed in this book are those of the author in his personal capacity and not as an office holder of any company or agency.

Sarfaraz K. Niazi, PhD, FRSB, SI, FPAMS, FACB
Chicago, Illinois

Chapter 1 Understanding proteins

Any fool can know. The point is to understand.

Albert Einstein

1.1 Background

Biopharmaceuticals are more complex and have larger molecular weight, variable structure, dynamic protein, and antibody molecules compared to pharmaceutical products wherein a fixed structure is always present. Some prominent examples include cytokines, antibodies, and hormones (Figure 1.1).

Cytokines are a broad and loose category of small proteins (~5–20 kDa) that are important in cell signaling. They are released by cells and they affect the behavior of other cells. Cytokines can also be involved in autocrine signaling. Cytokines include chemokines, interferons, interleukins, lymphokines, and tumor necrosis factor (TNF), but generally not hormones or growth factors (despite some terminology overlap). Cytokines are produced by a broad range of cells, including immune cells like macrophages, B lymphocytes, T lymphocytes, and mast cells, as well as endothelial cells, fibroblasts, and various stromal cells; a given cytokine may be produced by more than one type of cell. Cytokines act through receptors and are especially important in the immune system; cytokines modulate the balance between humoral and cell-based immune responses, and they regulate the maturation, growth, and responsiveness of particular cell populations. Some cytokines enhance or inhibit the action of other cytokines in complex ways. They are different from hormones, which are also important cell signaling molecules, in that hormones circulate in much lower concentrations and hormones tend to be made by specific kinds of cells.

An antibody, also known as an immunoglobulin, is a large, Y-shaped protein produced by plasma cells that are used by the immune system to identify and neutralize pathogens such as bacteria and viruses. The antibody recognizes an antigen, via the variable region. Each tip of the *Y* of an antibody contains a paratope that is specific for one particular epitope (analogous to a key) on an antigen, allowing these two structures to bind together with precision. Using this binding mechanism, an antibody can tag a microbe or an infected cell for attack by other parts of the immune system, or can directly neutralize its target (for example, by blocking

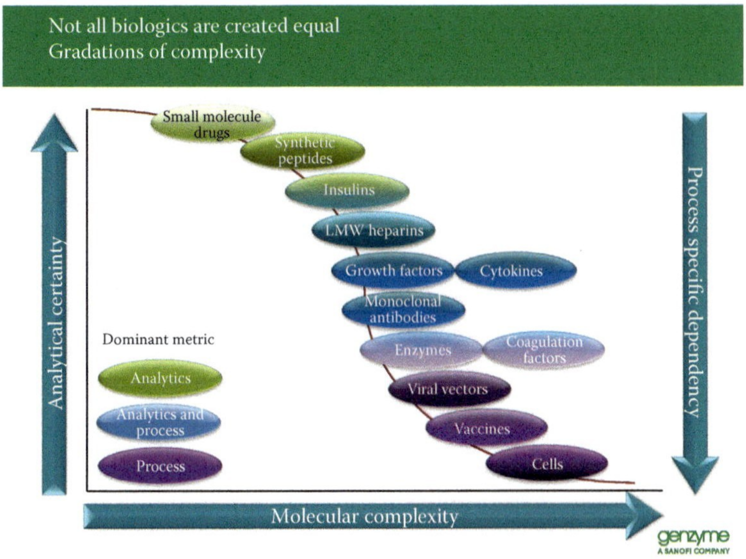

Figure 1.1 Analytics and process metrics. LMW: Low-molecular weight. (From http://www.fda.gov/downloads/AdvisoryCommittees/CommitteesMeetingMaterials/Drugs/AdvisoryCommitteeforPharmaceuticalScienceandClinicalPharmacology/UCM315764.pdf.)

a part of a microbe that is essential for its invasion and survival). The ability of an antibody to communicate with the other components of the immune system is mediated via its fragment crystallizable (Fc) region (located at the base of the *Y*), which contains a conserved glycosylation site involved in these interactions. The production of antibodies is the main function of the humoral immune system.

Although the general structure of all antibodies is very similar, a small region at the tip of the protein is extremely variable, allowing millions of antibodies with slightly different tip structures, or antigen-binding sites, to exist. This region is known as the hypervariable region. Each of these variants can bind to a different antigen. This enormous diversity of antibody paratopes on the antigen-binding fragments allows the immune system to recognize an equally wide variety of antigens.

Hormones are a class of signaling molecules produced by glands in multicellular organisms that are transported by the circulatory system to target distant organs to regulate physiology and behavior. Hormones have diverse chemical structures including eicosanoids, steroids, amino acid derivatives, peptides, and proteins. The glands that secrete hormones include the endocrine signaling system. The term *hormone* is sometimes extended to include chemicals produced by cells that affect the same cell (autocrine or intracrine signaling) or nearby cells (paracrine signaling).

The protein hormones are synthesized in cells from amino acids according to messenger ribonucleic acid (mRNA) transcripts, which are synthesized from deoxyribonucleic acid (DNA) templates inside the cell nucleus. Preprohormones, peptide hormone precursors, are then processed in several stages, typically in the endoplasmic reticulum, including the removal of the N-terminal signal sequence and sometimes glycosylation, resulting in prohormones. The prohormones are then packaged into membrane-bound secretory vesicles, which can be secreted from the cell by exocytosis in response to specific stimuli (e.g., an increase in Ca^{2+} and cyclic adenosine monophosphate concentration in the cytoplasm). These prohormones often contain superfluous amino acid residues that were needed to direct the folding of the hormone molecule into its active configuration but have no function once the hormone folds. Specific endopeptidases in the cell cleave the prohormone just before it is released into the bloodstream, generating the mature hormone form of the molecule. Mature peptide hormones then travel through the blood to all of the cells of the body, where they interact with specific receptors on the surfaces of their target cells.

The U.S. Food and Drug Administration (FDA) expects the sponsors to come up with a high level of scientific evaluation of their biosimilar candidate products, and it all begins with a full understanding of proteins as it is relevant to their development as biosimilar products. This chapter is not a primer on protein science, which I assume would be well understood by the sponsor, but a description of what is relevant to the development of biosimilars, as the FDA views it.

The first leg of establishing biosimilarity is a demonstration of structural similarity between a biosimilar candidate and the originator product. In this chapter, I describe the nature of the structural variants that are common, not necessarily always relevant, and the techniques available to establish this basic level of similarity. This is the step where we begin collecting evidence that will lead us to the totality of the evidence.

1.1.1 Developing biosimilars

If a new biological product development is akin to a horse running wild and reaching the goal post, biosimilar development is like running a horse on exactly the same track without any fences around the track. In one case, it is uncertain; in the other, extremely onerous. This chapter provides details of the critical aspects of protein and antibody structures that are relevant to establishing biosimilarity. This is not a primer on protein chemistry, as only those elements that are relevant to a regulatory development of biosimilar are provided here.

The nature of products that a biosimilar product developer will face greatly varies, even though they are all proteins. Our body cells exploit an enormous array of proteins, approximately 2000, to perform nearly every functional and structural role to stay alive. To date, more than 130 genuine and a similar number of modified therapeutic proteins are approved for clinical use in the European Union and the United States with sales into $100 billion plus, the monoclonal antibodies (mAbs) accounting for almost half of the sales volume.

Based on their pharmacological activity, therapeutic proteins can be divided into five groups: (a) replacing a protein that is deficient or abnormal; (b) augmenting an existing pathway; (c) providing a novel function or activity; (d) interfering with a molecule or organism; and (e) delivering other compounds or proteins, such as a radionuclide, a cytotoxic drug, or effector proteins. Therapeutic proteins can also be grouped based on their molecular types that include antibody-based drugs, Fc fusion proteins, anticoagulants, blood factors, bone morphogenetic proteins, engineered protein scaffolds, enzymes, growth factors, hormones, interferons, interleukins, and thrombolytics. They can also be classified based on their molecular mechanism of activity as (a) binding noncovalently to target, e.g., mAbs; (b) affecting covalent bonds, e.g., enzymes; and (c) exerting activity without specific interactions, e.g., serum albumin. Most protein therapeutics currently on the market are recombinant, and hundreds of them are in clinical trials for the therapy of cancers, immune disorders, infections, and other diseases. New engineered proteins, including bispecific mAbs and multispecific fusion proteins, mAbs conjugated with small molecule drugs, and proteins with optimized pharmacokinetics, are currently under development. Despite the remarkable growth in this category of drugs, the technology for their production remains genetic engineering–based recombinant production. Perhaps novel techniques of the future may make it possible to synthesize these drugs, which may reduce some complexity, but that seems far; the next generation of biosimilars, as reported in Chapter 2, will likely be recombinant proteins expressed in prokaryotic and eukaryotic systems, the living systems that inevitably and invariably introduce significant variability in the primary, secondary, tertiary, and quaternary structures of these proteins. A keen understanding of the possible differences and their source is essential to develop biosimilars; this chapter provides this discussion.

1.2 Protein structure

1.2.1 Building elements

The 20 different naturally occurring amino acids give a staggering number of different possible proteins, 20^n to be exact, where n is the number of amino acid units or residues (Figures 1.2 and 1.3).

Each amino acid has a carboxylic group and an amine group, and amino acids link to one another to form a chain by a dehydration reaction by joining the carboxyl group of one amino acid with the amino group of the next. Thus, polypeptide chains have an end with an unbound carboxyl group, the C-terminus, and begin with an amine group, the N-terminus.

Amino acid	Three-letter code	Single-letter code	Structure
Alanine	Ala	A	HOOC, ^2H_2N ≻ CH_3
Arginine	Arg	R	HOOC, H_2N ≻ $CH_2CH_2CH_2NHC(NH_2)=NH$
Asparagine	Asn	N	HOOC, H_2N ≻ CH_2CONH_2
Aspartic acid	Asp	D	HOOC, H_2N ≻ CH_2COOH
Cysteine	Cys	C	HOOC, H_2N ≻ CH_2SH
Glutamic acid	Glu	E	HOOC, H_2N ≻ CH_2CH_2COOH
Glutamine	Gln	Q	HOOC, H_2N ≻ $CH_2CH_2CONH_2$
Glycine	Gly	G	HOOC, H_2N ≻ H
Histidine	His	H	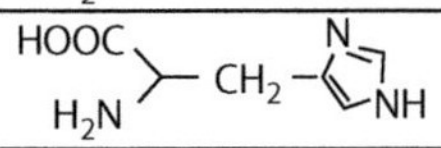
Isoleucine	Ile	I	HOOC, H_2N ≻ $CH(CH_3)CH_2CH_3$
Leucine	Leu	L	HOOC, H_2N ≻ $CH_2CH(CH_3)_2$
Lysine	Lys	K	HOOC, H_2N ≻ $CH_2CH_2CH_2CH_2NH_2$
Methionine	Met	M	HOOC, H_2N ≻ $CH_2CH_2SCH_3$
Phenylalanine	Phe	F	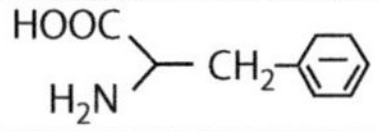
Proline	Pro	P	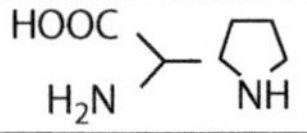
Serine	Ser	S	HOOC, H_2N ≻ CH_2OH
Threonine	Thr	T	HOOC, H_2N ≻ $CHCH_3$(OH)
Tryptophan	Trp	W	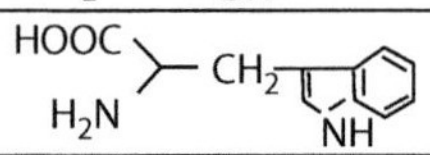
Tyrosine	Tyr	Y	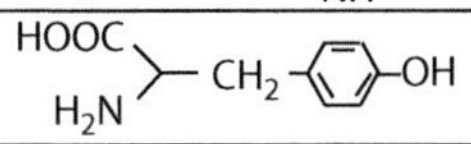
Valine	Val	V	HOOC, H_2N ≻ $CH(CH_3)_2$

Figure 1.2 The structures of the 20 essential amino acids.

Formula	MW	Middle unit residue ($-H_2O$) Formula	MW	Charge at pH 6.0–7.0	Hydrophobic (nonpolar)	Uncharged (polar)	Hydrophilic (polar)
$C_3H_7NO_2$	89.1	C_3H_5NO	71.1	Neutral	■		
$C_6H_{14}N_4O_2$	174.2	$C_6H_{12}N_4O$	156.2	Basic (−ve)			■
$C_4H_8N_2O_3$	132.1	$C_4H_6N_2O_2$	114.1	Neutral		■	
$C_4H_7NO_4$	133.1	$C_4H_5NO_3$	115.1	Acidic (−ve)			■
$C_3H_7NO_2S$	121.2	C_3H_5NOS	103.2	Neutral		■	
$C_5H_9NO_4$	147.1	$C_5H_7NO_3$	129.1	Acidic (−ve)			■
$C_5H_{10}N_2O_3$	146.1	$C_5H_8N_2O_2$	128.1	Neutral		■	
C_2H_5NO	275.1	C_2H_3NO	57.1	Neutral		■	
$C_6H_9N_3O_2$	155.2	$C_6H_7N_3O$	137.2	Basic (+ve)			■
$C_6H_{13}NO_2$	131.2	$C_6H_{11}NO$	113.2	Neutral	■		
$C_6H_{14}N_2O_2$	146.2	$C_6H_{12}N_2O$	128.2	Basic (+ve)			■
$C_5H_{11}NO_2S$	149.2	C_5H_9NOS	131.2	Neutral	■		
$C_9H_{11}NO_2$	165.2	C_9H_9NO	147.2	Neutral	■		
$C_5H_9NO_2$	115.1	C_5H_7NO	97.1	Neutral	■		
$C_3H_7NO_3$	105.1	$C_3H_5NO_2$	87.1	Neutral		■	
$C_4H_9NO_3$	119.1	$C_4H_7NO_2$	101.1	Neutral		■	
$C_{11}H_{12}N_2O_2$	204.2	$C_{11}H_{10}N_2O$	186.2	Neutral	■		
$C_9H_{11}NO_3$	181.2	$C_9H_9NO_2$	163.2	Neutral		■	
$C_5H_{11}NO_2$	117.1	C_5H_9NO	99.1	Neutral	■		

Figure 1.3 Properties of the 20 essential amino acids.

1.2.2 Translation

When a protein is translated from mRNA, it is created from N-terminus to C-terminus. The amino end of an amino acid (on a charged transfer RNA [tRNA]), during the elongation stage of translation, attaches to the carboxyl end of the growing chain. Since the start codon of the genetic code codes for the amino acid methionine, most protein sequences start with a methionine (or in bacteria, mitochondria, and chloroplasts, the modified version *N*-formylmethionine, fMet). However, some proteins are modified posttranslationally, for example, by cleavage from a protein precursor, and, therefore, may have different amino acids at their N-terminus.

1.2.3 Peptide bond

The chemical link between amino acids is called a *peptide bond.* It is formed between the carbonyl oxygen and carbon, with α-carbons on each side of the peptide bond, and the amide nitrogen and hydrogen, and is due to the partial double bond character that exists between the carbonyl carbon and the amide nitrogen atoms (Figure 1.4). The peptide bond has a planar structure that produces restrictions in the angular range of bond rotation around the Cα–N, expressed by ϕ (phi), and C–Cα, expressed as ψ (psi) bonds. These restrictions are summarized in a two-dimensional graphical plot called a Ramachandran plot; the plot graphically shows how certain structural features of proteins can only exist within limited ranges of angles, e.g., α-helix.

The ω angle at the peptide bond is normally 180° since the partial double bond character keeps the peptide planar. Because the dihedral angle values are circular, and 0° is the same as 360°, the edges of the Ramachandran plot "wrap" right to left and bottom to top (Figure 1.5).

The higher-order structure (HOS) of proteins includes secondary, tertiary, and quaternary structures as shown in Figure 1.6.

Figure 1.7 shows the three-dimensional (3D) structure of a filgrastim, a recombinant protein widely used for the treatment of neutropenia.

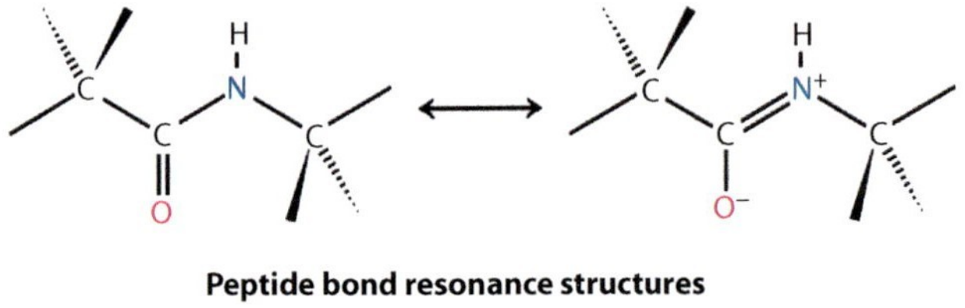

Figure 1.4 Peptide bond; the double bond character is about 40% due to resonance. (From Berg, J. M., J. L. Tymoczko, and L. Strye, *Biochemistry*, Seventh edition, W. H. Freeman and Co., New York, 2010.)

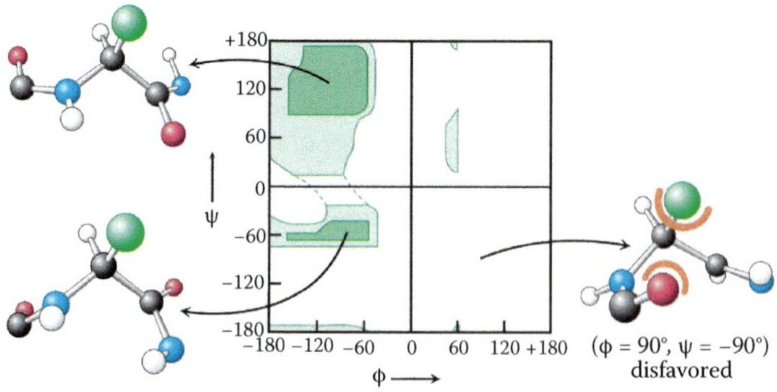

Figure 1.5 Ramachandran plot. (From Berg, J. M., J. L. Tymoczko, and L. Strye, *Biochemistry*, Seventh edition, W. H. Freeman and Co., New York, 2010. With permission.)

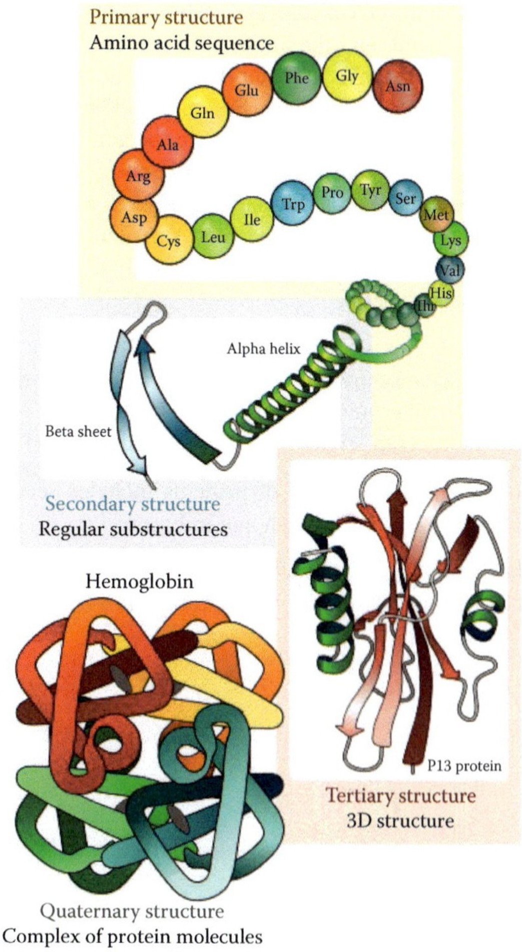

Figure 1.6 The four levels of protein structure.

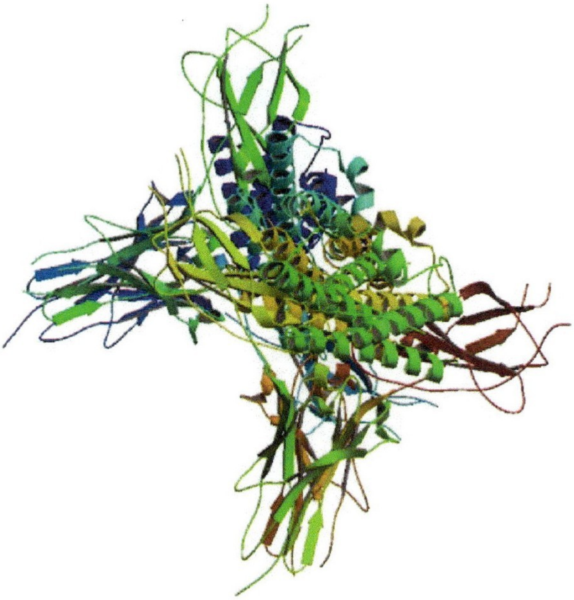

Figure 1.7 The 3D structure of filgrastim.

1.3 Motifs and domains

The primary and secondary structures are involved in a single polypeptide chain, the rest of the interaction of two or more identical or different polypeptide chains. The secondary structure leads to the formation of α-helices and β-sheets (Figure 1.6), which give rise to 3D structures, which are referred to as tertiary structures that provide the unique physicochemical and biological properties to proteins. The tertiary structures may acquire one or more peculiar folding patterns called *motifs* or supersecondary structure or complex folds, which are essentially "local tertiary structures" and should not be confused with the final or the global tertiary structure. The same applies to groups of motifs that are called domains, which are one or more independent compact regions of a protein. While motifs are structural elements, domains are functional elements, regardless of their size (Figure 1.8).

Proteins containing two or more domains are called multidomain proteins, wherein the domains may be covalently linked by highly flexible bonds called linkers. Despite the complexity of various HOSs, small changes in the amino acid sequence may not necessarily affect the HOS, a protein demonstrating the same activity. There can be more than one polypeptide chain, in which case, more than one tertiary structure is bonded to produce quaternary structures. Proteins can aggregate to form dimers, trimers, and tetramers; there is some confusion regarding the label used to describe these; a tetramer can be four polypeptide chains bonded through sulfur bonds, but that does not make a new monomer.

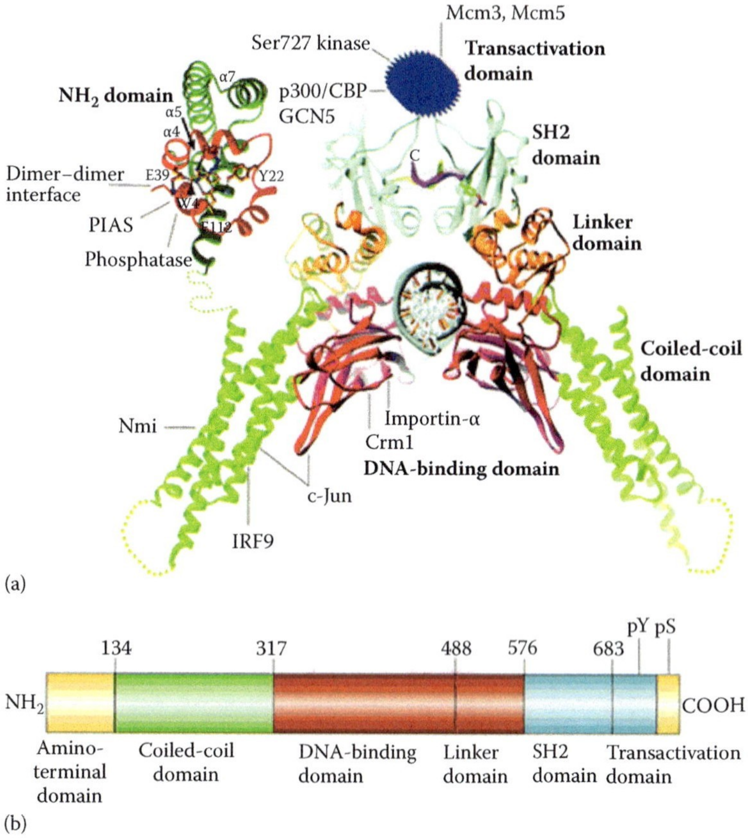

Figure 1.8 Domain structure of proteins. The core structure (amino acids approximately 130–712) shows binding of a STAT1 dimer to DNA and the location of binding sites of various proteins in various domains. The amino-terminal structure, the placement of which in the intact structure is undefined, also interacts with various partners, as does the carboxy-terminal transactivation domain, the structure of which is unknown. CBP, CREB binding protein; IRF, interferon regulatory factor; Mcm, minichromosome maintenance; Nmi, N-Myc interactor; PIAS, protein inhibitor of activated STAT; STAT, signal transducer and activator of transcription; SH2, Src-homology-2 domain; IRF9, interferon regulatory factor 9 gene; c-jun, protein encrypted by JUN gene; crm1, chromosomal maintenance 1, also known as Exportin 1; pS and pY, phosphorylation site and tyrosine phosphorylation site. (From D. E. Levy and J. E. Darnell, Jr, *Nature Reviews Molecular Cell Biology* 3, 651–662, September 2002. With permission.)

One domain may appear in a variety of different proteins. Molecular evolution uses domains as building blocks, and these may be recombined in different arrangements to create proteins with different functions. Domains vary in length from between about 25 amino acids up to 500 amino acids. The shortest domains such as zinc fingers are stabilized by metal ions or disulfide bridges. Domains often form functional units, such as the calcium-binding EF hand (helix-loop-helix) domain of calmodulin.

Because they are independently stable, domains can be swapped by genetic engineering between one protein and another to make chimeric proteins. It is independent because domains may often be cloned, expressed, and purified independently of the rest of the protein, and they may even show activity if there is any known activity associated with them. Some proteins contain only a single domain, while others may contain several domains. A protein domain is assigned a certain type of fold. Domains with the same fold may or may not be related to each other functionally because nature has used and reused the same fold many times in different contexts. The currently available protein 3D structures in the Protein Data Bank (PDB; http://www.wwpdb.org/) are a repository for the 3D structural data of large biological molecules, such as proteins and nucleic acids.

The domains can be divided into four main classes based on the secondary structural content of the domain:

- All-α domains have a domain core exclusively built from α-helices. This class is dominated by small folds, many of which form a simple bundle of helices running up and down.
- All-β domains have a core composed of antiparallel β-sheets, usually two sheets packed against each other. Various patterns can be identified in the arrangement of the strands, often giving rise to the identification of recurring motifs, for example, the Greek key motif.
- The α+β domains are a mixture of all-α and all-β motifs. The classification of proteins into this class is difficult because of overlaps between the other three classes and, therefore, is not used in the CATH (class, architecture, topology, homologous superfamily) domain database.
- The α/β domains are made from a combination of β–α–β motifs that are predominantly from a parallel β-sheet surrounded by amphipathic α-helices.

Domains have limits on the size and vary from 36 residues in E-selectin to 692 residues in lipoxygenase-1, but the majority, 90%, have less than 200 residues with an average of approximately 100 residues. Very short domains, less than 40 residues, are often stabilized by metal ions or disulfide bonds. Larger domains, greater than 300 residues, likely consist of multiple hydrophobic cores.

1.4 Association and aggregation

The HOS is stabilized through a large number of weak and strong bonds including weak noncovalent bonds formed ionic, dipoles (hydrogen bonds), nonpolar (hydrophobic), and van der Waals interactions. These bonds involve the interaction of amino acid side chains and the polypeptide chain. Since the transition from a polypeptide chain to HOS requires a significant loss of entry (structuring), it must be compensated for by enthalpy released from the forming of a bond (energy is released when a bond is formed); as a result, the protein structure can remain a dynamic state of structuring that may affect its activity as well as its stability. In most instances, the changes are transitory, and the protein returns to its native structure. However, the possibility of dynamic changes to a protein structure makes it possible for a molecule to have a different activity if its physicochemical properties are altered; additionally, if there is aggregation, this may lead to a loss of activity and a likely increase in the immunogenicity of the protein. Protein aggregation is caused by two factors: colloidal and conformational stabilities. The attractions on the surface of proteins can make colloidal dispersions that can be dynamic and significantly affect the safety and the effectiveness of proteins under stress conditions; the conformational changes are brought about by the hydrophobic interactions of the buried functional groups. There is a likelihood of both types of aggregates and, in some instances, one leads to another. So far, the regulatory authorities have not focused on these differentiations but over time, it is likely that these would be included as part of the risk analysis of the manufacturing process.

There is also a likelihood of aggregation due to molecular crowding when the drug is exposed to a high concentration of other proteins in the plasma. Would it ever be a requirement to study the nature of a circulating protein drug? This remains to be seen. However, a recent trend in the reformulation of proteins like adalimumab and rituximab in high-concentration formulations is an alarming trend; motivated by intellectual property (IP) protection as these drugs come off patent, the originators are reformulating their products, without fully realizing that the molecular crowding at the site of administration, if not in the vial or the syringe, is likely to increase the aggregation potential. The regulatory agencies should require a demonstration of safety at this level when a formula change request is made. This aspect of safety consideration is a topic of a citizen's petition filed by the author with the FDA.

The HOS a protein takes is intrinsically dictated by its primary structure and posttranslational modifications (PTMs). In the 1960s, Cyrus Levinthal proposed an interesting observation regarding protein folding. In a 100-residue protein, allowing 5×10^{47} conformations possible and if each confirmation takes 1 ps, it will take 10^{18} times as long as the age of the universe. It is truly amazing how a protein HOS is repeatedly formed approximately the same way, even if there are a few defects left in the primary structure. It is this possibility of variability that makes the development of biosimilar products challenging. Misfolded proteins often reach a stage of energy level that may be difficult to overcome and return them to their native state—the conditions under which proteins are manufactured can significantly alter this profile.

Protein synthesis involves a complex array of cellular machinery, primarily ribosomes. Proteins are synthesized from the N-terminus to the C-terminus in a sequential manner at a rate of 50–300 amino acids/minute; the folding begins once the chain has acquired 50–60 amino acids—cotranslational protein folding that constraints and limits the pathways a protein can take into HOS, and this may explain why Levinthal's Calculations come short.

Chaperones are proteins that help other proteins fold correctly in addition to proteolytic apparatus available in the cells.

There are some proteins that have no well-defined HOS. These are disordered or unstructured random coils, like the synthetic polymer chains or denatured proteins. This state may be a transitory state during the binding process and may be responsible for a multitude of protein actions in the cell. This intrinsic disorder creates a challenge to the demonstrate structure–function relationship, and whereas these aspects are not yet recognized by the regulatory authorities, it is only a matter of time when the biosimilar product developers may be required to demonstrate the disordered state comparisons as well—that will significantly raise the bar on the development of biosimilar products.

There are two types of proteins that can be labeled as *unnatural* construction—the fusion proteins or the conjugate (e.g., pegylated) proteins and very a large assembly of virus particles or nanoparticle delivery systems. The fusion of an Fc part of an antibody (typically an immunoglobulin G1 [IgG1] antibody) with that of another pharmaceutically relevant protein through recombinant genetic technology results in fusion proteins. The Fc portion of an antibody increases the circulation time just as does the pegylation; examples include fusion of Fc to the blood-clotting factor VIII and factor IX. In June 2014, the FDA approved Eloctate, antihemophilic factor (recombinant), Fc fusion protein, for use in adults and children who have hemophilia A. Eloctate is the first hemophilia A treatment designed to require less frequent injections when used to prevent or reduce the frequency of bleeding. In March 2014, the FDA approved Alprolix, coagulation factor IX (recombinant), Fc fusion protein, which is a recombinant DNA–derived coagulation factor IX concentrate. It temporarily replaces the missing coagulation factor IX needed for effective hemostasis. Etanercept is a fusion protein produced by recombinant DNA technology. It fuses the TNF receptor to the constant end of the IgG1 antibody. First, the sponsors isolated the DNA sequence that codes the human gene for soluble TNF receptor 2, which is a receptor that binds to TNF-alpha. Second, they isolated the DNA sequence that codes the human gene for the Fc end of IgG1. Third, they linked the DNA for TNF receptor 2 to the DNA for IgG1 Fc. Finally, they expressed the linked DNA to produce a protein that links the protein for TNF receptor 2 to the protein for IgG1 Fc.

The fusion of two relatively large proteins each being over 50 kDa raises the question whether this would impact the functionality of either protein. While there is a possible potential variance, the existing science reveals no significant impact. This comment is important as in the future, the regulatory authorities may raise this question.

The utility of pegylation is well understood and appreciated, as the popular products like Neulasta (pegylated granulocyte-colony stimulating factor) have established their safety and effectiveness while prolonging their disposition half-life. The two polyethylene glycol molecules protect the molecule from degradation in the body as well as reduce the immunogenicity.

1.5 Posttranslational modification

Biological products are complex structures, not only because of their basic protein structure, but also because of other modifications that they undergo during their maturation, generating a final form that is not a single and monomolecular entity (as could be expected of a chemical molecule with 99.9% purity) but rather a complex mix of the same protein molecule under various structurally close isoforms.

A protein is characterized by its primary to the quaternary structures as we often see and also by its additional characteristics acquired *during* the cellular process of protein synthesis. These are called posttranslational modifications, due to the fact that they occur once the gene (nucleic acid sequence) has been translated into the corresponding protein sequence (the amino acid chain). These modifications are also designated as the *maturation phase* essential before the release/

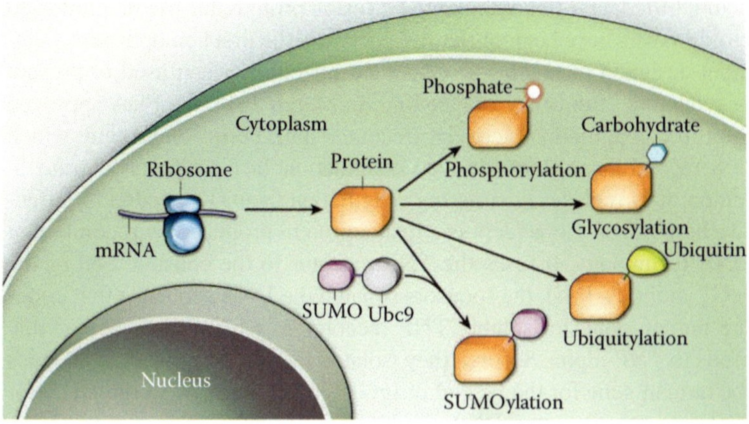

Figure 1.9 PTM of proteins.

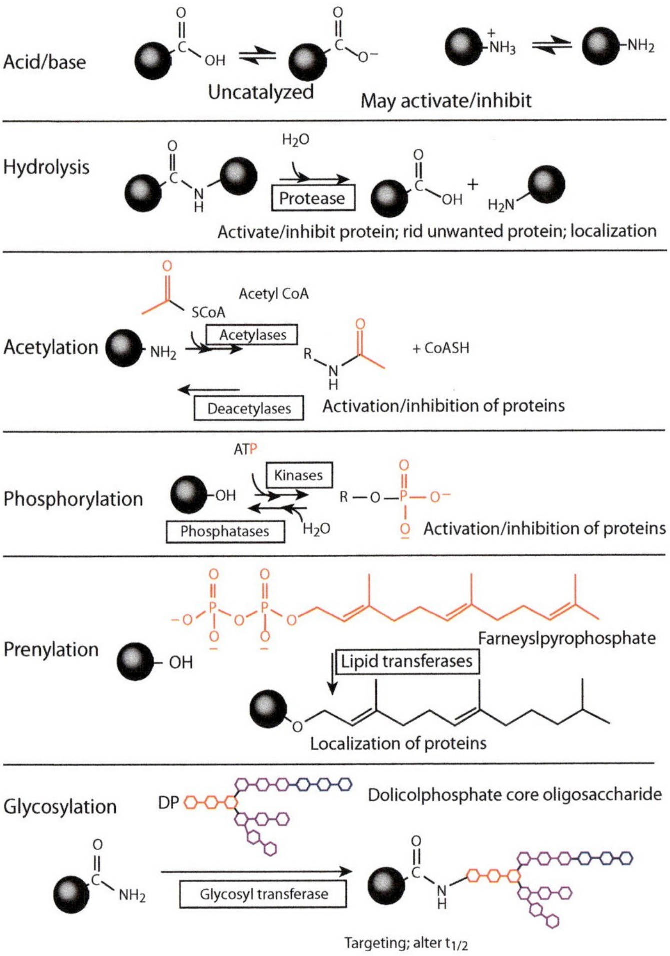

Figure 1.10 Common PTMs.

secretion of cell proteins. These modifications consist of the grafting on defined amino acids of one or several chemical/biological groups such as phosphate or sulfate groups or sugars (when it will be termed *glycosylation*) that modify the global charge and the physicochemical or biological characteristics of these *mature* proteins as the final active forms.

Figure 1.9 shows the process of PTM.

Figure 1.10 shows the various PTMs that are frequently encountered.

The impact of PTM on stability risk and functionality risk is demonstrated in Figure 1.11.

The PTMs that take place on specific sites of the protein are not controlled by the gene that expresses the protein sequence; instead,

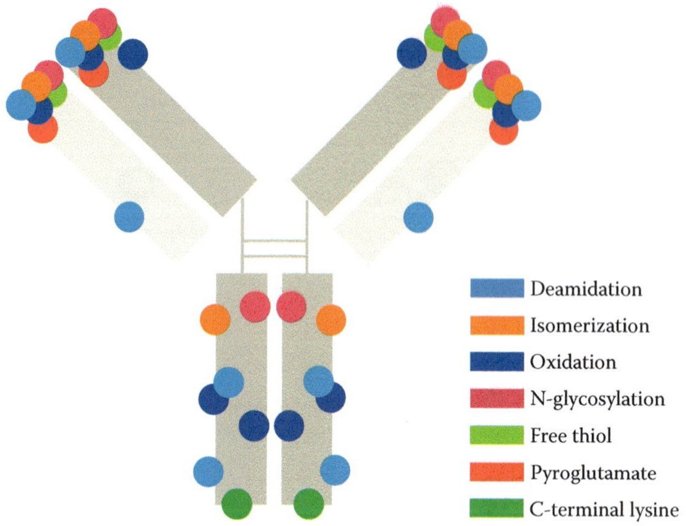

Figure 1.11 Possible sites of various PTMs.

they are specific to each cellular kind that presents a unique combination of milieu interior such as the presence of enzymes and the thermodynamic conditions during the reaction; it is for this reason that these complex chemical reactions are often not controllable by any alteration of the gene sequence, but only by mastering the production conditions during expression. However, this is not relevant to the expression inside prokaryotic organisms (bacteria), or to the very simple expression inside inferior eukaryotes such as yeasts, and PTMs are indigenous to *mammalian* cells like Chinese hamster ovary (CHO) cells.

Examples of PTMs include the following:

- PTMs involving the addition of an enzyme in vivo
  - PTMs involving the addition of hydrophobic groups for membrane localization
    - Myristoylation: The attachment of myristate, a C14 saturated acid
    - Palmitoylation: The attachment of palmitate, a C16 saturated acid
    - Isoprenylation or prenylation: The addition of an isoprenoid group (e.g., farnesol and geranylgeraniol)
      - Farnesylation
      - Geranylgeranylation
    - Glypiation: Glycosylphosphatidylinositol (GPI) anchor formation via an amide bond to C-terminal tail
  - PTMs involving the addition of cofactors for enhanced enzymatic activity

- Lipoylation: The attachment of a lipoate (C8) functional group
- The covalent attachment of a flavin moiety
- Heme C attachment via thioether bonds with cysteine
- Phosphopantetheine-lation: The addition of a 4′-phosphopantetheine moiety from coenzyme A, as in fatty acid, polyketide, nonribosomal peptide, and leucine biosynthesis
- Retinylidene Schiff base formation

- PTMs involving unique modifications of translation factors
  - Diphthamide formation (on a histidine found in eukaryotic translation elongation factor 2)
  - Ethanolamine phosphoglycerol attachment (on glutamate found ineukaryotic elongation factor 1α)
  - Hypusine formation (on conserved lysine of eukaryotic translation initiation factor 5A-1 (eukaryotic) and aIF5A gene (archeal)
- PTMs involving the addition of smaller chemical groups
  - Acylation, e.g., O-acylation (esters), N-acylation (amides), S-acylation (thioesters)
    - Acetylation: The addition of an acetyl group, either at the N-terminus of the protein or at the lysine residues; the reverse is called deacetylation
    - Formylation
  - Alkylation: The addition of an alkyl group, e.g., methyl and ethyl
    - Methylation by the addition of a methyl group, usually at lysine or arginine residues; the reverse is called demethylation
  - Amide bond formation
    - Amidation at C-terminus
    - Amino acid addition
      Arginylation: A tRNA-mediation addition
      Polyglutamylation: The covalent linkage of glutamic acid residues in the N-terminus of tubulin and some other proteins (see tubulin polyglutamylase)
      Polyglycylation: The covalent linkage of one to more than 40 glycine residues in the tubulin C-terminal tail
  - Butyrylation
  - Gamma carboxylation dependent on vitamin K
  - Glycosylation: The addition of a glycosyl group to either arginine, asparagine, cysteine, hydroxylysine, serine, threonine, tyrosine, or tryptophan, resulting in a glycoprotein; distinct from glycation, which is regarded as a nonenzymatic attachment of sugars
    - Polysialylation: The addition of polysialic acid to neural cell adhesion molecule

  - Malonylation
  - Hydroxylation
  - Iodination (e.g., of thyroglobulin)
  - Nucleotide addition such as ADP-ribosylation
  - Oxidation
  - Phosphate ester (O-linked) or phosphoramidate (N-linked) formation
    - Phosphorylation: The addition of a phosphate group, usually to serine, threonine, and tyrosine (O-linked), or histidine (N-linked)
    - Adenylylation: The addition of an adenylyl moiety, usually to tyrosine (O-linked), or histidine and lysine (N-linked)
  - Propionylation
  - Pyroglutamate formation
  - S-glutathionylation
  - S-nitrosylation
  - Succinylation: The addition of a succinyl group to lysine
  - Sulfation: The addition of a sulfate group to a tyrosine
- PTMs involving nonenzymatic additions in vivo
  - Glycation: The addition of a sugar molecule to a protein without the controlling action of an enzyme
- PTMs involving nonenzymatic additions in vitro
  - Biotinylation: The acylation of conserved lysine residues with a biotin appendage
  - Pegylation
- PTMs involving the addition of other proteins or peptides
  - ISGylation: The covalent linkage to the ISG15 protein (ISG: interferon-stimulated gene)
  - SUMOylation: The covalent linkage to the SUMO protein (SUMO: small ubiquitin-related modifier)
  - Ubiquitination: The covalent linkage to the protein ubiquitin
  - Neddylation: The covalent linkage to neural precursor cell expressed, developmentally down-regulated protein (nedd)
  - Pupylation: The covalent linkage to the prokaryotic ubiquitin-like protein
- PTMs involving the changing of the chemical nature of amino acids
  - Citrullination or deimination: The conversion of arginine to citrulline
  - Deamidation: The conversion of glutamine to glutamic acid or asparagine to aspartic acid
  - Elimination: The conversion of an alkene by beta-elimination of phosphothreonine and phosphoserine, or dehydration of threonine and serine, as well as by decarboxylation of cysteine
  - Carbamylation: The conversion of lysine to homocitrulline
- PTMs involving structural changes

- Disulfide bridges: The covalent linkage of two cysteine amino acids
- Proteolytic cleavage: The cleavage of a protein at a peptide bond
- Racemization
- Structural changes of proline by prolyl isomerase
- Structural changes of serine by a protein-serine epimerase
- Structural changes of alanine in dermorphin, a frog opioid peptide
- Structural changes of methionine in deltorphin, also a frog opioid peptide

1.5.1 Glycosylation

One of the more important PTMs is glycosylation; this is distinct from glycans. An example of how a glycosylation reaction occurs and its consequences upon protein characteristics and reproducibility of recombinant proteins is given in Figure 1.12.

Glycosylation is the most frequent PTM. The terms *glycan* and *polysaccharide* are defined by the International Union of Pure and Applied Chemistry as synonyms meaning "compounds consisting of a large number of monosaccharides linked glycosidically." However, in practice, the term *glycan* may also be used to refer to the carbohydrate portion of a glycol conjugate, such as a glycoprotein, glycolipid, or proteoglycan, even if the carbohydrate is only an oligosaccharide. Glycans usually solely consist of O-glycosidic linkages of monosaccharides. For example, cellulose is a glycan (or, to be more precise, a glucan) composed of β-1,4-linked D-glucose, and chitin is a glycan composed of β-1,4-linked *N*-acetyl-D-glucosamine.

Glycans can be homo- or heteropolymers of monosaccharide residues and can be linear or branched. The introduced chemical modifications

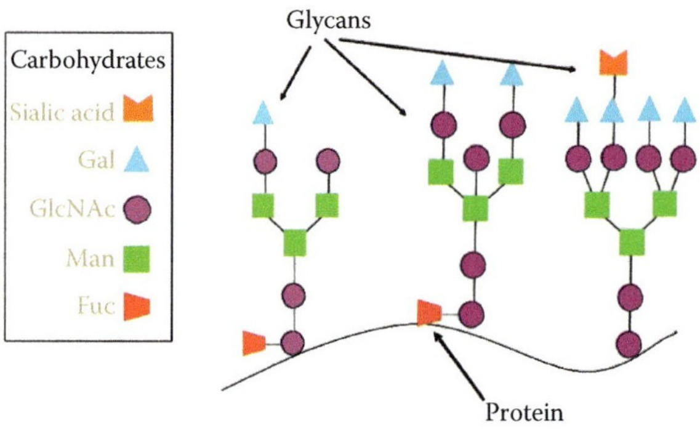

Figure 1.12 Schematic drawing of carbohydrate residues (or glycanic structures) present on some protein sequences (Gal = galactose, Man = mannose, Fuc = fucose, GlcNAc = N-acetyl glucosamine).

are very complex due to the glycan structures that are added to the protein skeleton. The protein glycosylation step occurs in the endoplasmic reticulum and the Golgi apparatuses. Glycosylation consists of branching on the protein, on determined amino acids (for instance, for N-glycosylation, asparagine [Asn] which is in the Asn–X–Thr sequence), sugar groups such as mannose, fructose, or galactose following well-determined orders. These glycosylation chemical reactions will lead to the making of *sugar chains*, more or less complex and diversified, considering all the possible attaching combinations (number of antenna(e) on a glycosylation site, and the nature of sugars making up this antenna), even if some mandatory sequences are found in each structure.

Finally, the end of the sugar chain is most often capped by a sialic acid in the form of neuraminic N-acetyl acid (NANA) in human cells; as for many mammals, a part of the sialic acid is in the form of neuraminic N-glycolyl acid (NGNA) because the gene which codes for the enzyme that allows the NANA form to become NGNA is muted and inactive in humans. This species specificity is important when choosing systems involving carbohydrate expression/production of the recombinant protein of interest, to ensure that the sialylation is as close as possible to the human form. The mature protein, so glycolyzed and more or less sialylated, gets some characteristics that are more or less acidic with a changed isoelectric point (pI). Consequently, at the end of PTMs, the protein appears not as a single entity but as a mix, a molecular population with the same basic protein structure (primary sequence imposed by gene sequence) on which various types of sugar chains will have been attached, giving each protein molecule its own pI. These series of isoforms are studied qualitatively and quantitatively using appropriate analytical techniques that separate the various isoforms such as based on their charge.

Since the glycosylation profile of a protein is critical in determining its activity, proteins are characterized by their pI value and by a series of visible and quantifiable bandwidths, by separation methods of isoelectrofocusing.

There are four types of glycosylation links:

- N-linked glycosylation: N-linked glycosylation is the most common type of glycosidic bond and is necessary for the folding of some eukaryotic proteins and for cell–cell and cell–extracellular matrix attachments. The N-linked glycosylation process occurs in eukaryotes in the lumen of the endoplasmic reticulum and widely in archaea, but very rarely in bacteria.
- O-linked glycosylation: O-linked glycosylation is a form of glycosylation that not only occurs in eukaryotes in the Golgi apparatus, but also occurs in archaea and bacteria. Xylose, fucose, mannose, and N-acetyl glucosamine (GlcNAc) phosphoserine glycans have been reported in the literature.

- C-mannosylation: A mannose sugar is added to the first tryptophan residue in the sequence W–X–X–W (*W* indicates tryptophan; *X* is any amino acid). Thrombospondins are one of the most commonly C-modified proteins, although this form of glycosylation appears elsewhere as well. C-mannosylation is unusual because the sugar is linked to a carbon rather than to a reactive atom such as nitrogen or oxygen. Recently, the first crystal structure of a protein containing this type of glycosylation has been determined to be that of human complement component 8, PDB ID 3OJY.
- Formation of GPI anchors (glypiation): A special form of glycosylation is the formation of a GPI anchor. In this kind of glycosylation, the protein is attached to a lipid anchor, via a glycan chain.

Glycanic structures are obtained by combining the sugar group's nature (Gal = galactose, Man = mannose, Fuc = fucose, GlcNAc = N-acetyl glucosamine) and its organization in antennae (mono-, bi-, even triantennae). Let us also note the presence of a "sialic acid" group that sometimes caps the antennae's ends. The sialic acid groups are notably contributing to the protein molecule's half-life.

PTMs, usually illustrated by the glycosylation profile, are intrinsic quality criteria of the protein as well as critical parameters to consider during the assessment of the production process and its reproducibility, notably when changes are introduced in the production method, and a fortiori when a new manufacturer offers a biosimilar version of a reference protein.

Indeed, for the new producer of a given glycosylated protein, one could fear an isoform distribution different from that of the original molecule. This different isoelectric profile, which is often difficult to distinguish by only the analytical methods offered by the manufacturer, will potentially have an impact on the pharmacokinetics or the biological activity of the therapeutic protein. Then, it will be the pharmacological and/or the clinical data that will reveal the sometimes subtle change in isoform distribution when the quality control analytical data are detecting no noticeable difference.

Although some studies suggest that the consequence of a different isoelectric profile mostly concerns the neoantigenicity risk, it seems that this phenomenon rather impacts the half-life of the molecule, which will be more or less rapidly eliminated by the receiving patient's body. Indeed, the sugar chains, notably depending on their sialic acid capping, protect the protein from capture and degradation by hepatic cells.

Thus, a recombinant protein will have to have an adapted glycosylation, as well as a correct sialic acid level (in the NANA form), to not be eliminated too quickly and keep a sufficient pharmacological activity and reduce any potential to generate a defense reaction in patients with the formation of antibodies to the protein of interest.

Whereas the molecules with PTM may have one species forming the majority of the protein component, the other glycans and components may be just as important in determining the final activity of the product.

1.6 Protein expression variability

A clear understanding of how the recombinant DNA technique works is necessary for the understanding of factors that may contribute to protein structure variability, besides the inherent properties as described earlier. The genes are DNA portions carrying a message that ultimately leads to the production of proteins. They are present in the genomes of all living creatures and are sequences of nucleotides (A, T, G, and C). Each of these genes' sequence is specific for a protein (Figure 1.13).

Cells transcribe the genes (DNA) into mRNA, which in turn are translated into proteins. These steps are represented in the sequence shown in Figure 1.14.

The living entities expressing cytokines and monoclonal antibodies have modified gene encoding to include the human protein sequence of interest. As the genetic code is universal, it will be read the same way by all cellular systems of the animal, plant, or bacterial kingdom (even as the existence of dominant codons per cell system is known). This universality is the basis of the production of recombinant therapeutic proteins of the human sequence into heterologous host systems (bacteria, yeast, plant, mammalian cell, and transgenic animals) to make that host system produce a protein of given sequence.

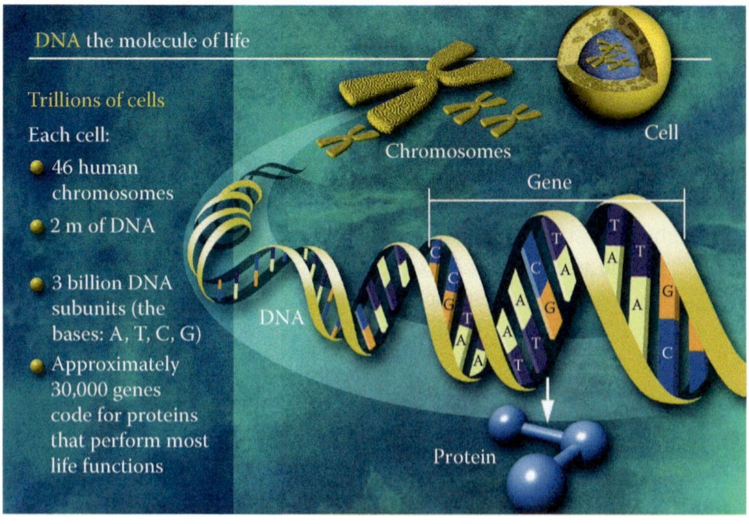

Figure 1.13 Structure of DNA. (From Office of Biological and Environmental Research of the U.S. Department of Energy Office of Science, https://science.energy.gov/ber/.)

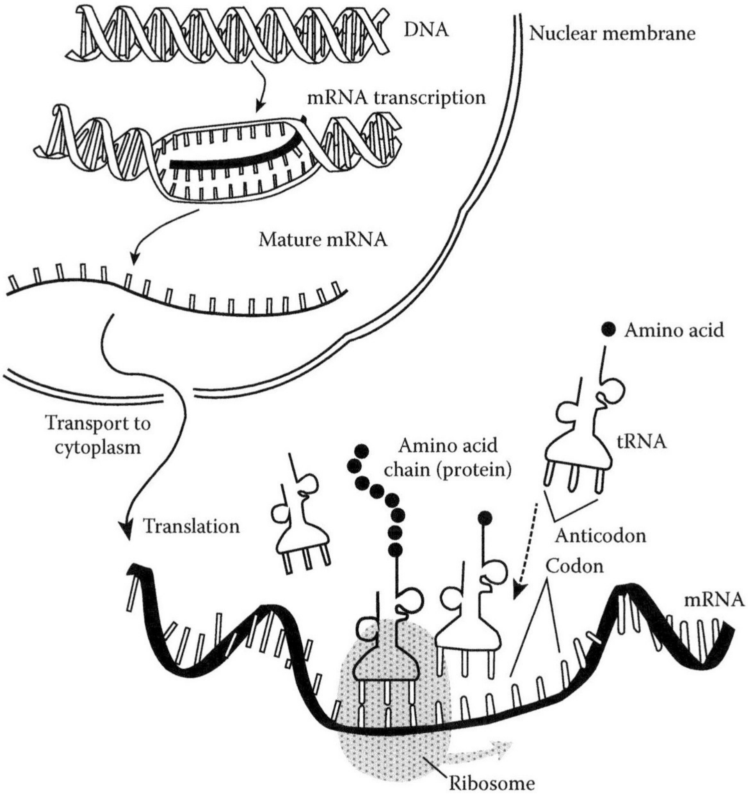

Figure 1.14 Gene expression system. (From https://mariakonovalenko.wordpress.com/2010/10/07/gene-expression-defined/. With permission.)

For the human protein to be correctly expressed by the producer-host organism, it is necessary to optimize the gene sequence in using for each amino acid the dominant codon of the species used. The optimized sequence is affixed to a promoter, which controls the protein expression by the genetically modified host system. Selecting the promoter depends on the host cell and leads to optimizing the expression yield.

For complex proteins, in necessitating posttranslation-specific reactions (such as specific conformations, oligomerization, proteolytic cleavages, phosphorylations, or glycosylation reactions), a eukaryotic system is needed wherein these reactions take place in the endoplasmic reticulum and in the Golgi apparatus. The following three levels of these organisms are used:

- Lower eukaryotes like yeasts and fungi are able to make relatively simple PTMs such as glycoproteins. Since yeasts produce N-glycosylations rich in mannose residues, which are strongly immunogenic to humans, the choice may be limited.

- Higher eukaryotes like mammalian cells or insect or plant cells provide much lower yields and are harder to manage. Mammalian cells such as ovarian cells of CHO are commonly used to produce complex glycoproteins.
- Plant and transgenic animals produce therapeutic proteins in a tissue (in the case of plants) or in a fluid (most often milk for transgenic animals) in large quantities that are highly practical sources of future biological products.

Given that living entities are involved in the expression of proteins, it is easy to see how a change in bioprocessing conditions can readily alter the structure of proteins. Harder to manage are the variance in the glycan patterns, the antibody-dependent cell-mediated cytotoxicity, and other similar variations that might not necessarily be clinically meaningful, yet to prove it otherwise may be impossible, resulting in a biosimilar product developer modifying the bioprocessing to assure that the structure of protein expressed is as close as possible to the originator molecule.

Bibliography

Anderson, C. L. (2012 June) Applications of imaged capillary isoelectric focussing technique in development of biopharmaceutical glycoprotein-based products. *Electrophoresis* 33 (11): 1538–1544.

Bártová, E., Krejcí, J., Harnicarová, A., Galiová, G., and Kozubek, S. (2008) Histone modifications and nuclear architecture: A review. *J Histochem Cytochem* 56 (8): 711–721.

Beck, A., Sanglier-Cianférani, S., and Van Dorsselaer, A. (2012 June 5) Biosimilar, biobetter, and next generation antibody characterization by mass spectrometry. *Anal Chem* 84 (11): 4637–4646.

Beck, A., Wurch, T., and Reichert, J. M. (2011 March–April 3) Sixth annual european antibody congress 2010: November 29–December 1, 2010, Geneva, Switzerland. *MAbs* 3 (2): 111–132.

Boubeva, R., Reichert, C., Handrick, R., Müller, C., Hannemann, J., and Borcharda, G. (2012) New expression method and characterization of recombinant human granulocyte colonystimulating factor in a stable protein formulation. *Chimia (Aarau)* 66 (5): 281–285.

Brennan, D. F. and Barford, D. (2009) Eliminylation: A post-translational modification catalyzed by phosphothreonine lyases. *Trends Biochem Sci* 34 (3): 108–114.

Cantor, C. R. and Schimmel, P. R., *Biophysical Chemistry Part 1: The Conformation of Biological Macromolecules*. New York: W. H. Freeman and Co.; 1980.

Cao, J., Sun, W., Gong, F., and Liu, W. (2014 May) Charge profiling and stability testing of biosimilar by capillary isoelectric focusing. *Electrophoresis* 35 (10): 1461–1468.

Chen, S. L., Wu, S. L., Huang, L. J., Huang, J. B., and Chen, S. H. (2013 June) A global comparability approach for biosimilar monoclonal antibodies using LC-tandem MS based proteomics. *J Pharm Biomed Anal* 80: 126–135.

Creighton, T. E., *Protein Structures and Molecular Properties*. Second ed., New York: W. H. Freeman and Co.; 1993.

Creighton, T. E., *The Biophysical Chemistry of Nucleic Acids and Proteins*. London: Helvetian Press; 2010.

Debaene, F., Wagner-Rousset, E., Colas, O., Ayoub, D., Corvaïa, N., Van Dorsselaer, A., Beck, A., and Cianférani, S. (2013 October 15) Time resolved native ion-mobility mass spectrometry tomonitor dynamics of IgG4 Fab arm exchange and "bispecific" monoclonal antibody formation. *Anal Chem* 85 (20): 9785–9792.

Declerck, P. J. (2013 February) Biosimilar monoclonal antibodies: A science-based regulatory challenge. *Expert Opin Biol Ther* 13 (2): 153–156.

Dorvignit, D., Palacios, J. L., Merino, M., Hernández, T., Sosa, K., Casaco, A., López-Requena, A., and Mateo de Acosta, C. (2012 July–August) Expression and biological characterization of an anti-CD20 biosimilar candidate antibody: A case study. *MAbs* 4 (4): 488–496.

Eddé, B., Rossier, J., Le Caer, J. P., Desbruyères, E., Gros, F., and Denoulet, P. (1990) Posttranslational glutamylation of alpha-tubulin. *Science* 247 (4938): 83–85.

Eichbaum, C. and Haefeli, W. E. (2011 November) Biologics—Nomenclature and classification. *Ther Umsch* 68 (11): 593–601.

Gadermaier, G. (2014) Non-specific lipid transfer proteins: A protein family in search of an allergenic pattern. *Int Arch Allergy Immunol* 164 (3): 169–170.

Gadermaier, G., Eichhorn, S., Vejvar, E., Weilnböck, L., Lang, R., Briza, P., Huber, C. G., Ferreira, F., and Hawranek, T. (2014 August) *Plantago lanceolata*: An important trigger of summerpollinosis with limited IgE cross-reactivity. *J Allergy Clin Immunol* 134 (2): 472–475.

Glozak, M. A., Sengupta, N., Zhang, X., and Seto, E. (2005) Acetylation and deacetylation of non-histone proteins. *Gene* 363: 15–23.

Guo, Q., Guo, H., Liu, T., Zheng, Y., Gu, P., Chen, X., Wang, H., Hou, S., and Guo, Y. (2014 November 2) Versatile characterization of glycosylation modification in CTLA4-Ig fusion proteins by liquid chromatography-mass spectrometry. *MAbs* 6 (6): 1474–1485.

Haselberg, R., de Jong, G. J., and Somsen, G. W. (2013 February 19) Low-flow sheathless capillary electrophoresis-mass spectrometry for sensitive glycoform profiling of intact pharmaceutical proteins. *Anal Chem* 85 (4): 2289–2296.

Hashii, N., Harazono, A., Kuribayashi, R., Takakura, D., and Kawasaki, N. (2014 April 30) Characterization of N-glycan heterogeneities of erythropoietin products by liquid chromatography/mass spectrometry and multivariate analysis. *Rapid Commun Mass Spectrom* 28 (8): 921–932.

Hassett, B., McMillen, S., and Fitzpatrick, B. (2013 September–October) Characterization and comparison of commercially available TNF receptor 2-Fc fusion protein products: Letter to the editor. *MAbs* 5 (5): 624–625.

Heringa, J. and Taylor, W. R., *Computational Protein Science: Methods in Structural Bioinformatics*. Hoboken, NJ: J. Wiley & Sons; 2016.

Jiang, H., Wu, S. L., Karger, B. L., and Hancock, W. S. (2010 July 15) Characterization of the glycosylation occupancy and the active site in the follow-on protein therapeutic: TNK-tissue plasminogen activator. *Anal Chem* 82 (14): 6154–6162.

Kessel, A. and Nir Ben-Tal, A., *Introduction to Proteins: Structure, Function, and Motion*. Boca Raton, FL: Chapman & Hall/CRC Mathematical and Computational Biology; 2010.

Khoury, G. A., Baliban, R. C., and Floudas, C. A. (2011) Proteome-wide post-translational modification statistics: Frequency analysis and curation of the swiss-prot database. *Sci Rep* 1 (90): 90.

Li, C., Rossomando, A., Wu, S. L., and Karger, B. L. (2013 July–August) Comparability analysis of anti-CD20 commercial (rituximab) and RNAi-mediated fucosylated antibodies by two LC-MS approaches. *MAbs* 5 (4): 565–575.

Lipiäinen, T., Peltoniemi, M., Sarkhel, S., Yrjönen, T., Vuorela, H., Urtti, A., and Juppo, A. (2015 February) Formulation and stability of cytokine therapeutics. *J Pharm Sci* 104 (2): 307–326.

Malakhova, O. A., Yan, M., Malakhov, M. P., Yuan, Y., Ritchie, K. J., Kim, K. I., Peterson, L. F., Shuai, K., and Zhang, D.-E. (2003) Protein ISGylation modulates the JAK-STAT signaling pathway. *Genes Dev* 17 (4): 455–460.

Mueller, D. A., Heinig, L., Ramljak, S., Krueger, A., Schulte, R., Wrede, A., Stuke, A. W. (2010 December) Conditional expression of full-length humanized anti-prion protein antibodies in Chinese hamster ovary cells. *Hybridoma (Larchmt)* 29 (6): 463–472.

Mydel, P. et al. (2010) Carbamylation-dependent activation of T cells: A novel mechanism in the pathogenesis of autoimmune arthritis. *J Immunol* 184 (12): 6882–6890.

Novo, J. B., Oliveira, M. L., Magalhães, G. S., Morganti, L., Raw, I., and Ho, P. L. (2010 November) Generation of polyclonal antibodies against recombinant human glucocerebrosidase produced in *Escherichia coli*. *Mol Biotechnol* 46 (3): 279–286.

Oh, M. J., Hua, S., Kim, B. J., Jeong, H. N., Jeong, S. H., Grimm, R., Yoo, J. S., and An, H. J. (2013 March) Analytical platform for glycomic characterization of recombinant erythropoietin biotherapeutics and biosimilars by MS. *Bioanalysis* 5 (5): 545–559.

Pan, J. and Borchers, C. H. (2014 May) Top–down mass spectrometry and hydrogen/deuterium exchange for comprehensive structural characterization of interferons: Implications for biosimilars. *Proteomics* 14 (10): 1249–1258.

Parnham, M. J., Schindler-Horvat, J., and Kozlović, M. (2007 February) Non-clinical safety studies on biosimilar recombinant human erythropoietin. *Basic Clin Pharmacol Toxicol* 100 (2): 73–83. Review. PubMed PMID: 17244255.

Polevoda, B. and Sherman, F. (2003) N-terminal acetyltransferases and sequence requirements for N-terminal acetylation of eukaryotic proteins. *J Mol Biol* 325 (4): 595–622.

Schellekens, H. (2004 August) When biotech proteins go off-patent. *Trends Biotechnol* 22 (8): 406–410. Review. PubMed PMID: 15283985.

Skrlin, A., Radic, I., Vuletic, M., Schwinke, D., Runac, D., Kusalic, T., Paskvan, I., Krsic, M., Bratos, M., and Marinc, S. (2010 September) Comparison of the physicochemical properties of a biosimilar filgrastim with those of reference filgrastim. *Biologicals* 38 (5): 557–566.

Sörgel, F., Lerch, H., and Lauber, T. (2010 December 1) Physicochemical and biologic comparability of a biosimilar granulocyte colony-stimulating factor with its reference product. *BioDrugs* 24 (6): 347–357.

Su, J., Mazzeo, J., Subbarao, N., and Jin, T. (2011 July) Pharmaceutical development of biologics: Fundamentals, challenges and recent advances. *Ther Deliv* 2 (7): 865–871. PubMed PMID: 22833901.

Tan, Q., Guo, Q., Fang, C., Wang, C., Li, B., Wang, H., Li, J., and Guo, Y. (2012 November–December) Characterization and comparison of commercially available TNF receptor 2-Fc fusion protein products. *MAbs* 4 (6): 761–774.

Thelwell, C. (2014 March) Biological standards for potency assignment to fibrinolytic agents used in thrombolytic therapy. *Semin Thromb Hemost* 40 (2): 205–213.

Toyama, A., Nakagawa, H., Matsuda, K., Sato, T. A., Nakamura, Y., and Ueda, K. (2012 November 20) Quantitative structural characterization of local N-glycan microheterogeneity in therapeutic antibodies by energy-resolved oxonium ion monitoring. *Anal Chem* 84 (22): 9655–9662.

Visser, J., Feuerstein, I., Stangler, T., Schmiederer, T., Fritsch, C., and Schiestl, M. (2013 October) Physicochemical and functional comparability between the proposed biosimilar rituximab GP2013 and originator rituximab. *BioDrugs* 27 (5): 495–507.

Walsh, G., *Post-Translational Modification of Protein Biopharmaceuticals*. Hoboken, NJ: Wiley-Blackwell; 2009.

Whiteheart, S. W. et al. (1989) Murine elongation factor 1 alpha (EF-1 alpha) is post-translationally modified by novel amide-linked ethanolamine-phosphoglycerol moieties: Addition of ethanolamine-phosphoglycerol to specific glutamic acid residues on EF-1 alpha. *J Biol Chem* 264 (24): 14334–14341.

Wilson, V. G. (Ed.), *Sumoylation: Molecular Biology and Biochemistry*. Oxford, UK: Horizon Bioscience; 2004. ISBN 0-9545232-8-8.
Xie, H., Chakraborty, A., Ahn, J., Yu, Y. Q., Dakshinamoorthy, D. P., Gilar, M., Chen, W., Skilton, S. J., and Mazzeo, J. R. (2010 July–August) Rapid comparison of a candidate biosimilar to an innovator monoclonal antibody with advanced liquid chromatography and mass spectrometry technologies. *MAbs* 2 (4): 379–394.
Yang, X. J. and Seto, E. (2008) Lysine acetylation: Codified crosstalk with other post-translational modifications. *Mol Cell* 31 (4): 449–461.

Chapter 2 The biosimilar landscape

In the landscape of extinction, precision is next to godliness.
Samuel Beckett

2.1 Background

Biopharmaceutical products constitute the newest category of products that will soon expand to constitute more than two-thirds of all new drugs over the next 20 years. Given the types of diseases and conditions, both rare and common, treated by biopharmaceutical products, which include cancer, diabetes, anemia, rheumatoid arthritis, multiple sclerosis, and many more to come, this category of products is indeed unique, the commercial returns astronomical and the service to humankind provided by lower-cost alternates to licensed biopharmaceuticals, biosimilars, unparalleled.

In 1902, Congress passed the Biologics Control Act, which applied to "any virus, therapeutic serum, toxin, antitoxin, or analogous product applicable to the prevention and cure of diseases of man" and required the licensure of facilities making these products. Over the next hundred plus years, Congress expanded this list of covered products to include, among other things, vaccines, blood, blood products, allergenic products, and proteins (except chemically synthesized polypeptides) and their analogs. Despite these amendments, Congress never defined the listed terms and, in particular, never defined *analogous*, so the scope of the biological product definition remained unclear. The overlapping definition of *drug* added to this complexity. The Food and Drugs Act of 1906 and the Federal Food, Drug, and Cosmetic Act of 1938 (FDCA) broadly define *drug* to include, among other things, substances intended for use in the cure, the mitigation, or the prevention of disease, and the latter statute mandated the submission of a nondisclosure agreement (NDA) before the marketing of a drug. Although these *drug* definitions encompassed many biologics, the statutes did not provide concrete parameters for distinguishing nonbiological drugs from biological products. In 1944, when Congress revised and codified the 1902 Public Health Service Act (PHSA), it clarified that the NDA requirement did not apply to biologics, but it did not elucidate the scope of the biological product definition. Regulators attempted to fill this gap by promulgating regulatory definitions of virus, therapeutic serum, toxin, antitoxin, and analogous product. For example, the 1947 regulations, which are essentially similar to the current ordinance, defined products analogous to a toxin or antitoxin as those intended for preventing, treating, or curing diseases or injuries "through specific immunization." The 1947 definition of products analogous to therapeutic serums excluded hormones. Hormones such as insulin and human growth hormone were licensed under the FDCA, not the PHSA. Despite the 1947 regulations, differentiating biologics from drugs remained challenging at the margins.

The advent of biotechnology, along with FDA organizational disputes, brought this issue to the forefront of the FDA's focus. In 1986, the FDA issued a policy statement stating that it would determine whether biotechnology products constituted biologics "based on the intended use of each product on a case-by-case basis." Thus, the FDA continued to make product-specific determinations informed by history and precedent, and different units of the FDA had to agree on the approval pathway for a given product. This proved to be difficult, with press reports of turf battles between the Center for Drug Evaluation and Research (CDER) and the Center for Biologics Evaluation and Research (CBER) for jurisdiction over blockbuster biotechnology products and claims that the decisions were inconsistent. For example, epidermal growth factors were regulated as drugs because their first licensed indications were traditionally drugged indications. Most mAbs were licensed as biologics because of their biological source material and immunologic function. Recombinant insulin and human growth hormone, similar to their naturally derived counterparts, were licensed pursuant to NDAs. CDER and CBER subsequently executed an intercenter agreement (ICA) that attempted to clarify the governing authorities for products derived from living material. The agreement provided that the following products, among others, were subject to licensure under the PHSA: vaccines; proteins, peptides, and carbohydrates produced by cell culture (other than hormones and products previously derived from human or animal tissue and licensed as drugs); proteins made in transgenic animals; blood and blood products; and allergenic products. NDAs were required for, among other things, hormones (regardless of method of manufacture), synthetic mononucleotide and polynucleotide products, and naturally derived products other than vaccines or allergens. Twelve years later, the FDA consolidated a review of most therapeutic proteins in CDER, but this transfer did not modify the governing statutory scheme for any ICA product, and the FDA continued to decide whether new products were biological products or nonbiologic drugs on a case-by-case basis using the principles of the ICA and the historical precedent.

In February 2012, the FDA issued a draft guidance aimed at implementing recent legislation that added "protein (except any chemically synthesized polypeptide)" to the biological product definition. In this draft guidance, the FDA proposed a bright-line rule distinguishing protein from "peptides" and "chemically synthesized polypeptide[s]" that the FDA proposes to approve under the FDCA. The FDA proposed to define *protein* as "any alpha amino acid polymer with a specifically defined sequence that is greater than 40 amino acids in size." According to the draft guidance, "peptides" have 40 or fewer amino acids and are not "proteins." The FDA also proposed to define *chemically synthesized polypeptide* as an alpha amino acid polymer that is entirely made by chemical synthesis and that has fewer than 100 amino acids. Until the draft guidance is finalized, these definitions must be considered proposals. Nevertheless, they signal that the FDA might be shifting from its traditional, ad hoc approach to jurisdictional decisions to a new approach guided by bright-line rules.

The differentiation of products from being therapeutically interchangeable pharmaceuticals to biosimilar biopharmaceuticals had its roots in the size of active molecules; compared with synthetic small molecules, biologics are 100 to 1000 times larger, having several hundred amino acids (average molecular weight of 150 per amino acid), which are biochemically joined together in a defined sequence by peptide bonds to form a polypeptide. Thus, structurally, biologics are more complex than low–molecular weight drugs, consisting of primary (amino acid sequence) and secondary (α-helix and β-pleated sheet) structures, which are folded into complicated 3D tertiary structures. In some biopharmaceuticals, stable associations of tertiary structures of individual proteins form a quaternary structure. After synthesis, these structures are often further modified by PTMs such as glycosylation or sialylation, which may be crucial for biological activity. Furthermore, due to a larger size and structural complexity, the characterization of a biopharmaceutical presents an enormous challenge.

2.2 The rise of biosimilars

The Patient Protection and Affordable Care Act (Affordable Care Act), signed into law by President Barack Obama on March 23, 2010, amends the PHSA to create an abbreviated licensure pathway for biological products that are demonstrated to be biosimilar to or interchangeable with an FDA-licensed biological product. This pathway is provided in the part of the law known as the Biologics Price Competition and Innovation Act (BPCI Act). Under the BPCI Act, a biological product may be demonstrated to be biosimilar if data show that, among other things, the product is "highly similar" to an already-licensed biological product.

2.2.1 Legislative history

The history of the developments leading to the signing of the agreement and the progress so far in implementing a biosimilar pathway are discussed in the following.

March 2009—Californian Democrat Henry Waxman introduces a bill in the House that would clear a regulatory path for generic manufacturers to produce biosimilars after a five-year period of market exclusivity. Major biotech companies were hoping for 14 years of exclusivity.

April 2009—Six senators introduce legislation in the Senate that cuts the time allowed before biosimilars could compete with the originals to five years. The present law calls for a 12-year period of exclusivity for biological drugs. The bill would give the FDA the discretion to approve biosimilars with less extensive testing.

July 2009—The Senate votes to give biologicals 12 years of market exclusivity. The White House had proposed seven years and Henry Waxman only five years.

November 2009—The proposed healthcare bill that will be brought before the House includes a provision creating a way for the FDA to approve biosimilars. The proposed bill gives brand name drug companies sales exclusivity for 12 years and allows them to extend that time frame, with minor changes to their formulas.

March 2010—President Obama signs the healthcare reform BPCI Act allowing the FDA to approve biosimilars to be marketed, with the FDA setting the rules as to what is required to gain approval.

October 2010—The FDA holds a two-day public meeting in order to obtain input on specific issues and challenges associated with the implementation of the BPCI Act.

January 2011—Debate continues over the fact that although the BPCI Act of 2010 provided for a 12-year period of exclusivity for biosimilar drugs, a controversy has arisen over the interpretation of the word *exclusivity* contained in the act.

October 2013—Biosimilar User Fee Act of 2012 (BsUFA)—The FDCA, as amended by the BsUFA, authorizes the FDA to assess and collect fees for biosimilar biological products from October 2012 through September 2017. The FDA dedicates these fees to expediting the review process for biosimilar biological products. Biosimilar biological products represent a significant public health benefit, with the potential to offer life-saving or life-altering benefits at reduced cost to the patient. BsUFA facilitates the development of safe and effective biosimilar products for the American public.

November 2014—The FDA Purple Book: Lists of Licensed Biological Products with Reference Product Exclusivity and Biosimilarity or Interchangeability Evaluations—The *Purple Book* lists biological products, including any biosimilar and interchangeable biological products licensed by the FDA under the PHSA. The lists include the date a biological product was licensed under Section 351(a) of the PHSA and whether the FDA evaluated the biological product for reference product exclusivity under Section 351(k)(7) of the PHSA. The Purple Book will also enable a user to see whether a biological product licensed under Section 351(k) of the PHSA has been determined by the FDA to be biosimilar to or interchangeable with a reference biological product (an already-licensed FDA biological product). Biosimilar and interchangeable biological products licensed under Section 351(k) of the PHSA will be listed under the reference product to which biosimilarity or interchangeability was demonstrated. Separate lists for those biological products regulated by the CDER and the CBER will be updated periodically.

2.2.2 Regulatory guidance

The FDA has struggled coming up with final guidelines for the development of biosimilars starting with the first installment in 2015 (Table 2.1).

2.2.3 The 351(k) Route

A 351(k) application must include information demonstrating the following:

- The biological product is biosimilar to a reference product.
- It utilizes the same mechanism(s) of action for the proposed condition(s) of use—only to the extent known for the reference product.

Table 2.1 FDA Guidance on Biosimilars

Category	Title	Type	Date
Procedural; biosimilarity	Reference Product Exclusivity for Biological Products Filed Under Section 351(a) of the PHS Act	Draft guidance	08/04/14
Biosimilarity	Scientific Considerations in Demonstrating Biosimilarity to a Reference Product	Final guidance	04/28/15
Biosimilarity	Quality Considerations in Demonstrating Biosimilarity of a Therapeutic Protein Product to a Reference Product	Final guidance	04/28/15
Biosimilars	Biosimilars: Questions and Answers Regarding Implementation of the Biologics Price Competition and Innovation Act of 2009 Guidance for Industry	Final guidance	04/28/15
Biosimilarity	Biosimilars: Additional Questions and Answers Regarding Implementation of the Biologics Price Competition and Innovation Act of 2009	Draft guidance	05/12/15
Biosimilarity; procedural	Formal Meetings Between the FDA and Biosimilar Biological Product Sponsors or Applicants	Final guidance	11/17/15
Biosimilarity	Clinical Pharmacology Data to Support a Demonstration of Biosimilarity to a Reference Product	Final guidance	12/28/16
Biosimilars naming	Nonproprietary Naming Guidance	Final guidance	01/12/2017
Biosimilars	Considerations in Demonstrating Interchangeability with a Reference Product Guidance for Industry	Draft guidance	01/17/17
Biosimilars	Statistical Approaches to Evaluate Analytical Similarity	Draft guidance	09/21/17

Source: https://www.fda.gov/Drugs/GuidanceComplianceRegulatoryInformation/Guidances/ucm290967.htm

- Conditions of the use proposed in labeling have been previously licensed for the reference product.
- It has the same route of administration, dosage form, and strength as the reference product that the biological product is highly similar to the reference product notwithstanding minor differences in clinically inactive components.
- There are no clinically meaningful differences between the biological product and the reference product in terms of the safety, purity, and potency of the product.

2.2.3.1 What interchangeable or interchangeability means

- The biological product is biosimilar to the reference product.
- It can be expected to produce the same clinical result as the reference product in any given patient.
- For a product administered more than once, the safety and the reduced efficacy risks of alternating or switching are not greater than with repeated use of the reference product without alternating or switching. Note that the interchangeable product may be substituted for the reference product without the authorization of the healthcare provider.

2.2.3.2 The totality-of-the-evidence approach

- The totality-of-the-evidence approach describes a stepwise approach to evidence development, ensuring that development include only those elements necessary to address residual uncertainty.
- It introduces a concept that only after a thorough review of data from structural and functional analyses can the FDA provide meaningful advice on scope and extent of necessary animal and human testing.
- It explains the general expectations for human clinical trials.
    - At least one study will be expected (immunogenicity/pharmacokinetic/pharmacodynamic [PK-PD]).
    - Comparative safety and effectiveness data may be necessary if residual uncertainty exists.

A *biosimilar* product is a biological product that is licensed based on a showing that it is highly similar to an FDA-licensed biological product, known as a reference product, and has no clinically meaningful differences in terms of safety and effectiveness of the reference product. Only minor differences in clinically inactive components are allowable in biosimilar products.

An *interchangeable* biological product is biosimilar to an FDA-licensed reference product and meets additional standards for interchangeability. An interchangeable biological product may be substituted for the reference product by a pharmacist without the intervention of the healthcare provider who prescribed the reference product.

The FDA requires licensed biosimilar and interchangeable biological products to meet the FDA's rigorous standards of safety and efficacy. That means patients and healthcare professionals will be able to rely on the safety and the effectiveness of the biosimilar or interchangeable product, just as they would for the reference product.

2.2.4 The FDA stance

The FDA has taken several bold steps in approving complex products. A case in point is the approval of the generic product enoxaparin; when challenged why no clinical studies were mandated for approval while European Medicines Agency (EMA) requires them, the FDA responded:

> "Although the EMA Guideline requires clinical studies to demonstrate comparable effectiveness to a similar LMWH [low–molecular weight heparin], the FDA notes that its approach (i.e., the five criteria) is more sensitive to differences between two enoxaparin products than the clinical studies recommended in the EMA guideline" (http://www.fda.gov/Drugs/DrugSafety/PostmarketDrugSafetyInformationforPatientsandProviders/ucm220037.htm).

While EMA has long established that a clinical trial is needed to establish biosimilarity, the most recent revision of EMA guidance now includes the following statement:

> "In specific circumstances, a confirmatory clinical trial may not be necessary. This requires that similar efficacy and safety can clearly be deduced from the similarity of physicochemical characteristics, biological activity/potency, and PK and/or PD profiles of the biosimilar and the reference product. In addition, it requires that the impurity profile and the nature of excipients of the biosimilar itself do not give rise to concern" (http://www.ema.europa.eu/docs/en_GB/document_library/Scientific_guideline/2014/10/WC500176768.pdf).

2.2.5 351(k) Terminology

2.2.5.1 Innovator versus originator

In the small chemical fields, when a new molecule is synthesized, isolated, or identified, the credit goes to the innovator—as many of them may end up getting a patent for the discovery. However, when it comes to biologics, there can be a differentiation. For example, filgrastim is an endogenous compound and a company discovering a gene to manufacture this product using recombinant technology will qualify as the originator, but not as an innovator. However, when filgrastim is pegylated (the form that does not exist in the body), this qualifies the sponsor as an innovator.

2.2.5.2 Authorized versus licensed

In Europe, biological drugs are authorized, not licensed. This difference goes back to the laws in the United States that considered biologics to be hazardous to produce, and a license was required to manufacture them. EMA requires a marketing authorization application (MAA), whereas the FDA requires a biological license application.

2.2.5.3 Medicines versus drugs

The EMA prefers to call the treatment modalities as medicines, and the FDA, drugs or biologics.

2.2.5.4 Similarity versus comparability

Comparability simply means comparing two products, but this vocabulary can be confusing because of the official exercise of Comparability Protocol (ICH [International Conference on Harmonisation] Q5E: Comparability of Biotechnological/Biological Products Subject to Changes in Their Manufacturing Process), which is a well-defined task for changing the manufacturing process of a licensed product. The change is made by filing specific documents with the regulatory authorities. The similarity is a demonstration of the extent of the sameness of the products being developed. Unfortunately, biosimilar guidelines in the EMA often refer to similarity as comparability, and this should be avoided. *Comparability* is frequently used in lieu of similarity testing. EMA explains: "If the biosimilar *comparability* exercise indicates that there are relevant differences between the intended biosimilar and the reference medicinal product making it unlikely that biosimilarity will eventually be established, a stand-alone development to support a full Marketing Authorisation Application (MAA) should be considered instead." Some have begun to differentiate between the two comparability exercises as internal (to comply with Q5E when the existing product is compared to a proposed changed product) or external, where a reference product is compared to a biosimilar candidate. The FDA does not condone this vocabulary, and the testing of biosimilar products is a similarity exercise. Also, it should be noted that biosimilarity is an assessment, not an exercise.

2.2.5.5 Effectiveness versus efficacy

Efficacy is a demonstration of clinical response in a controlled trial; effectiveness is a comparison of the clinical responses of two products. Unfortunately, both the EMA and the World Health Organization (WHO) got it wrong and used the word *efficacy* in describing the evaluation of biosimilars. The FDA did not. In the U.S. guidelines, *efficacy* is not the term used to compare the relative effectiveness, which is distinctly different from efficacy. See the comments of the FDA discussed earlier regarding enoxaparin approval.

2.2.5.6 One-size-fits-all versus case-by-case

The FDA has clearly enunciated that all evaluation of biosimilar products will be made on a case-by-case basis. The root of this decision lies in the extreme diversity in the type of molecules involved; for example, a simpler molecule like filgrastim that has little immunogenicity potential and presents an excellent pharmacodynamic modeling will be assessed differently than adalimumab, a 148 kDa molecule with variations in its glycoforms, antibody-dependent cell-mediated cytotoxicity (ADCC), and lysine components; also, the in vivo nonclinical testing can be significantly different, such as for adalimumab, wherein a suitable animal toxicology model does not exist.

2.2.5.7 Totality of the evidence

The FDA coined the phrase *totality of the evidence* in 2007 when it licensed Avonex stating in *Nature Reviews: Drug Discovery*:

> On the basis of these data, the FDA concluded that the totality of the evidence indicated that the Bioferon product and Avonex were sufficiently comparable to rely on the data from major efficacy study using Bioferon's product to support licensure of Avonex.

In 2011, the FDA stated in an article in *New England Journal of Medicine Nature Reviews*:

> The FDA has traditionally relied on integrating various kinds of evidence in making regulatory decisions. Such a "totality-of-the-evidence approach. . . ."

In 2012, when the FDA issued a draft guidance that was later formalized in 2015, the FDA continues to emphasize that the approval of biosimilars will be made based on the totality of the evidence, the burden of proof lying with the sponsor.

2.2.5.8 No clinically meaningful difference

Fully recognizing that lot-to-lot differences in the originator product demonstrate that some differences are not clinically meaningful since the originator product with these differences has gone into the patient without any adverse events associated with these differences. When a biosimilar product is evaluated and it demonstrates differences, a discussion ensues whether this difference is clinically meaningful or not. This consideration is an extremely sensitive issue since the FDA is privy to what constitutes a minor variation, which the biosimilar product developer may not know. It is for this reason that the FDA wants the sponsors to analyze a sufficient number of originator lots bearing different expiry dates, to fully evaluate the nature and the extent of variability in the originator product. Some variations are well known to be less meaningful such as the presence of norleucine in filgrastim, or the ADCC in the case of adalimumab. However, the FDA may require matching attributes that may not appear clinically meaningful. For most of the product-related components, where these match the originator, the discussion is not needed but if process-related impurities are found that are not present in the originator product, these may be clinically meaningful and will likely require complete identification and toxicology evaluation in some instances. The developer can make a good case by analyzing a large number of originator lots to avoid getting caught with observations that might be clinically meaningful.

2.2.5.9 Fingerprint-like similarity

The FDA has established four tiers of biosimilarity assessment: not similar, similar, highly similar, and fingerprint-like similar. The minimum entry level to be a biosimilar is highly similar, a vocabulary that is now also used by EMA. However, it is possible to develop fingerprint-like similarity that will further reduce the burden of proof on the sponsor to conduct any phase III trials. While the FDA has not provided specific guidance on what would constitute a fingerprint-like similarity, the scientific view of this assessment is known. Generally, a comparison of HOS using such standard techniques as ultraviolet, fluorescence, circular dichroism, Fourier transform infrared spectroscopy, size-exclusion chromatography, static and dynamic light scatterings, differential scanning calorimetry, area under the curve (AUC), and other similar techniques will not be considered providing fingerprint-like similarity assessment. While these techniques might provide sufficient characterization of the HOS, variability in the HOS as it might happen during use is not made evident by these techniques. There are two ways of escalating the evaluation. One is by using an orthogonal approach where the HOS is modified through thermodynamic stress applied to induce a change and then studied if similar changes take place in the originator and the biosimilar candidate product. Some of the stresses recommended include pH, ionic strength, temperature, agitation, freezing/thawing, concentration change, variations in surfactants, use of columbic forces, and magnetic field. All of these are proposed by the author and is a subject of several pending U.S. patents (e.g., United States Patent and Trademark Office Application No. 20140356968; inventor, Niazi).

Another approach to establishing fingerprint-like similarity involves using biophysical tools that can provide information with much higher spatial and temporal resolutions. Examples include hydrogen/deuterium exchange mass spectrometry, small-angle x-ray scattering, and nuclear magnetic resonance. The higher resolution of current instrumentation continues to make existing instruments more valuable. A good example is the increased sensitivity of mass spectrometry by a million times over the past decade; the higher utility of AUC using the program SEDFIT is another good example of improved instrumentation; the use of Orbitrap mass spectrometry further exemplifies the kind of studies that might qualify a biosimilar product to be labeled as fingerprint-like similar.

However, the FDA is not likely to designate products as fingerprint-like similarity—this is only useful for discussion with the FDA in reducing clinical study requirements. The reason why the FDA will not provide specific designation is to avoid developers claiming any superiority of their product over others.

2.2.5.10 Extrapolation

Extrapolation refers to the allowance of all indications licensed or a limited number of multiple indications licensed for the use of the originator product. The basis of this allowance resides in the importance given to structural and functional similarities, which, in turn, assures that the biosimilar product will have the same effectiveness and side effects. There is a huge hue and cry by the originator companies suggesting extraordinary scientific reasons why this should not be allowed; all of these arguments are driven to keep biosimilar products under the shadow of a doubt.

2.2.5.11 Label copy

The FDA has established that the label copy can be the same as that of the originator, somewhat similar to what is allowed for generic pharmaceutical products. There remains a differentiation of naming of the product; in its first approval, the FDA has required a four-letter suffix to the generic name but states that this issue is still not resolved. AbbVie has filed a citizen's petition protesting the use of identical label and states that whereas the FDA has presented alternate views, these views were retracted in the final guidance issued in 2015.

2.2.5.12 Interchangeable biosimilars

The BPCI Act allows for a designation of a biosimilar product as interchangeable if upon switching and alternating with the originator product, there is a reduction in clinical effectiveness and no increase in side effects as demonstrated in a clinical setting. The FDA anticipates reviewing two applications per year for interchangeable status. Before a product can be evaluated as interchangeable, it must first be a proven biosimilar product; it is for this reason that most developers are likely to achieve approval of their product as biosimilar first and then pursue an interchangeable status; the FDA is yet to provide any guidance on these protocols, but there is sufficient literature available to design these studies. EMA does not have any such category. However, several countries in Europe including France have declared that the government will only reimburse for a biosimilar product for new patients when an originator product is prescribed.

2.2.5.13 Pediatric waiver

For the purpose of pediatric use, biosimilar products are considered new drugs and the sponsor is required to submit pediatric study waiver and in all instances only those applications that are licensed for the originator will be allowed.

2.3.2.14 Impurity versus attributes

When a new pharmaceutical product is developed, any component other than the key element is suspected of being an impurity, which by definition is undesirable. ICH guidelines properly treat this subject, how the impurities are to be identified, what the critical levels are, and how to justify certain levels of these impurities. In the case of a biopharmaceutical product, the number of components is almost always more than what are found in pharmaceuticals; some of these are product-related impurities, some are process-related impurities, and some are structure-related components. For example, the various glycoforms are the variants, deamidation species, impurities, and the level of host-cell proteins and process-related components. When developing biosimilar products, the identification is further narrowed by the fingerprint provided by the originator product; the sponsor needs to replicate all attributes, components, and even in some cases impurities. Examples in point are the lysine variants found in adalimumab; scientific literature states that these are not clinically meaningful, and the FDA may agree with this. However, recent studies by the originator have begun to show that these components are significant, apparently to keep the competition out since there is an IP coverage on how to manage the lysine variants. The biosimilar developer is faced with the dilemma of going into the market with a product with a different profile, which may be acceptable to the FDA, but it will create a problem in marketing the product, as the originator will obviously make a big deal out of it.

2.3 Biosimilars in use

Biosimilar products have been in wide use in the developing countries, well before the regulated markets of the European Union (EU), Japan, or the United States came to recognize them. The early adoption of biosimilars in developing country markets was driven by the affordability issue, and in several global regions, these products were marketed despite IP protections in place. As a result, there is a long history of the use of biosimilars globally; whereas, in many of these countries, there may not be a formal system of properly reporting adverse events. The consensus is that there have not been any catastrophic results, the only major incidence being reported for erythropoietin in Europe. However, given that the adverse events to biological products may appear even years after their use in the form of compromised autoimmune disorders and the fact that these adverse events are tough to associate with the utilization of a particular product, the regulatory agencies in the developed world have taken a very conservative approach to approving biosimilar products. Many countries that had jumped the gun in approving these products are now adopting a new look at their approval process as the awareness about biosimilar products increases.

Europe has seen the most advanced penetration to date of true biosimilars, authorizing the first product in 2006. While developing nations have been using similar biologics longer, those products do not enjoy the structural similarity, the clinical equivalence, or the regulatory rigor that biosimilars in highly regulated markets do. Currently, there are 41 approved biosimilars in Europe, more than the combined biosimilars approved in the rest of the developed markets. India leads the biosimilar approval list in the developing countries. Table 2.2 shows the biosimilars licensed by the FDA as of mid-2018.

2.3.1 FDA-Approved biosimilar products

Biosimilar products are sold under their own brand names in Europe, but WHO and the United States have suggested differentiating the generic name with a suffix to differentiate it from the name of the generic form used by the originator. The debate still goes on in the United States, where the FDA has licensed its first product with a suffix but suggests that this is not finalized.

2.3.2 Future of biosimilars

Biosimilar biological products, a category of their own, have a great potential, as every biological product is subject to being developed as a biosimilar product. Table 2.3 shows a current listing of possible biosimilar products over the next two decades. Given that a majority of future regulatory filings in the United States are likely to be biological products, the

Table 2.2 Biosimilars Approved by FDA by 2017

Drug Name	Approval Date	FDA Information Link
Zarxio (Filgrastim-sndz)	March 2015	https://www.fda.gov/newsevents/newsroom/pressannouncements/ucm436648.htm
Inflectra (Infliximab-dyyb)	April 2016	https://www.fda.gov/newsevents/newsroom/pressannouncements/ucm494227.htm
Erelzi (Etanercept-szzs)	August 2016	https://www.fda.gov/newsevents/newsroom/pressannouncements/ucm518639.htm
Amjevita (Adalimumab-atta)	September 2016	https://www.fda.gov/newsevents/newsroom/pressannouncements/ucm522243.htm
Renflexis (Infliximab-abda)	May 2017	https://www.accessdata.fda.gov/scripts/cder/daf/index.cfm?event=overview.process&ApplNo=761054
Cyltezo (Adalimumab-adbm)	August 2017	https://www.accessdata.fda.gov/scripts/cder/daf/index.cfm?event=overview.process&applno=761058
Mvasi (Bevacizumab-awwb)	September 2017	https://www.accessdata.fda.gov/scripts/cder/daf/index.cfm?event=overview.process&applno=761028
Ogivri (trastuzumab-dkst)	December 2017	https://www.accessdata.fda.gov/scripts/cder/daf/index.cfm?event=overview.process&ApplNo=761074
Ixifi (infliximab-qbtx)	December 2017	https://www.accessdata.fda.gov/scripts/cder/daf/index.cfm?event=overview.process&ApplNo=761072

Table 2.3 Potential U.S. Biosimilar Candidates through 2024

Brand	Generic Name	Therapeutic Category	Worldwide Annual Sales (2015) ($millions)	Patent Expiry
Gonal-F	Follitropin alfa/beta	Genitourinary	767	Jun 2015
ReoPro	Abciximab	Blood	93	Jun 2015
Ovidrel	Choriogonadotropin alfa	Genitourinary	60	Jun 2015
Luveris	Lutropin alfa	Genitourinary	26	Jun 2015
Recothrom	Thrombin alfa	Blood	70	Jul 2015
Fabrazyme	Agalsidase beta	Various	602	Sep 2015
Neulasta	Pegfilgrastim	Oncology and immunomodulators	4,594	Oct 2015
Synagis	Palivizumab	Systemic antiinfectives	355	Oct 2015
Proleukin	Aldesleukin	Oncology and immunomodulators	124	Oct 2015
Thyrogen	Thyrotropin alfa	Oncology and immunomodulators	164	Nov 2015
Norditropin SimpleXx	Somatropin recombinant	Endocrine	1,112	Dec 2015
Helixate	Octocog alfa	Blood	396	Dec 2015
Puregon/Follistim	Follitropin beta	Genitourinary	335	Dec 2015
Provenge	Sipuleucel-T	Oncology and immunomodulators	268	Dec 2015
PEGIntron	Peginterferon alfa-2b	Oncology and immunomodulators	198	Dec 2015
Lemtrada	Alemtuzumab	Central nervous system	156	Dec 2015
Orgalutran/Antagon	Ganirelix acetate	Genitourinary	59	Dec 2015
Lantus	Insulin glargine recombinant	Endocrine	7,267	Jun 2016
Bexxar	Tositumomab; iodine I 131 tositumomab	Oncology and immunomodulators	9	Sep 2016
Humira	Adalimumab	Musculoskeletal	14,085	Dec 2016
Macugen	Pegaptanib sodium	Sensory organs	5	Jan 2017
Somavert	Pegvisomant	Endocrine	220	Mar 2017
NovoMix 30	Insulin aspart recombinant, insulin aspart protamine recombinant	Endocrine	1,633	Jun 2017
Replagal	Agalsidase alfa	Various	481	Sep 2017
Increlex	Mecasermin (rDNA origin)	Endocrine	20	Sep 2017
Pediarix	DTP; hepatitis B and polio vaccine	Systemic antiinfectives	1,268	Dec 2017
Erbitux	Cetuximab	Oncology and immunomodulators	704	Feb 2018
Kepivance	Palifermin	Gastrointestinal	11	Aug 2018
Remicade	Infliximab	Musculoskeletal	5,852	Sep 2018

(*Continued*)

Table 2.3 (Continued) Potential U.S. Biosimilar Candidates through 2024

Brand	Generic Name	Therapeutic Category	Worldwide Annual Sales (2015) ($millions)	Patent Expiry
Rituxan	Rituximab	Oncology and immunomodulators	7,153	Dec 2018
Xolair	Omalizumab	Respiratory	1,222	Dec 2018
	Omalizumab	Respiratory	803	Dec 2018
Forteo	Teriparatide recombinant human	Musculoskeletal	1,305	Dec 2018
Pegasys	Peginterferon alfa-2a	Oncology and immunomodulators	645	Dec 2018
Prochymal	Remestemcel-L	Oncology and immunomodulators	267	Dec 2018
Elonva	Corifollitropin alfa	Genitourinary	47	Dec 2018
Voraxaze	Glucarpidase	Oncology and immunomodulators	24	Jan 2019
RotaTeq	Rotavirus vaccine	Systemic antiinfectives	665	Feb 2019
Arcalyst	Rilonacept	Oncology and immunomodulators	17	May 2019
Herceptin	Trastuzumab	Oncology and immunomodulators	6,517	Jun 2019
Levemir	Insulin detemir recombinant	Endocrine	2,722	Jun 2019
Avastin	Bevacizumab	Oncology and immunomodulators	6,695	Jul 2019
Elaprase	Idursulfase	Various	586	Sep 2019
Orencia	Abatacept	Musculoskeletal	995	Oct 2019
Orencia SC	Abatacept	Musculoskeletal	770	Oct 2019
Actemra	Tocilizumab	Musculoskeletal	1,217	Nov 2019
	Tocilizumab	Musculoskeletal	225	Nov 2019
Aldurazyme	Laronidase	Various	206	Nov 2019
Advate	Factor VIII (procoagulant)	Blood	2,085	Dec 2019
Zevalin	Ibritumomab tiuxetan	Oncology and immunomodulators	23	Dec 2019
Vectibix	Panitumumab	Oncology and immunomodulators	589	Apr 2020
Lucentis	Ranibizumab	Sensory organs	1,770	Jun 2020
Afrezza	Insulin (human)	Endocrine	33	Jun 2020
Botox	Onabotulinumtoxina	Musculoskeletal	2,675	Jul 2020
Tysabri	Natalizumab	Central nervous system	2,094	Dec 2020
Recombivax HB	Hepatitis B vaccine	Systemic antiinfectives	184	Dec 2020
Cervarix	Human papillomavirus vaccine	Systemic antiinfectives	177	Dec 2020

(*Continued*)

Table 2.3 (Continued) Potential U.S. Biosimilar Candidates through 2024

Brand	Generic Name	Therapeutic Category	Worldwide Annual Sales (2015) ($millions)	Patent Expiry
Intron A	Interferon alfa-2b	Oncology and immunomodulators	120	Dec 2020
Simulect	Basiliximab	Oncology and immunomodulators	112	Dec 2020
Soliris	Eculizumab	Blood	2,613	Mar 2021
Myalept	Metreleptin	Endocrine	10	Mar 2021
Mircera	Methoxy polyethylene glycol-epoetin beta	Blood	265	Nov 2021
Cimzia	Certolizumab pegol	Musculoskeletal	1,161	Dec 2021
Entyvio	Vedolizumab	Gastrointestinal	438	Dec 2021
Cyramza	Ramucirumab	Oncology and immunomodulators	347	Dec 2021
Jetrea	Ocriplasmin	Sensory organs	26	Dec 2021
NovoThirteen	Catridecacog	Blood	23	Dec 2021
Nplate	Romiplostim	Blood	508	Jan 2022
Natpara	Parathyroid hormone	Endocrine	26	Jun 2022
V419	DTP; hepatitis B, hemophilus influenza type b, and polio vaccine	Systemic antiinfectives	12	Jun 2022
Simponi	Golimumab	Musculoskeletal	1,358	Jul 2022
Vpriv	Velaglucerase alfa	Various	370	Jul 2022
Zaltrap	Ziv-aflibercept	Oncology and immunomodulators	109	Jul 2022
Obizur	Susoctocog alfa	Blood	6	Jul 2022
Tanzeum	Albiglutide	Endocrine	118	Dec 2022
Actimmune	Interferon gamma-1b	Oncology and immunomodulators	102	Dec 2022
Ixiaro	Japanese encephalitis vaccine	Systemic antiinfectives	48	Dec 2022
Apidra	Insulin glulisine recombinant	Endocrine	437	Jan 2023
Myozyme	Alglucosidase alfa	Various	670	Feb 2023
Nulojix	Belatacept	Oncology and immunomodulators	66	Apr 2023
Imvamune	Smallpox vaccine	Systemic antiinfectives	8	May 2023
Kineret	Anakinra	Musculoskeletal	83	Jul 2023
Stelara	Ustekinumab	Oncology and immunomodulators	2,504	Sep 2023
Victoza	Liraglutide (rDNA origin)	Endocrine	2,516	Dec 2023

(Continued)

Table 2.3 (Continued) Potential U.S. Biosimilar Candidates through 2024

Brand	Generic Name	Therapeutic Category	Worldwide Annual Sales (2015) ($millions)	Patent Expiry
Yervoy	Ipilimumab	Oncology and immunomodulators	1,411	Dec 2023
Kadcyla	Ado-trastuzumab emtansine	Oncology and immunomodulators	806	Dec 2023
Benlysta	Belimumab	Oncology and immunomodulators	324	Dec 2023
Saxenda	Liraglutide (rDNA origin)	Gastrointestinal	86	Dec 2023
Elelyso	Taliglucerase alfa	Various	15	Feb 2024
Xgeva	Denosumab	Musculoskeletal	1,405	Mar 2024
Prolia	Denosumab	Musculoskeletal	1,280	Mar 2024
Aranesp	Darbepoetin alfa	Blood	1,891	May 2024
Blincyto	Blinatumomab	Oncology and immunomodulators	35	May 2024
ChondroCelect	Autologous-cultured chondrocytes	Musculoskeletal	5	Aug 2024
Kalbitor	Ecallantide	Blood	75	Sep 2024
Ilaris	Canakinumab	Oncology and immunomodulators	260	Dec 2024
Trulicity	Dulaglutide	Endocrine	189	Dec 2024

Note: rDNA: recombinant DNA.

pharmaceutical industry is ready for a major shift in its business strategy and biosimilars will play the most significant role in patient healthcare and the FDA will engage in a most significant manner with the industry.

2.3.2.1 Global mind-set

This chapter provided a vision of the current and the future landscape of biosimilar products; given the high cost of development, it will be economical for the sponsors to take a global approach to developing these products. It is likely that a developer will launch products in countries where the IP is not an issue first, and then move on to other jurisdictions. While the focus of this book is on U.S. regulatory expectations, it will be useful for the sponsors to carve out the most conservative specifications that will be globally admissible.

2.3.2.2 Immediate needs

The immediate focus of this book is to describe the concept of biosimilarity as viewed and practiced by the U.S. FDA. How this view has helped or hurt the entry of biosimilars was recently discussed and published by the author, where issues related to expediting entry of biosimilars in the

United States are presented. There is a need for both the FDA and the industry to change their practices, if we, in the United States, are able to catch up with the spread of biosimilars in Europe.

Bibliography

1. http://www.bioprocessintl.com/wp-content/uploads/2018/01/16-1-Biosimilars-eBook.pdf?submissionGuid=ba89dcc5-a456-4ef0-849d-bceda94f16a3
2. https://www.europeanpharmaceuticalreview.com/article/70987/obstacles-success-biosimilars-us-market/

Chapter 3 The FDA regulatory guidance

We have all a better guide in ourselves, if we would attend to it, than any other person can be.

Jane Austen
Mansfield Park

3.1 Background

A review of the existing guidelines, the differences in their approaches to approval of biosimilar products, and a futuristic view of the upcoming changes in the laws must be preceded by understanding the diverse terminology in place. Since the FDA has created a pathway for the approval of biosimilars based on their analytical and functional similarities and the fact that the initial pathway of 351(a) remains available for biosimilars, it is important to review the biological drug approval process in the United States as well. It is noteworthy that the first recombinant product granulocyte colony–stimulating factor (GCSF) in addition to the originator's product was approved under the 351(a) pathway.

Tables 3.1 and 3.2 list the guidance documents that are relevant to understanding the FDA perspective on how should the biosimilarity be demonstrated. Table 3.3 lists ICH guidance relevant to biosimilars. There are often overlaps between the two agencies. Note that many guidelines are frequently revised and promoted from draft to final, and new draft guidance documents added. The biosimilar sponsor is therefore directed to the FDA website to update this list.

Furthermore, the FDA is expected to release the following guidance documents in 2016:

- Considerations in demonstrating interchangeability with a reference product
- Labeling for biosimilar biological products
- Statistical approaches to the evaluation of analytical similarity data to support a demonstration of biosimilarity

Other guidances that are not directly addressing but relevant to the development of biosimilars are provided in Table 3.2.

Table 3.1 The FDA Guidance Relevant to Biosimilars

Guidance for Industry: Reference Product Exclusivity for Biological Products Filed under Section 351(a) of the PHSA (Draft Guidance)	http://www.fda.gov/downloads/Drugs/GuidanceComplianceRegulatoryInformation/Guidances/UCM407844.pdf
Guidance for Industry: Clinical Pharmacology Data to Support a Demonstration of Biosimilarity to a Reference Product (Draft Guidance)	http://www.fda.gov/downloads/Drugs/GuidanceComplianceRegulatoryInformation/Guidances/UCM397017.pdf
Guidance for Industry: Formal Meetings between the FDA and Biosimilar Biological Product Sponsors or Applicants (Draft Guidance)	http://www.fda.gov/downloads/Drugs/GuidanceComplianceRegulatoryInformation/Guidances/UCM345649.pdf
Guidance for Industry: Scientific Considerations in Demonstrating Biosimilarity to a Reference Product (Draft Guidance)	http://www.fda.gov/downloads/Drugs/GuidanceComplianceRegulatoryInformation/Guidances/UCM291128.pdf
Guidance for Industry: Quality Considerations in Demonstrating Biosimilarity to a Reference Protein Product (Draft Guidance)	http://www.fda.gov/downloads/Drugs/GuidanceComplianceRegulatoryInformation/Guidances/UCM291134.pdf
Biosimilars: Questions and Answers regarding Implementation of the Biologics Price Competition and Innovation Act of 2009 Guidance for Industry	http://www.fda.gov/downloads/Drugs/GuidanceComplianceRegulatoryInformation/Guidances/UCM444661.pdf

Table 3.2 The FDA Guidance for Biological Products Relevant to Biosimilars

FDA: Guidance for Industry: Comparability Protocols—Protein Drug Products and Biological Products—Chemistry, Manufacturing, and Controls Information	http://www.fda.gov/ucm/groups/fdagov-public/@fdagov-drugs-gen/documents/document/ucm070262.pdf
FDA: Guidance for Industry: Comparability Protocols—Chemistry, Manufacturing, and Controls Information	http://www.fda.gov/ucm/groups/fdagov-public/@fdagov-drugs-gen/documents/document/ucm070545.pdf
FDA: Points to Consider in the Manufacture and Testing of Monoclonal Antibody Products for Human Use	http://www.gpo.gov/fdsys/granule/FR-1997-02-28/97-5006
FDA: Guidance for Industry for the Submission of Chemistry, Manufacturing, and Controls Information for a Therapeutic Recombinant DNA–Derived Product or a Monoclonal Antibody Product for In Vivo Use	http://www.fda.gov/downloads/BiologicsBloodVaccines/GuidanceComplianceRegulatoryInformation/Guidances/General/UCM173477.pdf
FDA: Guidance for Industry: Cooperative Manufacturing Arrangements for Licensed Biologics	http://www.fda.gov/BiologicsBloodVaccines/GuidanceComplianceRegulatoryInformation/Guidances/General/ucm069883.htm
FDA: Guidance for Industry: Assay Development for Immunogenicity Testing of Therapeutic Proteins	http://www.fda.gov/downloads/Drugs/GuidanceComplianceRegulatoryInformation/Guidances/UCM192750.pdf
FDA: Guidance for Industry: Noninferiority Clinical Trials	http://www.fda.gov/downloads/Drugs/GuidanceComplianceRegulatoryInformation/Guidances/UCM202140.pdf

Table 3.3 ICH Guidance Relevant to Biosimilars

ICH Guidance for Industry M4Q: The Common Technical Document—Quality (ICH M4Q)	http://www.ich.org/fileadmin/Public_Web_Site/ICH_Products/CTD/M4_R1_Quality/M4Q__R1_.pdf
ICH Guidance for Industry Q1A(R2): Stability Testing of New Drug Substances and Products (ICH Q1A(R2))	http://www.ich.org/products/guidelines/quality/quality-single/article/stability-testing-of-new-drug-substances-and-products.html
ICH Guidance for Industry Q2(R1): Validation of Analytical Procedures: Text and Methodology (ICH Q2(R1))	http://www.ich.org/fileadmin/Public_Web_Site/ICH_Products/Guidelines/Quality/Q2_R1/Step4/Q2_R1__Guideline.pdf
ICH Guidance for Industry Q2B: Validation of Analytical Procedures: Methodology (ICH Q2B)	http://www.ich.org/fileadmin/Public_Web_Site/ICH_Products/Guidelines/Quality/Q2_R1/Step4/Q2_R1__Guideline.pdf
ICH Guidance for Industry Q3A: Impurities in New Drug Substances (ICH Q3A)	http://www.ich.org/products/guidelines/quality/quality-single/article/impurities-in-new-drug-substances.html
ICH Guidance for Industry Q5A: Viral Safety Evaluation of Biotechnology Products Derived from Cell Lines of Human or Animal Origin (ICH Q5A)	http://www.ich.org/products/guidelines/quality/quality-single/article/viral-safety-evaluation-of-biotechnology-products-derived-from-cell-lines-of-human-or-animal-origin.html
ICH Guidance for Industry Q5B: Quality of Biotechnological Products: Analysis of the Expression Construct in Cells Used for Production of r-DNA Derived Protein Products (ICH Q5B)	http://www.ich.org/products/guidelines/quality/quality-single/article/analysis-of-the-expression-construct-in-cells-used-for-production-of-r-dna-derived-protein-products.html
ICH Guidance for Industry Q5C: Quality of Biotechnological Products: Stability Testing of Biotechnological/Biological Products (ICH Q5C)	http://www.ich.org/products/guidelines/quality/quality-single/article/stability-testing-of-biotechnologicalbiological-products.html
ICH Guidance for Industry Q5D: Quality of Biotechnological/Biological Products: Derivation and Characterization of Cell Substrates used for Production of Biotechnological/Biological Products (ICH Q5D)	http://www.ich.org/products/guidelines/quality/quality-single/article/derivation-and-characterisation-of-cell-substrates-used-for-production-of-biotechnologicalbiologica.html
ICH Guidance for Industry Q5E: Comparability of Biotechnological/Biological Products Subject to Changes in Their Manufacturing Process (ICH Q5E)	http://www.ich.org/products/guidelines/quality/quality-single/article/comparability-of-biotechnologicalbiological-products-subject-to-changes-in-their-manufacturing-proc.html
ICH Guidance for Industry Q6B: Specifications: Test Procedures and Acceptance Criteria for Biotechnological/Biological Products (ICH Q6B)	http://www.ich.org/products/guidelines/quality/quality-single/article/specifications-test-procedures-and-acceptance-criteria-for-biotechnologicalbiological-products.html
ICH Guidance for Industry Q7(A): Good Manufacturing Practice Guidance for Active Pharmaceutical Ingredients (ICH Q7A)	http://www.ich.org/products/guidelines/quality/article/quality-guidelines.html
ICH Guidance for Industry Q8(R2): Pharmaceutical Development (ICH Q8(R2))	http://www.ich.org/products/guidelines/quality/quality-single/article/pharmaceutical-development.html
ICH Guidance for Industry Q9: Quality Risk Management (ICH Q9)	http://www.ich.org/products/guidelines/quality/quality-single/article/quality-risk-management.html
ICH Guidance for Industry Q10: Pharmaceutical Quality System (ICH Q10)	http://www.ich.org/products/guidelines/quality/quality-single/article/pharmaceutical-quality-system.html
ICH Guidance for Industry Q11: Development and Manufacture of Drug Substances (ICH Q11)	http://www.ich.org/products/guidelines/quality/quality-single/article/development-and-manufacture-of-drug-substances.html
ICH Guidance for Industry S6(R1): Preclinical Safety Evaluation of Biotechnology-Derived Pharmaceuticals (ICH S6(R1))	http://www.ich.org/products/guidelines/safety/safety-single/article/preclinical-safety-evaluation-of-biotechnology-derived-pharmaceuticals.html

The ICH guidelines that are often cross-referenced with the FDA guidance and are relevant to the development of biosimilars are listed in Table 3.3.

3.2 Overview of the FDA guidance

The BPCI Act was enacted as part of the Affordable Care Act on March 23, 2010. The BPCI Act creates an abbreviated licensure pathway for biological products shown to be biosimilar to, or interchangeable with, an FDA-licensed biological reference product. The objectives of the BPCI Act are conceptually similar to those of the Drug Price Competition and Patent Term Restoration Act of 1984 (Public Law 98-417) (commonly referred to as the *Hatch–Waxman Act*), which established abbreviated pathways for the approval of drug products under the FDCA. (See Sections 505(b)(2) and 505(j) of the FDCA [21 U.S. Code (U.S.C.) 355(b)(2) and 355(j)].)

The implementation of an abbreviated licensure pathway for biological products can present challenges given the scientific and technical complexities that may be associated with the larger and typically more complex structure of biological products, as well as the processes by which such products are manufactured. Most biological products are produced in a living system such as microorganism or plant or animal cells, whereas small-molecule drugs are typically manufactured by chemical synthesis.

Section 351(k) of the PHSA (42 U.S.C. 262(k)), added by the BPCI Act, sets forth the requirements for an application for a proposed biosimilar product and an application or a supplement for a proposed interchangeable product. Section 351(i) defines biosimilarity to mean

> that the biological product is highly similar to the reference product notwithstanding minor differences in clinically inactive components and that there are no clinically meaningful differences between the biological product and the reference product in terms of the safety, purity, and potency of the product. (see Section 351(i)(2) of the PHSA)

A 351(k) application must contain, among other things, information demonstrating that the biological product is biosimilar to a reference product based on data derived from analytical studies, animal studies, and a clinical study or studies, unless the FDA determines, in its discretion, that certain studies are unnecessary in a 351(k) application (see Section 351(k)(2) of the PHSA). To meet the additional standard of interchangeability, an applicant must provide sufficient information to demonstrate biosimilarity and also to demonstrate that the biological product can be expected to produce the same clinical result as the reference product in any given patient and, if the biological product is administered more than once to an individual, the risk in terms of safety or diminished efficacy of alternating or switching between the use of the biological product and the reference product is not greater than the risk of using the reference product without such alternation or switch (see Section 351(k)(4) of the PHSA). Interchangeable products may be substituted for the reference product without the intervention of the prescribing healthcare provider (see Section 351(i)(3) of the PHSA).

The BPCI Act also includes the following, among other provisions:

- A 12-year exclusivity period from the date of the first licensure of the reference product, during which the approval of a 351(k) application referencing that product may not be made effective (see Section 351(k)(7) of the PHSA)
- A four-year exclusivity period from the date of the first licensure of the reference product, during which a 351(k) application referencing that product may not be submitted (see Section 351(k)(7) of the PHSA)
- An exclusivity period for the first biological product determined to be interchangeable with the reference product for any condition of use, during which a second or a subsequent biological product may not be determined interchangeable with that reference product (see Section 351(k)(6) of the PHSA)
- An exclusivity period for certain biological products for which pediatric studies are conducted in accordance with a written request (see Section 351(m) of the PHSA)
- A transition provision for biological products that have been or will be approved under Section 505 of the FDCA (21 U.S.C. 355) before March 23, 2020 (see Section 7002(e) of the Affordable Care Act)
- A provision stating that a 351(k) application for a biosimilar product contains a "new active ingredient" for purposes of the Pediatric Research Equity Act (PREA) (see Section 505B(n) of the FDCA)

The BPCI Act also establishes procedures for identifying and resolving patent disputes involving applications submitted under Section 351(k) of the PHSA.

3.3 Formal meetings

There are five types of formal meetings that can occur between the sponsors or applicants and the FDA staff to discuss development of a biosimilar biological product.

3.3.1 Biosimilar initial advisory meeting

A biosimilar initial advisory meeting is an initial assessment limited to a general discussion regarding whether licensure under Section 351(k) of the PHSA may be feasible for a particular product, and, if so, a general advice on the expected content of the development program. This meeting type does not include any meeting that involves a substantive review of summary data or full study reports. However, preliminary comparative analytical similarity data should be provided with the meeting request to enable the FDA to make the initial determination as to whether licensure under Section 351(k) of the PHSA may be feasible for a particular product and to provide meaningful advice. An overview of the proposed development program also should be supplied.

3.3.2 Biosimilar biological product development (BPD) Type 1 meeting

A BPD Type 1 meeting is a meeting that is necessary for an otherwise stalled BPD program to proceed. Examples of a BPD Type 1 meeting include the following:

- Meetings to discuss clinical holds in which a response to hold issues has been submitted, but the FDA and the sponsor or applicant agree that the development is stalled, and a new path forward should be discussed
- Special protocol assessment meetings that are requested by sponsors or applicants after the receipt of the FDA evaluation of protocols under the special protocol evaluation procedures as described in Section VI of the Biosimilar User Fee Act of 2012 (BsUFA) goals letter
- Meetings to discuss an important safety issue, when such an issue is identified, and the FDA and the sponsor or applicant agree that the matter should be discussed
- Dispute resolution meetings as described in 21 Code of Federal Regulations (CFR) 10.75 and 312.48 and in Section 102 IV of the BsUFA goals letter and the draft guidance for industry and review staff (Formal Dispute Resolution: Appeals Above the Division Level 7, lines 104–105)

3.3.3 BPD Type 2 meeting

A BPD Type 2 meeting is a meeting to discuss a particular issue (e.g., proposed study design or end points) or questions where the FDA will provide targeted advice regarding an ongoing BPD program. This meeting type includes substantive reviews of summary data but does not include a review of full study reports.

3.3.4 BPD Type 3 meeting

A BPD Type 3 meeting is an in-depth data review and advice meeting regarding an ongoing BPD program. This meeting type includes a substantive consideration of full study reports, the FDA advice concerning the similarity between the proposed biosimilar biological product and the reference product, and the FDA advice concerning the need for additional studies, including design and analysis.

3.3.5 BPD Type 4 meeting

A BPD Type 4 meeting is a meeting to discuss the format and the content of a biosimilar biological product application or a supplement to be submitted under Section 351(k).

3.4 Scientific considerations

3.4.1 Background

Biosimilarity is defined in Section 351(i) of the PHSA to mean that the biological product is highly similar to the reference product notwithstanding minor differences in clinically inactive components and that there are no clinically meaningful differences between the biological product and the reference product in terms of the safety, the purity, and the potency of the product (see Section 351(i)(2) of the PHSA). Comparative analytical data provide the foundation for a development program for a proposed biosimilar product intended for submission under Section 351(k) of the PHSA. The BPCI Act also amended the definition of biological product to include "protein (except any chemically synthesized polypeptide)."

The three pillars of establishing biosimilarity include the following:

- Analytical studies that demonstrate that the biological product is highly similar to the reference product notwithstanding minor differences in clinically inactive components
- Animal studies (including the assessment of toxicity)
- A clinical study or studies (including the assessment of immunogenicity and pharmacokinetics [PK] or pharmacodynamics [PD]) that are sufficient to demonstrate safety, purity, and potency in one or more appropriate conditions of use for which the reference product is licensed and intended to be used and for which licensure is sought for the biological product

3.4.2 Complexities of protein products

The three pillars for establishing biosimilarity rest on heavy scientific foundation given the complexity of protein and antibody products. The FDA has provided extensive advice on how to approach understanding this complexity and what the FDA considers to be more critical factors.

3.4.2.1 Nature of protein products and related scientific considerations Unlike small-molecule drugs, whose structure can usually be completely defined and entirely reproduced, proteins are typically more complex and are unlikely to be shown to be structurally identical to a reference product. Many potential differences in the protein structure can arise. Because even minor structural differences (including certain changes in glycosylation patterns) can significantly affect a protein's safety and/or effectiveness, it is important to evaluate these differences.

In general, proteins can differ in at least three ways: (a) primary amino acid sequence; (b) modification of amino acids, such as sugar moieties (glycosylation) or other side chains; and (c) HOS (protein folding and protein–protein interactions). Modifications to amino acids may lead to heterogeneity and can be difficult to control. Protein modifications and HOS can be affected by formulation and environmental conditions, including light, temperature, moisture, packaging materials, container closure systems, and delivery device materials. Additionally, process-related impurities as well as product-related ones may increase the likelihood and/or the severity of an immune response to a protein product, and certain excipients may limit the ability to characterize the protein product.

Advances in analytical sciences enable some protein products to be extensively characterized with respect to their physicochemical and biological properties, such as HOSs and functional characteristics. These analytical methodologies have increasingly improved the ability to identify and characterize not only the drug substance of a protein product but also the excipients and product- and process-related impurities.

Despite such significant improvements in analytical techniques, however, the current analytical methodology may not be able to detect all relevant structural and functional differences between two protein products. In addition, there may be an incomplete understanding of the relationship between a product's structural attributes and its clinical performance. Thus, as set forth in the PHSA, data derived from analytical studies, animal studies, and a clinical study or studies are required to demonstrate biosimilarity unless the FDA determines an element unnecessary.

3.4.2.2 Manufacturing process considerations Different manufacturing processes may alter a protein product in a way that could affect the safety or the effectiveness of the product. For example, differences in biological systems used to manufacture a protein product may cause different PTMs, which in turn may affect the safety and/or the effectiveness of the product. Thus, when the manufacturing process for a marketed protein product is changed, the application holder must assess the effects of the change and demonstrate—through appropriate analytical testing, functional assays, and/or in some cases animal and/or clinical studies—that the change does not have an adverse effect on the identity, the strength, the quality, the purity, or the potency of the product as it relates to the safety or the effectiveness of the product.

Demonstrating that a proposed product is biosimilar to a reference product will be more complex than assessing the comparability of a product before and after the manufacturing changes made by the same manufacturer. This is because a manufacturer that modifies its own manufacturing process has extensive knowledge and information about the product and the existing process, including established controls and acceptance parameters. By contrast, the manufacturer of a proposed product is likely to have a different manufacturing process (e.g., different cell line, raw materials, equipment, processes, process controls, and acceptance criteria) from that of the reference product and no direct knowledge of the manufacturing process for the reference product. Therefore, even though some of the scientific principles described in ICH Q5E may also apply in the demonstration of biosimilarity, in general, the FDA anticipates that more data and information will be needed to establish biosimilarity than would be necessary to establish that a manufacturer's postmanufacturing change product is comparable to the premanufacturing change product.

3.4.3 U.S.-licensed reference product and other comparators

The licensing of a proposed product under Section 351(k) of the PHSA requires that the sponsor demonstrate that the proposed product is biosimilar to a single reference product that has been previously licensed by FDA. In general, a sponsor needs to provide information to demonstrate biosimilarity based on data directly comparing the proposed product with the reference product. As a scientific matter, analytical studies and at least one clinical PK study and, if appropriate, at least one PD study intended to support a demonstration of biosimilarity for purposes of Section 351(k) of the PHSA must include an adequate comparison of the proposed biosimilar product directly with the U.S.-licensed reference product unless it can be scientifically justified that such a study is not needed. However, a sponsor may seek to use data derived from animal or clinical studies comparing a proposed product with a non-U.S.-licensed comparator product to address, in part, the requirements of Section 351(k)(2)(A) of the PHSA. In such a case, the sponsor should provide adequate data or information to scientifically justify the relevance of these comparative data to an assessment of biosimilarity and establish an acceptable bridge to the U.S.-licensed reference product. Sponsors are encouraged to discuss with the FDA during the development program their plans to provide an adequate scientific justification and a bridge to the U.S.-licensed reference product. A final decision on the adequacy of such justification and bridge will be made by the FDA during the review of the 351(k) application.

3.4.4 Approaches to developing and assessing evidence to demonstrate biosimilarity

The FDA recommends that sponsors use a stepwise approach to developing the evidence needed to demonstrate biosimilarity. The FDA intends to consider the totality of the evidence provided by a sponsor when the Agency evaluates the sponsor's demonstration of biosimilarity, consistent with a long-standing agency approach to evaluating scientific evidence.

3.4.4.1 Using a stepwise approach to demonstrate biosimilarity The purpose of a biosimilar development program is to support a demonstration of biosimilarity between a proposed product and a reference product, including an assessment of the effects of any observed differences between the products, but not to independently establish the safety and the effectiveness of the proposed product. The FDA recommends that sponsors use a stepwise approach to developing the data and the information needed to support a demonstration of biosimilarity. At each step, the sponsor should evaluate the extent to which there is residual uncertainty about the biosimilarity of the proposed product and identify the next steps to try to address that uncertainty. Where possible, studies conducted should be designed to maximize their contribution to demonstrating biosimilarity. For example, a clinical immunogenicity study may also provide other useful information about the safety profile of the proposed product.

The stepwise approach should start with extensive structural and functional characterizations of both the proposed product and the reference product, which serves as the foundation of a biosimilar development program. The more comprehensive and robust the comparative structural and functional characterizations are—the extent to which these studies are able to identify (qualitatively or quantitatively) differences in relevant product attributes between the proposed product and the reference product (including the drug substance, excipients, and impurities)—the more useful such characterization will be in determining what additional studies may be needed. For example, rigorous structural and functional comparisons that show minimal or no difference between the proposed product and the reference product will strengthen the scientific justification for a selective and targeted approach to animal and/or clinical testing to support a demonstration of biosimilarity. It may be useful to further quantify the similarity or the differences between the two products using a meaningful fingerprint-like analysis algorithm that covers a large number of additional product attributes and their combinations with high sensitivity using orthogonal methods. Such a strategy may further reduce the possibility of undetected structural differences between the products and lead to a more selective and targeted approach to animal and/or clinical testing. A sufficient understanding of the mechanism of action (MOA) of the drug substance and the clinical relevance of any observed structural differences, the clinical knowledge of the reference product and its class that indicates low overall safety risks, and the availability of a relevant PD measure may provide further scientific justification for a selective and targeted approach to animal and/or clinical studies.

The sponsor should then consider the role of animal data in assessing toxicity and, in some cases, in providing additional support for demonstrating biosimilarity and in contributing to the immunogenicity assessment. The sponsor should then conduct comparative human PK and PD studies (if there is a relevant PD measure(s)) and compare the clinical immunogenicity of the two products in an appropriate study population. If there is residual uncertainty about biosimilarity after conducting structural analyses, functional assays, animal testing, human PK and PD studies, and clinical immunogenicity assessment, the sponsor should then consider what additional clinical data may be needed to adequately address that uncertainty. The FDA encourages sponsors to extensively consult with the Agency after completion of comparative structural and functional analyses (before finalizing the clinical program) and throughout development as needed.

The FDA recognizes that some of the aforementioned investigations could be performed in parallel; however, the Agency recommends that sponsors use a stepwise approach to better address residual uncertainty about biosimilarity that might remain at each step and incorporate FDA's advice provided after the FDA review of data and information collected at certain milestones.

3.4.4.2 Using a totality-of-the-evidence approach to assess a demonstration of biosimilarity In evaluating a sponsor's demonstration of biosimilarity, the FDA will consider the totality of the data and the information submitted in the application, including structural and functional characterizations, nonclinical evaluation, human PK and PD data, clinical immunogenicity data, and comparative clinical study data. The FDA intends to use a risk-based approach to evaluating all available data and information submitted in support of the biosimilarity of the proposed product.

Thus, a sponsor may be able to demonstrate biosimilarity, even though there are formulation or minor structural differences, provided that the sponsor provides sufficient data and information demonstrating that the differences are not clinically meaningful and the proposed product otherwise meets the statutory criteria for biosimilarity. For example, differences in certain PTMs or differences in certain excipients (e.g., human serum albumin) might not preclude a finding of biosimilarity if data and information provided by the sponsor show that the proposed product is highly similar to the reference product notwithstanding minor differences in clinically inactive components and that there are no clinically meaningful differences between the products in terms of safety, purity, and potency. In this example, because some excipients may affect the ability to characterize products, a sponsor should provide evidence that the excipients used in the reference product will not affect the capacity to characterize and compare the products.

Clinically meaningful differences could include a difference in the expected range of safety, purity, or potency of the proposed product and the reference product. By contrast, slight differences in rates of occurrence of certain adverse events between the two products would ordinarily not be considered clinically meaningful differences.

3.4.5 Demonstrating biosimilarity

This section discusses scientific considerations in the stepwise approach to developing data and information needed to support a demonstration of biosimilarity. To demonstrate biosimilarity, a sponsor must provide sufficient data and information to show that the proposed product and the reference product are highly similar notwithstanding minor differences in clinically inactive components and that there are no clinically meaningful differences between the two products in terms of safety, purity, and potency. The type and the amount of analyses and testings that will be sufficient to demonstrate biosimilarity will be determined on a product-specific basis.

3.4.5.1 Structural analyses The PHSA requires that a 351(k) application include information demonstrating biosimilarity based on data derived from, among other things, analytical studies that demonstrate that the biological product is highly similar to the reference product notwithstanding minor differences in clinically inactive components, unless the FDA determines that an element is unnecessary in a 351(k) application. The FDA expects that, first, a sponsor will extensively characterize the proposed product and the reference product with state-of-the-art technology because the extensive characterization of both products serves as the foundation for a demonstration of biosimilarity. It is expected that the expression construct for a proposed product will encode the same primary amino acid sequence as its reference product. However, minor modifications such as N- or C-terminal truncations that are not expected to change the product performance may be justified and should be explained by the sponsor. Additionally, sponsors should consider all relevant characteristics of the protein product (e.g., the primary, secondary, tertiary, and quaternary structures; PTMs; and biological activities) to demonstrate that the proposed product is highly similar to the reference product notwithstanding minor differences in clinically inactive components. The more comprehensive and robust the comparative structural and functional characterizations are, the stronger the scientific justification for a selective and targeted approach to animal and/or clinical testing.

Sponsors should use appropriate analytical methodologies with adequate sensitivity and specificity for structural characterization of the proteins. Generally, such tests include the following comparisons of the proposed product and the reference product:

- Primary structures, such as amino acid sequence
- HOSs, including secondary, tertiary, and quaternary structures (including aggregation)
- Enzymatic PTMs, such as glycosylation and phosphorylation
- Other potential variations, such as protein deamidation and oxidation
- Intentional chemical modifications, such as PEGylation sites and characteristics

Sponsors should conduct extensive structural characterizations of both the proposed product and the reference product in multiple representative lots to understand the lot-to-lot variability of both products in the manufacturing processes. Lots used for the analyses should support the biosimilarity of both the clinical material used in the clinical study intended to support a demonstration of biosimilarity and the to-be-marketed proposed product to the reference product. Characterization of lots manufactured during process development of the proposed product may also be useful. Sponsors should justify the selection of the representative lots, including the number of lots.

In addition, the FDA recommends that sponsors analyze the finished dosage form of multiple lots of the proposed product and the reference product, assessing excipients and any formulation effect on purity, product- and process-related impurities, and stability. Differences in the formulation between the proposed product and the reference product are among the factors that may affect the extent and the nature of subsequent animal or clinical testing. A sponsor considering manufacturing changes after completing the initial analytical similarity assessment or after completing clinical testing intended to support a 351(k) application should perform an additional analytical similarity assessment with lots manufactured by the new process and the reference product and establish comparability of the proposed product manufactured by the old and new manufacturing processes. The nature and the extent of the changes may determine the scope of the analytical similarity and comparability studies and any necessary additional studies.

If the reference product or the proposed product cannot be adequately characterized by state-of-the-art technology, the application for the proposed product may not be appropriate for submission under Section 351(k) of the PHSA, and the sponsor should consult the FDA for guidance on the proper submission pathway.

3.4.5.2 Functional assays The pharmacologic activity of protein products should be evaluated by in vitro and/or in vivo functional assays.

In vitro assays may include, but are not limited to, biological assays, binding assays, and enzyme kinetics. In vivo assays may include the use of animal models of disease (e.g., models that exhibit a disease state or symptom) to evaluate functional effects on PD markers or efficacy measures. A functional evaluation comparing a proposed product to the reference product that uses these types of assays is also an important part of the foundation that supports a demonstration of biosimilarity, and may be used to scientifically justify a selective and targeted approach to animal and/or clinical testing.

Sponsors can use functional assays to provide additional evidence that the biologic activity and the potency of the proposed product are highly similar to those of the reference product and/or to support a conclusion that there are no clinically meaningful differences between the proposed product and the reference product. Such assays also may be used to provide additional evidence that the MOAs of the two products are the same to the extent that the MOA of the reference product is known. Functional assays can be used to provide additional data to support results from structural analyses, investigate the consequences of observed structural differences, and explore structure–activity relationships. These assays are expected to be comparative so they can provide evidence of similarity or reveal differences in the performance of the proposed product compared to that of the reference product, especially the differences resulting from variations in structure that cannot be detected using current analytical methods. The FDA also recommends that sponsors discuss limitations of the assays they used when interpreting results in their submissions to FDA. Such discussions would be useful for the evaluation of analytical data and may guide whether additional analytical testing would be necessary to support a demonstration of biosimilarity.

Functional assays can also provide information that complements the animal and clinical data in assessing the potential clinical effects of minor differences in structure between the proposed product and the reference product. For example, cell-based bioactivity assays may be used to detect the potential for inducing cytokine release syndrome in vivo. The available information about these assays, including sensitivity, specificity, and extent of validation, can affect the amount and the type of additional animal or clinical data that may be needed to establish biosimilarity. As is the case for the structural evaluation, sponsors should justify the selection of the representative lots, including the number of lots.

3.4.5.3 Animal data The PHSA also requires that a 351(k) application include information demonstrating biosimilarity based on data derived from animal studies (including the assessment of toxicity) unless the FDA determines that such studies are not necessary for a 351(k) application. Results from animal studies may be used to support the safety evaluation of the proposed product and more generally to support the demonstration of biosimilarity between the proposed product and the reference product.

3.4.5.3.1 Animal toxicity studies As a scientific matter, animal toxicity data are considered useful when, based on the results of extensive structural and functional characterizations, uncertainties remain about the safety of the proposed product that need to be addressed before the initiation of clinical studies in humans (assuming that results from animal studies can meaningfully address the remaining uncertainties).

The scope and the extent of any animal toxicity studies will depend on the information about the reference product, the information about the proposed product, and the extent of known similarities or differences between the two. The FDA encourages sponsors to initiate early discussions with the Agency with regard to their biosimilar development plans, including identifying appropriate scientific justifications for not conducting an animal toxicity study or for the scope and the extent of such a study. The steps to meeting the FDA are laid out in the listing of the types of meeting the FDA has created for the development of biosimilar products.

If comparative structural and functional data using the proposed product provide strong support for analytical similarity to a reference product, then limited animal toxicity data may be sufficient to support the initial clinical use of the proposed product. Such a study may be nonsacrificial and include end points that measure in life parameters, PD, and PK (with an assessment of immunogenicity).

If the structural and functional data are limited in scope, or there are concerns about the proposed product quality, a general toxicology study may be needed that includes full animal pathology, histopathology, PD, PK, and immunogenicity assessments. When animal toxicology studies are conducted, it will be useful to perform a comparative study with the proposed product and the reference product (i.e., comparative bridging toxicology studies). The selection of dose, regimen, duration, and test species for these studies should provide a meaningful toxicological comparison between the two products. It is important to understand the limitations of such animal studies (e.g., small sample size and intraspecies variations) when interpreting results comparing the proposed product and the reference product. For a detailed discussion on the design of animal toxicology studies relevant to biological products, see the ICH guidance for industry *S6(R1): Preclinical Safety Evaluation of Biotechnology-Derived Pharmaceuticals* (ICH S6(R1)).

Safety data derived from animal toxicity studies are generally not expected if clinical data (e.g., from studies or marketing experience outside the United States) using the proposed product are available (with the same proposed route of administration and formulation) that provide sufficient evidence for its safe use, unless animal toxicity studies are otherwise needed to address a particular product quality concern.

Animal toxicity studies are generally not useful if there is no animal species that can provide pharmacologically relevant data for the product (i.e., no species in which the biologic activity of the product mimics the human response). For a detailed discussion about demonstrating species relevance, see the criteria described in ICH S6(R1). However, there may be some instances when animal data from a pharmacologically nonresponsive species (including rodents) may be useful to support clinical studies with a proposed product that has not been previously tested in human subjects, for example, comparative PK and systemic tolerability studies. If animal toxicity studies are not warranted based on an acceptable scientific justification, additional comparative in vitro testing (using human cells or tissues when appropriate) is encouraged. Data derived using human cells can provide valuable comparative information between the proposed product and the reference product regarding potential clinical effects, particularly in situations where there are no animal species available for safety testing.

In general, nonclinical safety pharmacology, reproductive and developmental toxicities, and carcinogenicity studies are not warranted when the proposed product and the reference product have been demonstrated to be highly similar through extensive structural and functional characterizations and animal toxicity studies (if such studies were conducted).

3.4.5.3.2 Inclusion of animal PK and PD measures Under certain circumstances, a single-dose study in animals comparing the proposed product and the reference product using PK and PD measures may contribute to the totality of evidence that supports a demonstration of biosimilarity. Specifically, sponsors can use results from animal studies to support the degree of similarity based on the PK and PD profiles of the proposed product and the reference product. PK and PD measures can also be incorporated into a single animal toxicity study, where appropriate. Animal PK and PD assessments will not negate the need for human PK and PD studies.

3.4.5.3.3 Interpreting animal immunogenicity results Animal immunogenicity assessments are conducted to assist in the interpretation of the animal study results and generally do not predict potential immune responses to protein products in humans. However, when differences in manufacturing (e.g., impurities or excipients) between the proposed product and the reference product may result in differences in immunogenicity, a measurement of antitherapeutic protein antibody responses in animals may provide useful information. Additionally, differences observed in animal immunogenicity assessments may reflect potential structural or functional differences between the two products not captured by other analytical methods.

3.4.5.4 Clinical studies—General considerations The sponsor of a proposed product must include in its submission to the FDA information demonstrating that "there are no clinically meaningful differences between the biological product and the reference product in terms of the safety, purity, and potency of the product" (Section 7002(b)(3) of the Affordable Care Act and Section 351(i)(2)(B) of the PHSA). To support a demonstration of biosimilarity, the statute also requires a clinical study or studies (including the assessment of immunogenicity and PK or PD) sufficient to demonstrate safety, purity, and potency in one or more appropriate conditions of use for which the reference product is licensed and intended to be used and for which licensure is sought for the biological product, unless the FDA determines an element unnecessary (Section 7002(a)(2) of the Affordable Care Act and Section 351(k)(2)(A)(i)(I)(cc) of the PHSA). As a general matter, the FDA anticipates that the recommendations described in this guidance designed to demonstrate that the proposed product is highly similar to its reference product notwithstanding minor differences in clinically inactive components and to show that no clinically meaningful differences exist between the two products will provide data sufficient to demonstrate the safety, the purity, and the potency of the proposed product. The FDA recommends that sponsors identify which study or studies will provide data regarding no clinically meaningful differences prior to starting clinical studies.

The nature and the scope of the clinical study or studies will depend on the nature and the extent of residual uncertainty about biosimilarity after conducting structural and functional characterizations and, where relevant, animal studies. The frequency and the severity of safety risks and other safety and effectiveness considerations (e.g., the poor relationship between pharmacologic effects and effectiveness) for the reference product may also affect the design of the clinical program. The scope of the clinical program and the type of clinical studies (i.e., comparative human PK, PD, clinical immunogenicity, or clinical safety and effectiveness) should be scientifically justified by the sponsor.

As a scientific matter, the FDA expects a sponsor to conduct comparative human PK and PD studies (if there is a relevant PD measure(s)). Note that a PD study may also incorporate PK measures (i.e., a combined PK/PD study) and a clinical immunogenicity assessment. In certain cases, the results of these studies may provide adequate clinical data to support a conclusion that there are no clinically meaningful differences between the proposed biosimilar product and the reference product. However, if residual uncertainty about biosimilarity remains after conducting these studies, an additional comparative clinical study or studies would be needed to further evaluate whether there are clinically meaningful differences between the two products. PK and PD studies provide quite different types of information. In simple terms, a PK study measures how the body acts on a drug (how the drug is absorbed, distributed, metabolized, and eliminated), and a PD study measures how the drug acts on the body (typically assessing a measure related to the drug's biochemical and physiologic effects on the body). Therefore, one type of study does not duplicate or substitute for the information provided by the other. Both PK studies and PD studies provide valuable information for assessing biosimilarity; and, therefore, as a scientific matter, comparative human PK studies and PD studies (where there is a relevant PD measure(s)) will be generally expected.

3.4.5.4.1 Human pharmacology data Human PK and PD profiles of a protein product cannot often be adequately predicted from functional assays and/or animal studies alone. Therefore, human PK and PD studies comparing a proposed product to the reference product are generally fundamental components in supporting a demonstration of biosimilarity. Both PK and PD studies (where there is a relevant PD measure(s)) will generally be expected to establish biosimilarity, unless a sponsor can scientifically justify that such a study is not needed. Even if relevant PD measures are not available, sensitive PD end points may be assessed if such assessment may help reduce residual uncertainty about biosimilarity.

Sponsors should provide a scientific justification for the selection of the human PK and PD study populations (e.g., patients versus healthy subjects) and parameters, taking into consideration the relevance and sensitivity of such population and parameters, the population and parameters studied for the licensure for the reference product, as well as the current knowledge of the intrasubject and intersubject variability of human PK and PD for the reference product. For example, comparative human PK and PD studies should use a population, a dose, and a route of administration that are adequately sensitive to allow for the detection of differences in PK and PD profiles. The FDA recommends that, to the extent possible, the sponsor selects PD measures that (a) are relevant to clinical outcomes (e.g., on mechanistic path of MOA or disease process related to effectiveness or safety); (b) are measurable for a sufficient period after dosing to ascertain the full PD response and with appropriate precision; and (c) have the sensitivity to detect clinically meaningful differences between the proposed product and the reference product. The use of multiple PD measures that assess different domains of activities may also be of value.

When there are established dose–response or systemic exposure–response relationships (response may be PD measures or clinical end points), it is important to select, whenever possible, a dose for a study on the steep part of the dose–response curve for the proposed product. Studying doses that are on the plateau of the dose–response curve is unlikely to detect clinically meaningful differences between the two products. Sponsors should predefine and justify the criteria for PK and PD parameters for studies included in the application to demonstrate biosimilarity.

A human PK study that demonstrates similar exposure (e.g., serum concentration over time) for the proposed product and the reference product may provide support for a demonstration of biosimilarity. A human PK study may be particularly useful when the exposure correlates with clinical safety and effectiveness. A human PD study that demonstrates a similar effect on a relevant PD measure related to effectiveness or specific safety concerns (except for immunogenicity, which is evaluated separately) represents even stronger support for a biosimilarity determination.

In certain cases, establishing similar clinical PK, PD, and immunogenicity profiles may provide sufficient clinical data to support a conclusion that there are no clinically meaningful differences between the two products. PK and PD parameters are generally more sensitive than clinical efficacy end points in assessing the similarity of two products. For example, an effect on thyroid-stimulating hormone levels would provide a more sensitive comparison of two thyroxine products than an effect on clinical symptoms of euthyroidism.

In cases where there is a meaningful correlation between PK and PD results and clinical effectiveness, convincing PK and PD results may make a comparative efficacy study unnecessary. For example, similar dose–response curves of the proposed product and the reference product on a relevant PD measure, combined with a similar human PK profile and clinical immunogenicity profile, could provide sufficient evidence to support a conclusion of no clinically meaningful differences. Even if there is still residual uncertainty about biosimilarity based on PK and PD results, establishing similar human PK and PD profiles may provide a scientific basis for a selective and targeted approach to subsequent clinical testing.

For PD studies using products with a short half-life (e.g., shorter than five days), a rapid PD response, and a low incidence of immunogenicity, a crossover design is appropriate, when feasible. For products with a longer half-life (e.g., more than five days), a parallel design will usually be needed. Sponsors should provide a scientific justification for the selection of study dose (e.g., one dose or multiple doses) and route of administration. The FDA recommends that sponsors consider the time it takes for a PD measure to change and the possibility of nonlinear PK. The FDA also encourages consideration of the role of modeling and simulation in designing comparative human PK and PD studies.

3.4.5.4.2 Clinical immunogenicity assessment The goal of the clinical immunogenicity assessment is to evaluate potential differences between the proposed product and the reference product in the incidence and the severity of human immune responses. Immune responses may affect both the safety and the effectiveness of the product by, for example, altering PK, inducing anaphylaxis, or promoting the development of neutralizing antibodies that neutralize the product as well as its endogenous protein counterpart. Thus, establishing that there are no clinically meaningful differences in immune response between a proposed product and the reference product is a fundamental element in the demonstration of biosimilarity. Structural, functional, and animal data are generally not adequate to predict immunogenicity in humans. Therefore, at least one clinical study that includes a comparison of the immunogenicity of the proposed product to that of the reference product will be expected. The FDA encourages that, where feasible, sponsors collect immunogenicity data in any clinical study, including human PK or PD studies.

The extent and the timing of the clinical immunogenicity assessment will vary depending on a range of factors, including the extent of analytical similarity between the proposed product and the reference product and the incidence and clinical consequences of immune responses for the reference product. For example, if the clinical consequence is severe (e.g., when the reference product is a therapeutic counterpart of an endogenous protein with a critical, nonredundant biological function or is known to provoke anaphylaxis), a more extensive immunogenicity assessment will likely be needed to support a demonstration of biosimilarity. If the immune response to the reference product is rare, a premarketing evaluation to assess apparent differences in immune responses between the two products may be adequate to support biosimilarity. In addition, in some cases, certain safety risks may need to be evaluated through postmarketing surveillance or studies.

The overall immunogenicity assessment should consider the nature of the immune response (e.g., anaphylaxis, neutralizing antibody), the clinical relevance and severity of consequences (e.g., loss of efficacy of life-saving therapeutic and other adverse effects), the incidence of immune responses, and the population being studied. The FDA recommends the use of a comparative parallel design (i.e., a head-to-head study) in treatment-naive patients with the most sensitive design for a premarketing study to assess potential differences in the risk of immunogenicity. However, depending on the clinical experience of the reference and proposed products (taking into consideration the conditions of use and patient population), a sponsor may need to evaluate a subset of patients to provide a substantive descriptive assessment of whether a single crossover from the reference product to the proposed biosimilar would result in a major risk in terms of hypersensitivity, immunogenicity, or other reactions. The design of any study to assess immunogenicity and acceptable differences in the incidence and other parameters of immune response should be discussed with the FDA before initiating the study. Differences in immune responses between a proposed product and the reference product in the absence of observed clinical sequelae may be of concern and may warrant further evaluation (e.g., extended period of follow-up evaluation).

The study population used to compare immunogenicity should be justified by the sponsor and agreed to by the Agency. If a sponsor is seeking to extrapolate immunogenicity findings for one condition of use to other conditions of use, the sponsor should consider using a study population and a treatment regimen that are adequately sensitive for predicting a difference in immune responses between the proposed product and the reference product across the conditions of use. Usually, this will be the population and the regimen for the reference product for which development of immune responses with adverse outcomes is most likely to occur (e.g., patients on background immunosuppressants would be less liable to develop immune responses than patients who are not immunosuppressed).

The selection of clinical immunogenicity end points or PD measures associated with immune responses to therapeutic protein products (e.g., antibody formation and cytokine levels) should take into consideration the immunogenicity issues that have emerged from the use of the reference product. Sponsors should prospectively define the clinical immune response criteria (e.g., definitions of significant clinical events such as anaphylaxis), using established criteria where available, for each type of potential immune response and should obtain agreement from the FDA on these criteria before initiating the study.

The duration of follow-up evaluation should be determined based on (a) the time course of the generation of immune responses (such as the development of neutralizing antibodies, cell-mediated immune responses) and expected clinical sequelae (informed by experience with the reference product), (b) the time course of the disappearance of the immune responses and the clinical sequelae following cessation of therapy, and (c) the length of administration of the product. For example, for chronically administered agents, the follow-up period is recommended to be one year unless a shorter duration can be scientifically justified based on the totality of the evidence to support biosimilarity.

As a scientific matter, a sponsor should evaluate the following antibody parameters in the clinical immunogenicity assessment:

- Titer, specificity, relevant isotype distribution, time course of development, persistence, disappearance, impact on PK, and association with clinical sequelae
- Neutralization of product activity: Neutralizing capacity to all relevant functions (e.g., uptake and catalytic activities, neutralization for replacement enzyme therapeutics)

The sponsor should develop assays capable of sensitively detecting immune responses, even in the presence of the circulating drug product (proposed product and reference product). The proposed product and the reference product should be assessed in the same assay with the same patient sera whenever possible. The FDA recommends that immunogenicity assays be developed and validated early in development, and the validation should consider both the proposed product and the reference product. Sponsors should consult with the FDA on the sufficiency of assays before initiating any clinical immunogenicity assessment.

3.4.5.4.3 Comparative clinical studies As a scientific matter, a comparative clinical study will be necessary to support a demonstration of biosimilarity if there is residual uncertainty about whether there are clinically meaningful differences between the proposed product and the reference product based on structural and functional characterizations, animal testing, human PK and PD data, and clinical immunogenicity assessment. A sponsor should provide a scientific justification if it believes that a comparative clinical study is not necessary.

The following are examples of factors that may influence the type and the extent of the comparative clinical study data needed:

- The nature and the complexity of the reference product, the extensiveness of structural and functional characterizations, and the findings and limitations of comparative structural, functional, and nonclinical testings, including the extent of observed differences
- The degree to which differences in structure, function, and nonclinical pharmacologies and toxicologies predicts differences in clinical outcomes, in conjunction with the degree of understanding of the MOA of the reference product and the disease pathology
- The extent to which human PK or PD is known to predict clinical outcomes (e.g., PD measures known to be relevant to effectiveness or safety)
- The scope of clinical experience with the reference product and its therapeutic class, including the safety and risk–benefit profiles (e.g., whether there is a low potential for off-target adverse events), and the appropriate end points and biomarkers for safety and effectiveness (e.g., availability of established, sensitive clinical end points)
- The extent of any other clinical experience with the proposed product (e.g., if the proposed product has been marketed outside the United States)

A sponsor should provide a scientific justification for how it intends to use these factors to determine what type of a clinical study is needed and the design of any necessary study. For example, if a comparative clinical study is needed, a sponsor should explain how these factors were considered in determining the design of such a study, including the end point, the population, the similarity margin, and the statistical analyses.

Additionally, specific safety or effectiveness concerns regarding the reference product and its class (including the history of manufacturing or source-related adverse events) may warrant more comparative clinical data. Alternatively, if there is information regarding other biological products that could support a biosimilarity determination (with marketing histories that demonstrate no apparent differences in clinical safety and effectiveness profiles), such information may be an additional factor supporting a selective and targeted approach to the clinical program.

3.4.5.4.4 End points A sponsor should use end points that can assess clinically meaningful differences between the proposed product and the reference product in a comparative clinical study. The end points may be different from those used as primary end points in the reference product's clinical studies if they are scientifically supported. Certain end points (such as PD measures) are more sensitive than clinical end points and, therefore, may enable more precise comparisons of relevant therapeutic effects. There may be situations when the assessment of multiple PD measures in a comparative clinical study will enhance the sensitivity of the study. The adequacy of the end points depends on the extent to which the PD measures correlate with the clinical outcome; the extent of structural and functional data support for biosimilarity, the understanding of the MOA, and the nature or seriousness of outcome are affected.

3.4.5.4.5 Study population The choice of study population should allow for an assessment of clinically meaningful differences between the proposed product and the reference product. Often, the study population will have characteristics consistent with those of the population studied for the licensure of the reference product for the same indication. However, there are cases where a study population could be different from that in the clinical studies that supported the licensure of the reference product. For example, if a genetic predictor of response was developed following licensure of the reference product, it may be possible to use patients with the response marker as the study population.

3.4.5.4.6 Sample size and duration of study The sample size for and the duration of the comparative clinical study should be adequate to allow for the detection of clinically meaningful differences between the two products. Certain end points, such as PD measures, may be more sensitive than clinical end points and facilitate the conduct of a smaller study of limited duration. In such cases where the size and the length of the comparative clinical study may not be adequate for the detection of relevant safety signals, a separate assessment of safety and immunogenicity may be needed.

3.4.5.4.7 Study design and analyses A comparative clinical study of a biosimilar development program should be designed to investigate whether there are clinically meaningful differences between the proposed product and the reference product. The design should take into consideration the nature and the extent of residual uncertainty that remains about biosimilarity based on data generated from comparative structural and functional characterizations, animal testing, human PK and PD studies, and clinical immunogenicity assessment.

Generally, the FDA expects a clinical study or studies designed to establish statistical evidence that the proposed product is neither inferior to the reference product by more than a specified margin nor superior to the reference product by more than a (possibly different) specified margin. Typically, an equivalence design with symmetric inferiority and superiority margins would be used. Symmetric margins would be reasonable when, for example, there are dose-related toxicities.

In some cases, it would be more appropriate to use an asymmetric interval with a larger upper bound to rule out superiority than lower bound to rule out inferiority. An asymmetric interval could be reasonable, for example, if the dose used in the clinical study is near the plateau of the dose–response curve, and there is little likelihood of dose-related effects (e.g., toxicity). In most cases, the use of an asymmetric interval would generally allow for a smaller sample size than would be needed with symmetric margins. However, if there is a demonstration of clear superiority, then further consideration should be given as to whether the proposed product can be considered biosimilar to the reference product.

In some cases, depending on the study population and the end point, ruling out only inferiority may be adequate to establish that there are no clinically meaningful differences between the proposed product and the reference product. For example, if it is well established that doses of a reference product pharmacodynamically saturate the target at the clinical dose level, and it would be unethical to use the lower than clinically approved doses, a noninferiority (NI) design may be sufficient. If an NI design is considered appropriate, sponsors are encouraged to refer to the draft guidance for industry.

3.4.5.4.8 Noninferiority clinical trials A sponsor should provide adequate scientific justification for the choice of study design, study population, study end point, estimated effect size for the reference product, and margin (how much difference to rule out). Sponsors should discuss their study proposals and overall clinical development plan with the FDA before initiating the comparative clinical study. Differences between conditions of use with respect to the factors described above do not necessarily preclude extrapolation. A scientific justification should address these differences in the context of the totality of the evidence supporting a demonstration of biosimilarity.

In choosing which condition of use to study that would permit subsequent extrapolation of clinical data to other conditions of use, the FDA recommends that a sponsor consider choosing a condition of use that would be adequately sensitive to detect clinically meaningful differences between two products.

3.4.5.4.9 Extrapolation of clinical data across indications If the proposed product meets the statutory requirements for licensure as a biosimilar product under Section 351(k) of the PHSA based on, among other things, data derived from a clinical study or studies sufficient to demonstrate safety, purity, and potency in an appropriate condition of use, the applicant may seek licensure of the proposed product for one or more additional terms of use for which the reference product is licensed. However, the applicant would need to provide sufficient scientific justification for extrapolating clinical data to support a determination of biosimilarity for each condition of use for which licensure is sought.

Such scientific justification for extrapolation should address, for example, the following issues for the tested and extrapolated conditions of use:

- The MOA in each condition of use for which licensure is sought; this may include the following:
  - The target/receptors for each relevant activity/function of the product
  - The binding, the dose/concentration–response, and the pattern of molecular signaling upon engagement of target/receptors
  - The relationships between product structure and target/receptor interactions
  - The location and expression of the target/receptors
- The PK and biodistribution of the product in different patient populations (relevant PD measures may also provide important information on the MOA)
- The immunogenicity of the product in different patient populations
- Differences in expected toxicities in each condition of use and patient population (including whether expected toxicities are related to the pharmacological activity of the product or to off-target activities)
- Any other factor that may affect the safety or the efficacy of the product in each condition of use and patient population for which licensure is sought

The sponsor of a proposed product may obtain licensure only for a condition of use that has been previously licensed as the reference product. If a reference product has a condition of use that was licensed under Section 506(c) of the FDCA and 21 CFR part 601, subpart E (accelerated approval), and the reference product's clinical benefit in this condition of use has not yet been verified in postmarketing studies, the proposed product sponsor should consider studying another condition of use for which the reference product is licensed to avoid potential complications in the event that postmarketing studies fail to verify the clinical benefit of the reference product for the condition of use.

3.5 Postmarketing safety monitoring considerations

Robust postmarketing safety monitoring is an important component in ensuring the safety and the effectiveness of biological products, including biosimilar therapeutic protein products.

Postmarketing safety monitoring should first take into consideration any particular safety or effectiveness concerns associated with the use of the reference product and its class, the proposed product in its development and clinical uses (if marketed outside the United States), the specific condition of use and patient population, and patient exposure in the biosimilar development program. Postmarketing safety monitoring for a proposed product should also have adequate mechanisms in place to differentiate between the adverse events associated with the proposed product and those associated with the reference product, including the identification of adverse events associated with the proposed product that have not been previously associated with the reference product. Rare, but potentially serious, safety risks (e.g., immunogenicity) may not be detected during preapproval clinical testing because the size of the population exposed will likely not be large enough to assess rare events. In particular cases, such risks may need to be evaluated through postmarketing surveillance or studies. In addition, as with any other biological product, the FDA may take any appropriate action to ensure the safety and the effectiveness of a proposed product, including, for example, requiring a postmarketing study or clinical trial to evaluate certain safety risks.

Because some aspects of postmarketing safety monitoring are product specific, the FDA encourages sponsors to consult with appropriate FDA divisions to discuss the sponsor's proposed approach to postmarketing safety monitoring.

3.5.1 Consultation with the FDA

Many product-specific factors can influence the components of a product development program intended to establish that a proposed product is biosimilar to a reference product. Therefore, the FDA will ordinarily provide feedback on a case-by-case basis on the components of a development program for a proposed product. In addition, it may not be possible to identify in advance all the necessary components of a development program, and the assessment of one element (e.g., structural analyses) at one step can influence decisions about the type and the amount of subsequent data for the next step. For these reasons, the FDA recommends that sponsors use a stepwise approach to establish the *totality of the evidence* that supports a demonstration of biosimilarity.

The FDA also advises sponsors intending to develop biosimilar products to meet with the FDA to present their product development plans and establish a schedule of milestones that will serve as landmarks for future discussions with the Agency. The FDA anticipates that early discussions with the FDA about product development plans and about the approaches to providing adequate scientific justifications will facilitate biosimilar development.

3.6 Quality considerations in demonstrating biosimilarity

3.6.1 Background

In the 1980s, the FDA began to receive marketing applications for biotechnology-derived protein products, mostly for recombinant DNA–derived versions of naturally sourced products. Consequently, the FDA established a regulatory approach for the approval of recombinant DNA–derived protein products, which was announced in the Federal Register (FR) (51 FR 23302, June 26, 1986), in conjunction with a 1985 document titled *Points to Consider in the Production and Testing of New Drugs and Biologicals Produced by Recombinant DNA Technology.* This approach addresses the submission of an investigational NDA (IND) to the FDA for evaluation before initiation of clinical investigations in human subjects and the submission and approval of an NDA or biologics license application (BLA) for marketing the products made with recombinant DNA technology, even if the active ingredient in the product is thought to be identical to a naturally occurring substance or a previously approved product. The policy set forth in those documents was developed in part because of the challenges in evaluating protein products solely by physicochemical and functional testings and because the biological system in which a protein product is produced can have a significant effect on the structure and the function of the product itself. Because of the complexities of protein products, the FDA has, as a matter of policy, generally required submission of an NDA (in accordance with Section 505(b)(1) of FDCA) or a BLA (in accordance with Section 351(a) of the PHSA) containing product-specific full safety and efficacy data for recombinant DNA–derived protein products. The FDA has recognized, however, that "[i]n some instances complete new applications may not be required" (51 FR 23309, June 26, 1986).

Improvements in manufacturing processes, process controls, materials, and product testing, as well as characterization tests and studies, have led to a gradual evolution in the regulation of protein products. For example, in 1996, the FDA provided recommendations in its *The FDA Guidance Concerning Demonstration of Comparability of Human Biological Products, including Therapeutic Biotechnology Products*, which explains how a sponsor may demonstrate, through a combination of analytical testing, functional assays (in vitro and/or in vivo), assessment of PK, and/or PD, and toxicity in animals, and clinical testing (clinical pharmacology, safety, and/or efficacy), that a manufacturing change does not adversely affect the identity, the purity, or the potency of its FDA-approved product.

Since 1996, the FDA has approved many manufacturing process changes for licensed biological products based on a demonstration of product comparability before and after the process change, as supported by quality criteria and analytical testing and without the need for additional nonclinical data and clinical safety and/or efficacy studies. In some cases, uncertainty about the effect of the change and/or the results of the biochemical/functional comparability studies has necessitated assessment of additional data, including nonclinical and/or clinical testing, to demonstrate product comparability. These concepts were further developed by the ICH of Technical Requirements for Registration of Pharmaceuticals for Human Use and resulted in the ICH guidance for industry *Q5E: Comparability of Biotechnological/Biological Products Subject to Changes in Their Manufacturing Process.*

Although the scope of ICH Q5E is limited to an assessment of the comparability of a biological product before and after a manufacturing process change made by the same manufacturer, certain general scientific principles described in ICH Q5E are applicable to an assessment of biosimilarity between a proposed product and its reference product. However, demonstrating that a proposed product is biosimilar to an FDA-licensed reference product manufactured by a different manufacturer will typically be more complex and will likely require more extensive and comprehensive data than assessing the comparability of a product before and after a manufacturing process change made by the product's sponsor. A manufacturer that modifies its own manufacturing process has extensive knowledge and information about the product and the existing process, including established controls and acceptance parameters. By contrast, the manufacturer of a proposed product will likely have a different manufacturing process (e.g., different cell line, raw materials, equipment, processes, process controls, and acceptance criteria) from that of the reference product and no direct knowledge of the manufacturing process for the reference product.

In October 1999, the FDA issued the draft guidance for industry *Applications Covered by Section 505(b)(2)*, which, among other things, states that the FDA may accept an application submitted through the approval pathway described by Section 505(b)(2) of the FDCA for a drug product containing an active ingredient derived from natural sources or recombinant DNA technology. For example, the FDA approved a 505(b)(2) application for a follow-on recombinant DNA–derived human growth hormone product in May 2006. Greater knowledge as a result of advances in science and technology and improvements in manufacturing processes, process controls, materials, and product testing, as well as characterization tests and studies, may support the use of an abbreviated pathway for the approval of a protein product.

The BPCI Act was enacted as part of the Affordable Care Act on March 23, 2010. The BPCI Act creates an abbreviated licensure pathway for biological products demonstrated to be biosimilar to or interchangeable with a reference product. Section 351(k) of the PHSA (42 U.S.C. 262(k)), added by the BPCI Act, sets forth the requirements for a biosimilar product application.

3.6.2 Scope

The scientific advice from the FDA heavily dwells on analytical studies that are relevant to assessing whether the proposed product and a reference product are highly similar to support a demonstration of biosimilarity. Although the FDA guidance specifically applies to therapeutic protein products, the general scientific principles may be informative for the development of other protein products, such as in vivo protein diagnostic products. If the reference product or the proposed product cannot be adequately characterized with state-of-the-art technology as recommended by this guidance, the application may not be appropriate for submission under Section 351(k) of the PHSA. The FDA recommends that the sponsor consult the FDA for guidance on the proper submission pathway.

The FDA provides detailed guidance for additional chemistry, manufacturing, and controls (CMC) information that are relevant to assessing whether the proposed product and the reference product are highly similar. All product applications should contain a complete and thorough CMC section that provides the necessary and appropriate information (e.g., characterization, adventitious agent safety, process controls, and specifications) for the product to be adequately reviewed. The FDA encourages early interactions to discuss specific CMC issues that may arise for a sponsor's proposed product. For CMC requirements for submission of a marketing application, sponsors should consult current regulations and see the guidance for industry *Submission on Chemistry, Manufacturing, and Controls Information for a Therapeutic Recombinant DNA–Derived Product or a Monoclonal Antibody Product for In-Vivo Use*, as well as other applicable FDA guidance documents.

The use of the terms *product-related substances* and *product-* and *process-related impurities* is consistent with their use and meaning in the ICH guidance for industry Q6B Specifications: Test Procedures and Acceptance Criteria for Biotechnological/Biological Products.

In addition to comparative analytical studies, an assessment of whether a proposed product is biosimilar to a reference product will include animal studies (including the assessment of toxicity) and a clinical study or studies (including the assessment of immunogenicity and PK and/or PD).

3.6.3 General principles

Advances in analytical sciences (both physicochemical and biological) enable some protein products to be extensively characterized in terms of their physicochemical and biological properties. These analytical procedures have improved the ability to identify and characterize not only the desired product but also the product-related substances and the product- and process-related impurities. Advances in manufacturing science and production methods, as well as advances in analytical sciences, may enhance the likelihood that a proposed product can be demonstrated to be highly similar to a reference product by better targeting the reference product's physicochemical and functional properties. In addition, advances in analytical sciences may enable detection and characterization of the differences between the protein products. These differences should be further assessed to understand the impact on product performance.

Despite improvements in analytical techniques, the current analytical methodology may not be able to detect or characterize all relevant structural and functional differences between the two protein products. A thorough understanding of each analytical method's limitations will be critical to a sponsor's successful identification of residual uncertainties and, in turn, to the design of subsequent testing. In addition, there may be an incomplete understanding of the relationship between a product's structural attributes and its clinical performance. Sponsors should use an appropriate analytical methodology that has adequate sensitivity and specificity to detect and characterize the differences between the proposed product and the reference product. Accordingly, the FDA encourages the use of widely available state-of-the-art technology.

In addition to a complete CMC data submission as required under Section 351(a) of the PHSA, an application submitted under Section 351(k) of the PHSA is needed to include data supporting the analytical similarity of the proposed biosimilar product to the reference product. The rationale for the analytical similarity assessment should be clearly described with consideration for the known quality attributes and performance characteristics of the specific reference product.

Comparative analytical data provide the foundation for a biosimilar development program and can influence decisions about the type and the amount of animal and clinical data needed to support a demonstration of biosimilarity. Such analytical data should be available early in product development and will permit more detailed discussion with the Agency because known quality attributes can be used to shape biosimilar development and to justify certain development decisions. Thus, in addition to the preliminary comparative analytical similarity data that should be submitted to support an initial advisory meeting, the FDA encourages sponsors to submit comprehensive analytical similarity data early in the development process: at the pre-IND stage, with the original IND submission, or with the submission of data from the initial clinical studies, such as PK and PD studies. The FDA will best be able to provide meaningful input on the extent and the scope of animal and additional clinical studies for a proposed biosimilar development program once the Agency has considered the analytical similarity data.

Extensive, robust comparative physicochemical and functional studies (these may include biological assays, binding assays, and enzyme kinetics) should be performed to evaluate whether the proposed product and the reference product are highly similar. A meaningful assessment as to whether the proposed product is highly similar to the reference product depends on, among other things, the capabilities of available state-of-the-art analytical assays to assess, for example, the molecular weight of the protein, the complexity of the protein (HOS and PTMs), the degree of heterogeneity, the functional properties, the impurity profiles, and the degradation profiles denoting stability. The capability of the methods used in these analytical assessments, as well as their limitations, should be described by the sponsor. Physicochemical and functional characterization studies should be sufficient to establish relevant quality attributes including those that define a product's identity, quantity, safety, purity, and potency. The product-related impurities, product-related substances, and process-related impurities should be identified, characterized as appropriate, quantified, and compared with multiple lots of the proposed product to multiple lots of the reference product, to the extent feasible and relevant, as part of an assessment of the potential impact on the safety, the purity, and the potency of the product.

The primary structure of some protein products can be highly heterogeneous, which could affect the expected clinical performance of a protein product. Protein heterogeneity may arise in a number of ways. Replication errors in the DNA encoding the protein sequence and amino acid misincorporation may occur during translation, although the level of these errors is typically small. In addition, most protein products undergo some PTM that can alter the functions of the protein by attaching other biochemical groups such as phosphate and various lipids and carbohydrates; by proteolytic cleavage following translation; by changing the chemical nature of an amino acid (e.g., formylation); or by many other mechanisms. Such modifications can result from intracellular activities during cell culture or by deliberate modification of the protein, for example, PEGylation. Other PTMs can be a consequence of manufacturing process operations; for instance, glycation may occur with exposure to the product to reducing sugars. Also, storage conditions may be permissive for certain degradation pathways such as oxidation, deamidation, or aggregation. All of these product-related variants may alter the biological properties of the expressed recombinant protein. Therefore, identification and determination of the relative levels of these protein variants should be included in the comparative analytical characterization studies.

The 3D conformation of a protein is a major factor in its biological function. Proteins generally exhibit complex 3D conformations (tertiary structure and, in some cases, quaternary structure) because of their large size and the rotational characteristics of protein alpha carbons. The resulting flexibility enables dynamic, but subtle, changes in protein conformation over time, some of which may be required for functional activity. These rotations are often dependent on low energy interactions, such as hydrogen bonds and van der Waals forces, which may be very sensitive to environmental conditions. Current analytical technology is capable of evaluating the 3D structure of many proteins. Using multiple, relevant, state-of-the-art methods can help define protein tertiary structure and, to varying extents, quaternary structure and can add to the body of information supporting biosimilarity. At the same time, a protein's 3D conformation can often be difficult to precisely define using current physicochemical analytical technology. Any differences HOS between a proposed product and a reference product should be evaluated in terms of a potential effect on protein function and stability. Thus, functional assays are also critical tools for assessing the integrity of the HOSs.

A scientifically sound characterization that provides a comprehensive understanding of the chemical, physical, and biological characteristics of the proposed product is essential to the design of the manufacturing process and to the conduct of development studies. The body of knowledge that emerges will serve to support a demonstration of product quality and the effectiveness of a suitable control system during development and approval of the product.

Manufacturers should perform in-depth chemical, physical, and bioactivity comparisons with side-by-side analyses of an appropriate number of lots of the proposed product and the reference product and, where available and adequate, a comparison with a reference standard for suitable attributes (e.g., potency). The evaluation of multiple lots of a reference product and multiple lots of a proposed product enables estimation of product variability across lots. The number of lots needed to understand and estimate the lot-to-lot variability of both the reference and proposed products may differ on a case-by-case basis, and should be scientifically justified by the sponsor. The FDA encourages sponsors to consult to ensure that an appropriate number of lots are evaluated. Identification of specific lots of a reference product used in analytical similarity studies, together with expiration dates and time frames and when the lots were analyzed and used in other types of studies, should be provided. This information will be useful in justifying acceptance criteria to ensure product consistency, in addition to assessing similarity. However, the acceptance criteria should be based on the totality of the analytical data and not simply on the observed range of product attributes of the reference product. This is because some product attributes act in combination to affect a product's safety, purity, and potency profile; therefore, their potential interaction should be considered when evaluating similarity and setting specifications. For example, for some glycoproteins, the content and the distribution of tetra-antennary and *N*-acetyl-lactosamine repeats can affect in vivo potency and should not be evaluated independently of each other. Additionally, the data obtained from lots used in nonclinical and clinical studies and relevant information on the relationship between an attribute and the performance of the drug product (see ICH Q8 (R2)) suitable attributes (e.g., potency).

An extensive analytical characterization may also reveal differences between the reference product and the proposed product, especially when using analytical techniques capable of discriminating qualitative or quantitative differences in product attributes. Emphasis should be placed on developing orthogonal quantitative methods to distinguish any differences in product attributes. Based on the results of analytical studies assessing functional and physicochemical characteristics, including, for example, HOS, PTMs, and impurity and degradation profiles, the sponsor may have an appropriate scientific basis for a selective and targeted approach to subsequent animal and/or clinical studies to support a demonstration of biosimilarity. It may be useful to compare differences in the quality attributes of the proposed product with those of the reference product using a meaningful fingerprint-like analysis algorithm that covers a large number of additional product attributes and their combinations with high sensitivity using orthogonal methods. Enhanced approaches in manufacturing science, as discussed in ICH Q8(R2), may facilitate production processes that can better match a reference product's fingerprint. Such a strategy could further quantify the overall similarity between two molecules and may lead to additional bases for a more selective and targeted approach to subsequent animal and/or clinical studies.

The type, the nature, and the extent of any differences between the proposed product and the reference product, introduced by design or observed from the comprehensive analytical characterization of multiple manufacturing lots, should be clearly described and discussed. The discussion should include identification and comparison of relevant quality attributes from product characterization, as this is an important factor in assessing whether the proposed product is highly similar to the reference product. The potential clinical effects of observed structural and functional differences between the two products should be evaluated and supported by animal or clinical studies, if necessary.

The type and the extent of animal or clinical studies that are needed to demonstrate biosimilarity of the proposed product can be influenced by several factors, especially the ability to discern differences between the proposed product and the reference product and their potential effect on safety, purity, and potency. For example, factors such as the ability to robustly characterize the proposed product or the reference product (e.g., lack of suitable or sufficiently discriminative analytical techniques) or the availability of a relevant drug substance derived from the reference product could affect the nature and the extent of subsequent animal or clinical studies.

In general, a sponsor needs to provide information to demonstrate biosimilarity based on data directly comparing the proposed product with the reference product. Under certain circumstances, a sponsor may use a non-U.S.-licensed comparator product in certain studies to support a demonstration that the proposed product is biosimilar to the U.S.-licensed reference product. However, as a scientific matter, analytical studies and at least one clinical PK study and, if appropriate, at least one PD study intended to support a demonstration of biosimilarity must include an adequate comparison of the proposed product directly with the U.S.-licensed reference product unless it can be scientifically justified that such a study is not needed. If a sponsor seeks to use data from an animal study or a clinical study comparing its proposed product to a non-U.S.-licensed product to address, in part, the requirements of Section 351(k)(2)(A) of the PHSA, the sponsor should provide adequate data or information to scientifically justify the relevance of these comparative data to an assessment of biosimilarity and establish an acceptable bridge to the U.S.-licensed reference product.

As a scientific matter, the type of bridging data needed will always include data from analytical studies (e.g., structural and functional data) that directly compares all three products (i.e., the proposed product, the U.S.-licensed reference product, and the non-U.S.-licensed comparator product) and is likely to also include bridging clinical PK and/or PD study data for all three products. All three pairwise comparisons should meet the prespecified acceptance criteria for analytical and PK and/or PD similarity. The acceptability of such an approach will be evaluated on a case-by-case basis and should be discussed in advance with the Agency. For certain complex biological products, a modified approach may be needed.

The issues that a sponsor may need to address to use a non-U.S.-licensed comparator product in a biosimilar development program include, but are not limited to, the scientific bridge between the non-U.S.-licensed comparator product and the U.S.-licensed reference product, including comparative physicochemical characterization, biological assays/functional assays, degradation profiles under stressed conditions, and comparative clinical PK and, when appropriate, PD data, to address the impact of any differences in formulation or primary packaging on product performance.

3.7 Factors for consideration in assessing whether products are highly similar

When assessing whether products are highly similar, manufacturers should consider a number of factors, including the following.

3.7.1 Expression system

Therapeutic protein products can be produced in microbial cells (prokaryotic or eukaryotic), cell lines (e.g., mammalian, avian, insect, plant), or tissues derived from animals or plants. It is expected that the expression construct for a proposed product will encode the same primary amino acid sequence as its reference product. However, minor modifications, such as N- or C-terminal truncations (e.g., the heterogeneity of C-terminal lysine of a mAb) that are not expected to change the product performance, may be justified and should be explained by the sponsor. Possible differences between the chosen expression system (i.e., the host cell and the expression construct) of the proposed product and that of the reference product should be carefully considered because the type of expression system will affect the types of process- and product-related substances, impurities, and contaminants (including potential adventitious agents) that may be present in the protein product. For example, the expression system can have a significant effect on the types and the extent of translational modifications and PTMs that are imparted to the proposed product, which may introduce additional uncertainty into the demonstration that the proposed product is highly similar to the reference product.

Minimizing the differences between the proposed and reference expression systems to the extent possible can enhance the likelihood of producing an extremely similar protein product. The use of different expression systems will be evaluated on a case-by-case basis.

3.7.2 Manufacturing process

A comprehensive understanding of all the steps in the manufacturing process for the proposed product should be established during product development. Characterization tests, process controls, and specifications that will emerge from information gained during the process development must be specific for the proposed product and the manufacturing process. The use of enhanced approaches in manufacturing is described in guidances for industry such as ICH Q8(R2), ICH Q9, ICH Q10, and ICH Q11. A type II Drug Master File (DMF) may, however, be used to support an IND for a biosimilar product. Assurance of product quality should be provided for each lot of material produced by the DMF holder. Procedures should also be in place to ensure that the IND sponsor is notified by the DMF holder of significant changes to the DMF potentially affecting product quality. The sponsor is expected to provide notification to the Agency of any relevant change in the IND in order to initiate a reevaluation of the DMF.

A sponsor considering manufacturing changes after completing the initial analytical similarity assessment or after completing clinical studies intended to support a 351(k) application will need to demonstrate comparability between the pre- and the postchange proposed product and may need to conduct additional analytical studies. The nature and the extent of the changes may determine the magnitude of these additional similarity studies. The analytical similarity studies should include a sufficient number of lots from the proposed biosimilar product used in clinical studies as well as from the proposed commercial process if the process used to produce the material utilized in the clinical studies is different.

3.7.3 Assessment of physicochemical properties

Physicochemical evaluation of the proposed product and the reference product should consider all relevant characteristics of the protein product (e.g., the primary, secondary, tertiary, and quaternary structures; PTMs; and functional activities). The objective of this assessment is to maximize the potential for detecting differences in quality attributes between the proposed product and the reference product.

The sponsor should address the concept of the desired product (and its variants) as discussed in ICH Q6B when designing and conducting the characterization studies. Thus, it will be significant to understand the heterogeneity of the proposed product and the reference product (e.g., nature, location, and levels of glycosylation) and the ranges of variability of different isoforms, including those that result from PTMs.

Particular analytical methodologies can be used to assess specific physicochemical characteristics of proteins. These methodologies are described in published documents, including scientific literature, regulatory guidelines, and pharmacopoeial compendia. Some techniques provide information on multiple characteristics. It is expected that appropriate analytical test methods will be selected based on the nature of the protein being characterized and the knowledge regarding the structure and the heterogeneity of the reference product and the proposed product, as well as those characteristics that are critical to product performance.

To adequately address the full range of physicochemical properties or biological activities, it is often necessary to apply more than one analytical procedure to evaluate the same quality attribute. Methods that use different physicochemical or biological principles to assess the same attribute are especially valuable because they provide independent data to support the quality of that attribute (e.g., orthogonal methods to assess aggregation). In addition, the use of complementary analytical techniques in series, such as peptide mapping or capillary electrophoresis combined with mass spectrometry of the separated molecules, should provide a meaningful and sensitive method for comparing products.

Unlike routine quality control assays, the tests used to characterize the product do not necessarily need to be validated. But the tests used to characterize the product should be scientifically sound, be fit for their intended use, and provide results that are reproducible and reliable. In selecting these tests, it is important to consider the characteristics of the protein product, including known and potential impurities. Information regarding the ability of a method to discern relevant differences between a proposed product and a reference product should be submitted as part of the comparison.

The tests chosen to detect and characterize posttranslational protein modifications should be demonstrated to be of appropriate sensitivity and specificity to provide meaningful information as to whether the proposed product and the reference product are highly similar.

3.7.4 Functional activities

Functional assays serve multiple purposes in the characterization of protein products. These tests act to complement physicochemical analyses and are a qualitative measure of the function of the protein product.

Depending on the structural complexity of the protein and the available analytical technology, the physicochemical analysis may be unable to confirm the integrity of the HOSs. Instead, the integrity of such structures can usually be inferred from the product's biological activity. If the clinically relevant MOAs are known for the reference product or can be reasonably determined, the functional assays should reflect these MOAs to the extent possible. Multiple functional assays should, in general, be performed as part of the analytical similarity assessments. The assessment of functional activity is also useful in providing an estimate of the specific activity of a product as an indicator of manufacturing process consistency, as well as product purity, potency, and stability.

If a reference product exhibits multiple functional activities, the sponsors should perform a set of appropriate assays designed to evaluate the range of relevant activities for that product. For example, with proteins that possess multiple functional domains expressing enzymatic and receptor-mediated activities, the sponsors should evaluate both activities. For products where functional activity can be measured by more than one parameter (e.g., enzyme kinetics or interactions with blood-clotting factors), the comparative characterization of each parameter between products should be assessed.

The sponsor should recognize the potential limitations of some types of functional assays, such as high variability, that might preclude detection of small but significant differences between the proposed product and the reference product. Because an extremely variable assay may not provide a meaningful assessment as to whether the proposed product is highly similar to the reference product, the sponsors are encouraged to develop assays that are less variable and are sensitive to changes in the functional activities of the product. In addition, in vitro bioactivity assays may not fully reflect the clinical activity of the protein. For example, these assays do not generally predict the bioavailability (PK and biodistribution) of the product, which can affect PD and clinical performance. Also, bioavailability can be dramatically altered by subtle differences in glycoform distribution or other PTMs. Thus, these limitations should be taken into account when assessing the robustness of the quality of data supporting biosimilarity and the need for additional information that may address residual uncertainties. Finally, functional assays are important in evaluating the occurrence of neutralizing antibodies in nonclinical and clinical studies.

3.7.5 Receptor-binding and immunochemical properties

When binding or immunochemical properties are part of the activity attributed to the protein product, analytical tests should be performed to characterize the proposed product in terms of these particular properties (e.g., if binding to a receptor is inherent to protein function, this property should be measured and used in comparative studies) (see ICH Q6B for additional details). Various methods such as surface plasmon resonance, microcalorimetry, or classical Scatchard analysis can provide information on the kinetics and the thermodynamics of binding. Such information can be related to the functional activity and the characterization of the proposed product's HOS.

3.7.6 Impurities

The sponsor should characterize, identify, and quantify impurities in the proposed product and the reference product, to the extent feasible. A risk-based assessment should be performed on any differences in process-related impurities identified between the proposed product and the reference product. If a comparative physicochemical analysis reveals comparable product-related impurities at similar levels between the two products, pharmacological/toxicological studies to characterize potential biological effects of specific impurities may not be necessary. However, if the manufacturing process used to produce the proposed product introduces different impurities or higher levels of impurities than those present in the reference product, additional pharmacological/toxicological or other studies may be necessary. See the ICH guidance for industry *S6(R1): Preclinical Safety Evaluation of Biotechnology-Derived Pharmaceuticals*, which states: "[i]t is preferable to rely on purification processes to remove impurities … rather than to establish a preclinical testing program for their qualification."

The use of the terms *product-* and *process-related impurities* is consistent with their use and meaning in ICH Q6B. Process-related impurities arising from cell substrates (e.g., host cell DNA, host cell proteins), cell culture components (e.g., antibiotics, media components), and downstream processing steps (e.g., reagents, residual solvents, leachable, endotoxin, bioburden) should be evaluated. The process-related impurities in the proposed product are not expected to match those observed in the reference product. However, process-related impurities in the proposed product should be assessed side by side with the impurities in the reference product. The potential impact of the differences in the impurity profile on safety should be addressed and supported by appropriate data. The FDA will apply a product-specific evaluation approach toward differences in impurities between the proposed product and the U.S.-licensed reference product and will consider and evaluate the sponsor's assessment of the potential impact of these differences for biosimilar products. In all cases, the chosen analytical procedures should be adequate to detect, identify, and accurately quantify biologically significant levels of impurities (see the ICH guidance for industry *Q2B: Validation of Analytical Procedures: Methodology*). In particular, results of immunological methods used to detect host cell proteins depend on the assay reagents and the cell substrate used. Such assays should be validated using the product cell substrate and the orthogonal methodologies to ensure accuracy and sensitivity. This should be done across both products to the extent relevant and feasible. (This may be limited by the availability of high levels of reference product host cell proteins or differences in product and reference substrate.)

The safety of the proposed product, as with any biological product, with regard to adventitious agents or endogenous viral contamination, should be ensured by screening critical raw materials and confirmation of robust virus removal and inactivation achieved by the manufacturing process (see the ICH guidance for industry *Q5A: Viral Safety Evaluation of Biotechnology Products Derived from Cell Lines of Human or Animal Origin*).

3.7.7 Reference product and reference standards

A thorough physicochemical and biological assessment of the reference product should provide a base of information from which to develop the proposed product and to justify the reliance on certain existing scientific knowledge about the reference product. Sufficient evidence that the proposed product is highly similar to the reference product must be provided in an appropriate time frame to support a selective and targeted approach to early product development (e.g., selected animal studies and/or additional clinical studies).

The analytical similarity assessment submitted with the marketing application should support the demonstration of biosimilarity of the proposed product used in the principal clinical study, as well as the proposed commercial product, to the reference product. The biosimilar marketing application should include a thorough analytical comparison between the proposed product and a single reference product previously licensed by FDA. A sponsor considering manufacturing changes after completing the initial analytical similarity assessment or after completing clinical studies intended to support a 351(k) application may need to conduct additional analytical similarity studies. The nature and the extent of the changes may determine the scope of these additional similarity studies.

If the drug substance has been extracted from the reference product to assess analytical similarity, the sponsor should describe the extraction procedure and provide support that the procedure itself does not alter relevant product quality attributes. This undertaking would include consideration of alteration or loss of the desired products and impurities and relevant product-related substances, and it should include appropriate controls to ensure that the relevant product characteristics of the reference product are not significantly altered by the extraction procedure.

If there is a suitable, publicly available, and well-established reference standard for the protein, a physicochemical and/or functional comparison of the proposed product with this standard may also provide useful information. Although studies with such a reference standard may be helpful, they do not satisfy the BPCI Act's requirement to demonstrate the biosimilarity of the proposed product to the U.S.-licensed reference product. For example, if an international standard for calibration of potency is available, a comparison of the relative potency of the proposed product with this potency standard should be performed. As recommended in ICH Q6B, an in-house reference standard should always be qualified and used for the control of the manufacturing process and the product.

In summary, analytical studies carried out to support the approval of a proposed product should not focus solely on the characterization of the proposed product in isolation. Rather, these studies should be part of a broad comparison that includes, but is not limited to, the proposed product, the reference product, the applicable reference standards, and the consideration of relevant publicly available information.

3.7.8 Finished drug product

Product characterization studies should be performed on the most downstream intermediate best suited for the analytical procedures used. The attributes evaluated should be stable through any further processing steps. For these reasons, characterization studies are often performed on a bulk drug substance. However, if a bulk drug substance is reformulated and/or exposed to new materials in the finished dosage form, the impact of these changes should be considered. Whenever possible, if the finished drug product is best suited for a particular analysis, the sponsors should analyze the finished drug product. The characterization should compare the proposed finished product and the finished reference product. If an analytical method more sensitively detects specific attributes in the drug substance but the attributes it measures are critical and/or may change during the manufacture of the finished drug product, comparative characterization may be called for on both the extracted protein and the finished drug product.

The sponsors should clearly identify the excipients used in the proposed product that differ from those in the reference product. The acceptability of the type, the nature, and the extent of any differences between the proposed finished product and the finished reference product should be evaluated and supported by appropriate data and rationale. Additionally, different excipients in the proposed product should be supported by existing toxicology data for the excipient or by additional toxicity studies with the formulation of the proposed product. Excipient interactions, as well as direct toxicities, should be considered. Proteins are very sensitive to their environment. Therefore, differences in excipients or primary packaging may affect product stability and/or clinical performance. Differences in the formulation and primary packaging between the proposed product and the reference product are among the factors that may affect whether or how subsequent clinical studies may take a selective and targeted approach. (See ICH Q8(R2): Pharmaceutical Development.)

3.7.9 Stability

As part of an appropriate physicochemical and functional comparison of the stability profile of the proposed product with that of the reference product, accelerated and stress stability studies, as well as forced degradation studies, should be used to establish degradation profiles and to provide a direct comparison of the proposed product with the reference product. These comparative studies should be conducted under multiple stress conditions (e.g., high temperature, freeze–thaw, light exposure, and agitation) that can cause incremental product degradation over a defined period. Results of these studies may reveal product differences that warrant additional evaluations and also identify conditions under which additional controls should be employed in manufacturing and storage (see ICH guidances for industry *Q5C: Quality of Biotechnological Products: Stability Testing of Biotechnological/Biological Products* and *Q1A(R2): Stability Testing of New Drug Substances and Products*). Sufficient real-time, real-condition stability data from the proposed product should be provided to support the proposed shelf life.

3.7.10 Conclusion

The foundation for assessment and demonstration of biosimilarity between a proposed product and its reference product includes analytical studies that demonstrate that the proposed product is highly similar to the reference product notwithstanding minor differences in clinically inactive components. The demonstration that the proposed product is highly similar to the reference product involves robust characterization of the proposed product, including comparative physicochemical and functional studies with the reference product. The information gained from these studies is critical to the overall product assessment that, as a scientific matter, is necessary for the development of a proposed product as a biosimilar. In addition, a 351(k) application for a proposed product must contain, among other things, information demonstrating biosimilarity based on data derived from animal studies (including the assessment of toxicity) and a clinical study or studies (including the assessment of immunogenicity and pharmacokinetics or pharmacodynamics), unless the Agency determines that an element is unnecessary in a particular 351(k) application.

3.8 Clinical pharmacology data to support biosimilarity

3.8.1 Background

Clinical pharmacology studies play a critical role in the development of biosimilar products. These studies are part of a stepwise process for demonstrating biosimilarity between a proposed biosimilar product and the reference product and add to the totality of the evidence to support an overall demonstration of biosimilarity between the proposed biosimilar product and the reference product through the demonstration of no clinically meaningful differences. Data gathered from clinical pharmacology studies may also support a selective and targeted approach to the design of any necessary subsequent clinical studies to support a demonstration of biosimilarity.

In May 2014, the U.S. agency issued draft guidance for industry to assist sponsors with the design and the use of clinical pharmacology studies to support a decision that a proposed therapeutic biological product is biosimilar to its reference product. This guidance pertains to those products—such as therapeutic biological products—for which PK and PD data are required as part of a stepwise approach to developing the data and the information necessary to support a demonstration of biosimilarity. Specifically, the guidance discusses some of the overarching concepts related to the clinical pharmacology testing for biosimilar products, the approaches for developing the appropriate clinical pharmacology database, and the utility of modeling and simulation for designing clinical trials. Structurally difficult to characterize, these products have side effects like immunogenic responses and stability profiles that are difficult to predict, and structure–activity relationship ill defined, all leading to the realization that the bioequivalence of these products cannot be demonstrated by the currently used methods used for chemically-derived drugs (small molecule).

3.8.2 The role of clinical pharmacology studies

The BPCI Act, which was enacted as part of the Patient Protection and Affordable Care Act (Affordable Care Act), established an abbreviated pathway for agency licensure of biological products that are demonstrated to be biosimilar to or interchangeable with an agency-licensed reference product. The term *biosimilarity* is defined in Section 351(i) of the PHSA to mean that the biological product is "highly similar to the reference product notwithstanding minor differences in clinically inactive components" and that there are "no clinically meaningful differences between the biological product and the reference product in terms of the safety, purity, and potency of the product." Under Section 351(k)(2) of the PHSA, a 351(k) application must contain, among other things, information demonstrating that the biological product is biosimilar to a reference product (a biological product already licensed under Section 351(a) of the PHSA) based on data derived from analytical studies; animal studies; and a clinical study or clinical studies, including the assessment of immunogenicity and PK and PD, unless the Agency determines, in its discretion, that certain studies are unnecessary in a 351(k) application.

Clinical pharmacology studies are normally a critical part of demonstrating biosimilarity by supporting a demonstration that there are no clinically meaningful differences between the proposed biosimilar and the reference product. These studies provide the data that describe the degree of similarity in drug exposure between the proposed biosimilar and the reference product. In addition, clinical pharmacology studies often include PD end points (both therapeutic and toxic) and pharmacometric analysis to assess whether or not there are clinically meaningful differences between the proposed biosimilar and the reference product. If done well, they can add to the totality of the evidence, reduce residual uncertainty, and thus guide the need for the design of subsequent clinical testing to successfully support a demonstration of no clinically meaningful differences in the overall demonstration of biosimilarity. Clinical pharmacology data may be an important component of the scientific justification supporting extrapolation of clinical data to one or more additional conditions of use.

The types of clinical pharmacology studies to be conducted will depend on the residual uncertainties about biosimilarity that these studies are capable of addressing in the context of the overall program for biosimilar product development.

3.8.3 Critical considerations in the use of clinical pharmacology studies to support biosimilarity

Three key concepts, exposure and response assessment, evaluation of residual uncertainty, and assumptions about analytical quality and similarity, are especially relevant to the development of proposed biosimilar products.

3.8.3.1 Exposure and response assessment to support a demonstration of biosimilarity The objective of a well-designed clinical PK and PD study in a biosimilar development program is to evaluate the similarities and the differences in the PK and PD profiles between the proposed biosimilar product and the reference product. Exposure–response information is necessary for the determination of safety, purity, and potency of any biological product, as well as for the identification of any potential clinically meaningful difference between two products. Determining the response to exposure to a biological product is particularly challenging because the active product is not a single chemical and/or its active metabolites; rather, it is a mixture of closely related, complex biological substances that, in the aggregate, make up the active component.

The FDA uses the broad term *exposure* to refer to PK variables, including input of all active components of the biological product as measured by dose (drug input to the body) and various measures of single or integrated drug concentrations in plasma and other biological fluid, e.g., peak concentration (C_{max}), lowest concentration measured following dosing (C_{min}), concentration prior to the next dose during multiple dosing ($C_{trough\ ss}$), and area under the plasma/blood concentration–time curve (AUC). The response, referred to here as PD, is a direct measure of the pharmacological or toxicological effect of a drug. Clinical pharmacology similarity may include assessments of PK similarity and PD similarity.

The PD markers used to measure response may be a single biomarker or a composite of markers that effectively demonstrate the characteristics of the product's target effects. Use of a single, scientifically acceptable, established PD marker or a composite of more than one relevant PD marker can reduce residual uncertainty with respect to clinically meaningful differences between products and significantly add to the overall demonstration of biosimilarity. Using broader panels of biomarkers (e.g., by conducting a protein or an mRNA microarray analysis) that capture multiple pharmacological effects of the product may be of additional value. When determining which markers should be used to measure response, it is important to consider the following:

- The time of onset of the PD marker relative to dosing.
- Sensitivity of the PD marker to differences between the proposed biosimilar product and the reference product.
- The relevance of the PD marker to the MOA of the drug.
- The relationship between changes in the PD marker and the clinical outcomes. If these criteria are addressed, through the submission of convincing PK and PD results, the extent of the clinical development program can be refined in both the design and the scope of additional clinical trials necessary to assess whether there are clinically meaningful differences between the proposed biosimilar product and the reference product. It is important to note that, in some instances, PD markers with the relevant characteristics listed earlier have not

been identified, but the sponsor is encouraged to incorporate PD biomarkers that correlate well with drug exposure over a wide concentration range as these represent potentially orthogonal tests that may be supportive of clinical pharmacology similarity. When PD markers are not sensitive or specific enough to be used to assess for clinically meaningful differences, the derived PK parameters should be used as the primary basis for evaluating similarity from a clinical pharmacology perspective, and the PD markers may be used to augment the PK data.
- A combination of PK and PD similarities representing orthogonal biosimilarity may be an important assessment in demonstrating no clinically meaningful differences.

3.8.3.2 Evaluation of residual uncertainty In evaluating a sponsor's data to support a demonstration of biosimilarity, using a risk-based approach, the Agency will consider the totality of the data and the information submitted, including, for example, data from the structural and functional characterizations, nonclinical evaluations, human PK and PD studies, clinical immunogenicity testing, and investigation of clinical safety and, when necessary, clinical effectiveness. These data should be collected in a stepwise manner. Especially pertinent to the Agency's clinical pharmacology evaluation is the clinical PK and PD data and safety data obtained in conjunction with the clinical pharmacology studies. The need for additional studies at each step in this progressive approach will be determined by the degree of residual uncertainty that remains at each step regarding the similarity of the products and whether or not the study can address these uncertainties.

3.8.3.3 Assumptions about analytical quality and similarity In a stepwise assessment of biosimilarity, extensive and robust comparative structural and functional studies (e.g., bioassays, binding assays, and studies of enzyme kinetics) should be performed to evaluate whether the proposed biosimilar product and the reference product are highly similar. A meaningful assessment depends on, among other things, the capabilities of available state-of-the-art analytical assays to assess, for example, the protein's molecular weight, HOS and PTMs, heterogeneity, functional properties, impurity profiles, and degradation profiles denoting stability. The sponsor should describe the capabilities and the limitations of the methods used in the analytical assessment.

An extensive analytical characterization may reveal differences between the proposed biosimilar product and the reference product. The type, the nature, and the extent of any differences between the two products should be clearly identified, and the potential effect of these differences should be addressed and supported by appropriate data. In some cases, additional studies may demonstrate that the identified difference is within an acceptable range to consider the proposed biosimilar product to be highly similar to the reference product. However, certain differences in the results of the analytical characterization may preclude a determination by the Agency that the proposed biosimilar product is highly similar to the reference product and, therefore, its further development through the 351(k) regulatory pathway is not recommended.

It may be useful to compare the quality attributes of the proposed biosimilar product with those of the reference product by using a meaningful fingerprint-like analysis algorithm that covers a large number of product attributes and their combinations with high sensitivity using orthogonal methods. Such a strategy can further quantify the overall similarity between two products and it may provide a basis for a more selective and targeted approach to subsequent animal and/or clinical studies.

The result of the comparative analytical characterization may lead to one of four assessments within a development phase continuum:

- Not similar: Certain differences in the outcome of the analytical characterization may lead to an assessment of "not similar" and further development through the 351(k) regulatory pathway is not recommended unless, for example, modifications are made to the manufacturing process for the proposed biosimilar product that is likely to lead to a highly similar biological product.
- Similar: Further information is needed to determine if the product is highly similar to the reference product. Additional analytical data or other studies are necessary to determine if the observed differences are within an acceptable range to consider the proposed biosimilar product to be highly similar to the reference product. As an example, glycosylation plays a significant role in the PK of certain protein products. Manufacturing process conditions may impact glycosylation. Comparative PK and PD studies of the proposed biosimilar product and the reference product help resolve that some differences in glycosylation identified in the analytical studies would be within an acceptable range to consider the proposed biosimilar product to be highly similar to the reference product.
- Highly similar: The proposed biosimilar product meets the statutory standard for analytical similarity. The results of the comparative analytical characterization permit high confidence in the analytical similarity of the proposed biosimilar and the reference product, and it would be appropriate for the sponsor to conduct targeted and selective animal and/or clinical studies to resolve residual uncertainty and support a demonstration of biosimilarity.
- Highly similar with fingerprint-like similarity: The proposed biosimilar product meets the statutory standard for analytical similarity based on integrated, multiparameter approaches that are extremely sensitive in identifying analytical differences. The results of these fingerprint-like analyses permit a very

high level of confidence in the analytical similarity of the proposed biosimilar and the reference product, and it would be appropriate for the sponsor to use a more targeted and selective approach to conducting animal and/or clinical studies to resolve residual uncertainty and support a demonstration of biosimilarity.

The outcome of the comparative analytical characterization should inform the next steps in the demonstration of biosimilarity.

3.8.4 Integrity of the bioanalytical methods used in PK and PD studies

When performing an evaluation of clinical pharmacology similarity, it is critical to use the appropriate bioanalytical methods to evaluate the PK and PD properties of a proposed biosimilar product and its reference product. Because of the complex molecular structure of biological products, conventional analytical methods used for chemical drugs may not be suitable for biological products. The bioanalytical methods used for PK and PD evaluations should be accurate, precise, specific, sensitive, and reproducible. The scientific requirements of bioanalytical methods have been described in a separate guidance document.

3.8.4.1 General PK assay considerations A sponsor should design or choose an assay based on a thorough understanding of the MOA and/or structural elements of the proposed biosimilar product and the reference product critical for activity. Analytical assays should be able to detect the active and/or the free product instead of the total product, particularly if binding to a soluble ligand is a necessary step for activity and clinical effect. The inability to develop such an assay should be supported with a justification as to why failure to detect free and/or active forms does not compromise the PK similarity assessment.

3.8.4.2 General PK and PD assay considerations Sponsors should make every effort to employ the most suitable assays and methodologies with the aim of obtaining data that are meaningful and reflective of the drug exposure, the biological activity, and/or the PD effect of the proposed biosimilar product and the reference product. Furthermore, the sponsor should provide a rationale for the choice of the assay and the relevance of the assay to drug activity in submissions to the Agency.

3.8.4.3 Specific assays Three types of assays are of particular importance for biosimilar product development: ligand-binding assays, concentration and activity assays, and PD assays.

3.8.4.3.1 Ligand-binding assays Currently, the concentration of most biological products in circulation is measured using ligand-binding assays. These assays are analytical methods in which quantification is based on macromolecular interactions with assay reagents, such as antibodies, receptors, or ligands, that bind with adequate affinity and selectivity for the biological product. The ligand-binding assay reagents chosen for capturing and detecting the biological product should be carefully evaluated with the goal of producing concentration product data that are meaningful to, and reflective of, the pharmacological activity and/or the PD effect of the biological product of interest. Some biological products exert pharmacological effects only after multiple molecular interactions. In some cases, mAbs, bispecific antibodies, or fusion proteins bind to ligand or receptor proteins through the target antigen-binding (Fab) epitope of the molecule and to FcγR with the Fc portion of the molecule. A sponsor should choose the most appropriate interactions to measure.

Generally, assays for mAb product concentrations rely on molecular interactions involving the Fab region, in particular, epitopes in the complementarity-determining regions. Antibody-based assays for biological products that rely on epitopes involved in pharmacological/biochemical interactions with targets are most likely to produce concentration data that are meaningful with respect to target binding activity.

3.8.4.3.2 Concentration and activity assays Bioanalytical methods that are not based on ligand binding can be used for quantification of the proposed biosimilar product and the reference product concentrations. For some biological products, such as those that are used to achieve enzyme replacement, the drug availability measurements may rely on activity and it should be captured through an appropriate activity assay. Depending on the complexity of the structural features, some biological products may need more than one assay to fully characterize the systemic exposure of the proposed biosimilar product and the reference product. In such cases, mass spectrometry and other assays may be useful in distinguishing the structures of product variants.

3.8.4.3.3 PD assays Relevant PD markers may not always be available to support a proposed biosimilar product's development through clinical pharmacology studies. However, when PD assessment is a component of the biosimilarity evaluation, sponsors should provide a rationale for the selection of the PD end points and/or markers, as well as data to demonstrate the quality of the assay, in written communications to the Agency. PD assays should be sensitive to a product or a product class and designed to quantitatively evaluate the pharmacologic activity of the biologic product. Ideally, the activity measured by the PD assay should be relevant to a clinical outcome; however, the PD assay should at least be of interest to a pharmacological effect of the biologic product. If the selected PD end points are not closely related to the clinical outcome, the use of multiple complementary PD assays may be most useful. Because the PD assay is highly dependent on the pharmacological activity of the product, the approach for assay validation and the characteristics of the assay performance may differ depending on the specific PD assay. However, the general guiding principles for choosing PK assays (i.e., demonstration of specificity, reliability, and robustness) also apply to PD assays. Sponsors should provide supporting data for the choice of the assay and the justification of PD markers in submissions to the Agency.

3.8.4.4 Safety and immunogenicity In the context of this guidance, *immunogenicity* refers to an immune response to the biological product that may result in immune-mediated toxicity and/or lack of effectiveness. Safety and immunogenicity data from the clinical pharmacology studies should be collected and evaluated. The Agency recognizes that safety and immunogenicity data derived from these studies may need to be supplemented by additional evaluations either preapproval or postapproval. However, as part of their role in the overall assessment of biosimilarity, clinical pharmacology studies may sometimes suggest that there are clinically meaningful differences between the products that may inform the design and the details of additional investigations and/or clinical studies conducted to further investigate these potential differences. It is important to note that depending on the extent of such potential differences, it may not be appropriate for additional studies to be conducted in the context of a biosimilar development program.

Publicly available information on the safety and immunogenicity profile of a reference product should be considered when incorporating safety and immunogenicity measurements in the clinical pharmacology studies. For example, when a reference product is known to have the potential for immune-mediated toxicity, assays capable of detecting binding antibodies (and their neutralizing potential) should be developed in advance to analyze samples obtained from PK and PD studies, so that immunogenicity may be evaluated in real time. Generally, samples can be stored for future analysis if such assays are not yet developed. In either approach, sponsors should carefully consider assay confounders, such as the systemic presence of the proposed biosimilar or reference product. Recommendations for immunogenicity assay development have been described in a separate guidance document.

When evaluating data (e.g., safety, immunogenicity) collected during the PK and PD studies, sponsors should have an understanding of the time course of the appearance and the resolution of safety signals or immune responses. The PK profile of the proposed biosimilar product and/or the publicly available PK data for the reference product can be used to inform the duration of follow-up for safety signals or immunogenicity.

3.8.5 Developing clinical pharmacology data for supporting a demonstration of biosimilarity

Sponsors are encouraged to discuss the crucial aspects of their clinical pharmacology development plan with the Agency in the early stages of the biosimilar development program. Some critical study design issues that should be discussed with the Agency are set forth below.

3.8.5.1 Study design To evaluate clinical PK and PD similarities for the development of proposed biosimilar products, two study designs are of particular relevance: crossover designs and parallel study designs.

3.8.5.1.1 Crossover design For PK similarity assessments, a single-dose, randomized, crossover study is generally the preferred design. A crossover study is recommended for a product with a short half-life (e.g., shorter than five days), a rapid PD response (e.g., onset, maximal effect, and disappearance in conjunction with drug exposure), and a low incidence of immunogenicity. This design is considered the most sensitive to assess PK similarity, and it can provide reliable estimates of differences in exposure with a minimum number of subjects. For PD similarity assessments, multiple doses may be appropriate when the PD effect is delayed or is otherwise not parallel to the single-dose drug PK profile. The time course of appearance and disappearance of immunogenicity and its relation to the washout period is an issue for consideration for studies using a crossover design.

3.8.5.1.2 Parallel design Many biological products have a long half-life and elicit immunogenic responses. A parallel group design is appropriate for products that have a long half-life or for which repeated exposures can lead to an increased immune response that can affect the PK and/or PD similarity assessments. This design is also appropriate for diseases that exhibit time-related changes associated with exposure to the drug.

3.8.5.2 Reference product The BPCI Act defines the reference product for a proposed biosimilar product as the single biological product licensed under Section 351(a) of the PHSA against which a proposed biosimilar product is evaluated in a 351(k) application. As a scientific matter, analytical studies and at least one clinical PK and, if appropriate, PD study, intended to support a demonstration of biosimilarity must include an adequate comparison of the proposed biosimilar product directly with the U.S.-licensed reference product. However, a sponsor may use a non-U.S.-licensed comparator product in certain studies to support a demonstration that the proposed biological product is biosimilar to the U.S.-licensed reference product. If a sponsor seeks to use data from a clinical study comparing its proposed biosimilar product to a non-U.S.-licensed product to address, in part, the requirements of Section 351(k)(2)(A) of the PHSA, the sponsor should provide adequate data or information to scientifically justify the relevance of these comparative data to an assessment of biosimilarity and to establish an acceptable bridge to the U.S.-licensed reference product. As a scientific matter, the type of bridging data needed will always include data from analytical studies (e.g., structural and functional data) that directly compare all three products (i.e., the proposed biosimilar product, the U.S.-licensed reference product, and the non-U.S.-licensed product) and are also likely to include PK and, if appropriate, PD study data for all three products.

3.8.5.3 Study population

- Healthy volunteer versus patient: The study population selected should be the most informative for detecting and evaluating differences in PK and PD profiles between the proposed biosimilar product and the reference product. Human PK and PD studies should be conducted in healthy volunteers if the product can be safely administered to this population. A study in healthy volunteers is considered to be more sensitive in evaluating the product similarity because it is likely to produce less PK variability compared with that in patients with potentially confounding factors such as underlying and/or concomitant disease and concomitant medications. If safety or ethical considerations preclude the participation of healthy volunteers in human PK and PD studies for certain products (e.g., immunogenicity or known toxicity from the reference product), or if PD markers would be relevant only in patients with the condition or disease, the clinical pharmacology studies should be conducted in patients. In cases where PK and/or PD will be the full assessment for clinically meaningful differences, a population that is representative of the patient population to which the drug is targeted will be appropriate for the study.
- Demographic group: Clinical pharmacology studies should be conducted in the subject or patient demographic group most likely to provide a sensitive measure of differences between the proposed biosimilar product and the reference product. The sponsor should provide justification for why the subject or patient group chosen for clinical pharmacology studies will provide the most sensitive measure of the difference between the proposed biosimilar and reference products. The total number of subjects should provide adequate power for similarity assessment. Analysis of the data from all subjects as one group represents the primary study end point, and a statistical analysis of the data from the subgroups would be exploratory only.

3.8.5.4 Dose selection See Section 351(i)(4) of the PHSA. As in the selection of the study population, the dose selected should be the most sensitive to detect and evaluate differences in the PK and PD profiles between the proposed biosimilar product and the reference product. The dose selected should be the one most likely to provide clinically meaningful and interpretable data. If a study is conducted in a patient population, the approved dose for the reference product may be the appropriate choice because this may best demonstrate the pharmacological effects in a clinical setting. However, a lower dose on the steep part of the exposure–response curve may be appropriate when PD is being measured or when healthy subjects are selected for evaluation.

In certain cases, a dose selected from a range of doses may be useful for a clinical PK and PD similarity assessment. For example, if the concentration–effect relationship of the reference product is known to be highly variable or nonlinear, a range of doses can be used to assess dose–response.

If the product can be administered only to patients, an alternative dosing regimen, such as a single dose for a chronic indication or a lower dose than the approved dose, may be acceptable if the approved dose results in nonlinear PK or exceeds the dose required for maximal PD effect and therefore will not allow the detection of differences. However, the appropriateness of an alternative dosing regimen will depend on certain factors, e.g., the lower dose is known to have the same effect as the approved dose, or if it is ethically acceptable to give lower doses notwithstanding differences in effect. Adequate justification for the selection of an alternative dosing regimen should be provided in written communication to the Agency.

When appropriate, PD markers should be used to assess PK/PD similarity between a proposed biosimilar product and the reference product. Development of a dose–response profile that includes the steep part of the dose–response curve is a sensitive test for similarity between products, and if clinical pharmacology similarity between products is demonstrated, in some instances, this may complete the clinical evaluation, and in others it may support a more targeted clinical development program.

3.8.5.5 Route of administration Human PK and PD studies should be conducted using the same route of administration for the proposed biological product and the reference product. If more than one route of administration (e.g., both intravenous and subcutaneous) is approved for the reference product, the route selected for the assessment of PK and PD similarity should be the one most sensitive for detecting clinically meaningful differences. In most cases, this is likely to be the subcutaneous or other extravascular routes of administration, because extravascular routes can provide insight into potential PK differences during the absorption phase in addition to the distribution and elimination phases.

3.8.5.6 PK measures All PK steps should be obtained for the proposed biosimilar product and the reference product. The sponsor should obtain measures of C_{max} and total exposure (AUC) in a relevant biological fluid. For single-dose studies, total exposure should be calculated as the area under the biological product concentration–time curve from time zero to time infinity ($AUC_{0-\infty}$), where $AUC_{0-\infty} = AUC_{0-t} + C_t/k_{el}$

(C_t—concentration at the last measurable time point—divided by k_{el}—elimination rate constant) is calculated based on an appropriate method. C_{max} should be determined from the data without interpolation. For intravenous studies, $AUC_{0-\infty}$ will be considered the primary end point. For subcutaneous studies, C_{max} and AUC will be considered coprimary study end points. For multiple-dose studies, the measurement of total exposure should be the area under the concentration–time profile from time zero to time τ over a dosing interval at steady state ($AUC_{0-\tau}$), where τ is the length of the dosing interval, and this is considered the primary end point. The steady-state $C_{trough\ ss}$ should be measured at the end of a dosing interval before initiating the next dose and the C_{max} and these are considered secondary end points. Population PK data will not provide an adequate assessment for PK similarity.

3.8.5.7 PD measures In certain circumstances, human PK and PD data that demonstrate similar exposure and response between a proposed biosimilar product and the reference product may be sufficient to assess completely clinically meaningful differences between the products. This would be based on similar PDs using a PD measure that reflects the MOA in cases where the PD measure has a wide dynamic range over the range of drug concentrations achieved during the PK study. In such instances, a full evaluation of safety and immunogenicity would still be necessary, either before or after approval. When human PD data in a PK/PD study are insufficient to assess completely for clinically meaningful differences, obtaining such data may support a more targeted approach for the collection of subsequent clinical safety and effectiveness data. The selection of appropriate time points and durations for the measure of PD markers will depend on the characteristics of the PD markers (e.g., timing of PD response with respect to product administration based on the half-life of the product and the anticipated duration of effect). When a PD response lags after initiation of product administration, it may be important to study multiple-dose and steady-state conditions, especially if the proposed therapy is intended for long-term use. Comparison of the PD markers between the proposed biosimilar product and the reference product should be by determination of the area under the effect curve. If only one PD measurement is available due to the characteristics of the PD marker, it should be linked to a simultaneous drug concentration measurement, and this should be used as a basis for comparison between products.

The use of a single, scientifically acceptable, established PD marker as described above, or a composite of more than one relevant PD markers, can reduce residual uncertainty with respect to clinically meaningful differences between products and significantly add to the overall demonstration of biosimilarity. Using broader panels of biomarkers (e.g., by conducting a protein or an mRNA microarray analysis) that capture multiple pharmacological effects of the product may be of additional value.

When available and appropriate, clinical end points in clinical pharmacology studies may also provide useful information about the presence of clinically meaningful differences between two products.

3.8.5.8 Defining the appropriate PD time profile The optimal sampling strategy for determining PD measures may differ from the strategy used for PK measures. For PK sampling, frequent sampling at early time points following product administration with decreased frequency later is generally the most effective to characterize the concentration–time profile. However, the PD–time profile may not mirror the PK–time profile. In such cases, the PD sampling should be well justified. When both PK and PD data are to be obtained during a clinical pharmacology study, the sampling strategy should be optimized for both PK and PD measures.

3.8.5.9 Statistical comparison of PK and PD results The assessment of clinical pharmacology similarity of a proposed biosimilar product and the reference product in PK and PD studies is based on the statistical evaluation. The recommended clinical pharmacology similarity assessment relies on (a) a criterion to allow the comparison, (b) a confidence interval for the criterion, and (c) an acceptable limit. The Agency recommends that log transformation of the exposure measures be performed before the statistical analysis. Sponsors should use an average equivalence statistical approach to compare PK and PD parameters for both replicate and nonreplicate design studies. This approach involves a calculation of a 90% confidence interval for the ratio between the means of the parameters of the proposed biosimilar product and the reference product. To establish PK and/or PD similarity, the calculated confidence interval should fall within an acceptable limit. The selection of the confidence interval and the acceptable limits may vary among products. An appropriate starting point for an acceptable limit for the confidence interval of the ratio may be 80%–125%; however, this is not a default range, and the sponsor should justify the limits selected for the proposed biosimilar product. There may be situations in which the results of the PK and/or the PD study fall outside the predefined limits. Although such results may suggest the existence of underlying differences between the proposed biosimilar product and the reference product that may preclude development under the 351(k) pathway, the Agency encourages sponsors to analyze and explain such findings. If such differences do not translate into clinically meaningful differences and the safety, the purity, and the potency of the product are not affected, it may be possible to continue the development under the 351(k) pathway.

3.8.5.10 Utility of simulation tools Modeling and simulation tools can be useful when designing a PK and/or a PD study. For instance, such tools can contribute to the selection of an optimally informative dose or doses for evaluating PD similarity. When a biomarker-based comparison is used, it is preferable that the selected dose be on the steep portion of the dose–response curve of the reference product. Sponsors should provide data to support the claim that the selected dose is on the steep part of the dose–response curve and not on the plateau of the dose–response curve where it is not likely to result in observed differences between two products. Publicly available data for the dose (or exposure)–response relationship of the reference product can be analyzed using model-based simulations to justify the dose selected for the PK and/or the PD study.

If the exposure–response data for the reference product are not available, the sponsor may decide to generate this information using a small study to determine an optimally informative dose (e.g., representing the median effective dose of the reference product). Such a study may involve evaluating PK/PD at multiple dose levels (e.g., low, intermediate, and highest approved doses) to obtain dose–response and/or exposure–response data. Alternatively, when possible, sponsors can conduct a similarity study between the reference product and the proposed biosimilar product with low, intermediate, and highest approved doses where a clear dose–response is observed. If multiple doses are studied, PK/PD parameters such as half maximum activity response, E_{max}, and slope of the concentration effect relationship should be evaluated for similarity. Such studies would be useful for the demonstration of PK, PK/PD, and PD similarities when the clinical pharmacology evaluation is likely to be the major source of information to assess clinically meaningful differences. Publicly available information on biomarker–clinical end point relationships accompanied with modeling and simulation can also be used to define the acceptable limits for PD similarity.

3.9 Regulatory exclusivities

Regulatory exclusivities are automatically granted upon new drug approval by the regulatory agency that licenses the product for commercial distribution. (In its draft guidance document entitled *Reference Product Exclusivity for Biological Products Filed under Section 351(a) of the PHSA* [http://www.fda.gov/downloads/Drugs/GuidanceCompliance RegulatoryInformation/Guidances/UCM407844.pdf], the FDA has proposed that the applicant include in its 351(a) application a request for reference product exclusivity. More specifically, the FDA recommends that the applicant provide an explanation how the biological product meets the statutory requirements for exclusivity, and submits adequate data and information to support the request.) These exclusivities provide pharmaceutical companies with an incentive to undertake the risk and the capital investment required to develop and obtain regulatory approval for drug and biologic products. Innovator companies requested this type of exclusivity during the negotiations that accompanied the enactment of the 1984 Drug Price Competition and Patent Term Restoration Act (more commonly known as the Hatch–Waxman Act), which defined the approval pathway that created the generic pharmaceutical market in the United States (§ 505(j) of the FDCA). Innovator companies grounded their request on the premise that the award of an exclusivity period would provide greater certainty that the financial investments required to develop a new drug would be repaid. Congress has characterized the regulatory exclusivities as a quid pro quo for the practice of allowing generic companies to file an abbreviated approval package focused on establishing that the proposed generic is a "bioequivalent" to the originator's product and making reference to, and relying on, the clinical package of the originator's product to establish safety and efficacy. Note that generic manufacturers obtain regulatory approval by filing an abbreviated NDA and by submitting data establishing the bioequivalence of the generic drug, without additional safety or efficacy data.

The type of regulatory exclusivity that is granted, and the length of time that it provides exclusivity depends on the nature of the therapeutic agent and varies from country to country. Pharmaceutical companies that obtain approval for new chemical entities, pursuant to the provisions of Section 505 of the FDCA by filing an NDA, are granted five years of data exclusivity. Data exclusivity has the effect of creating a limited monopoly for the originator who sponsored the clinical studies, by defining a period during which generic manufacturers cannot make reference to the originator's data package, and, therefore, cannot seek approval for launching a generic product.

The BPCI Act grants originator biologic products a period of 12 years of reference product exclusivity, beginning on the date the FDA first licenses the product. An additional six months of exclusivity is available for biologic products approved for pediatric use. (If the FDA believes that studies relating to the use of a biologic in a pediatric population could benefit public health, it makes a written request for pediatric studies. If the applicant completes the pediatric studies then, regardless of the outcome of the studies, the term of the regulatory exclusivities can be extended by six months.) The 12 years of exclusivity comprises four years of data exclusivity followed by eight years of market exclusivity. During the data exclusivity period, biosimilar applicants (for both proposed biosimilar and interchangeable products) are barred from making reference to the reference drug's clinical package as a basis for licensing their product. In fact, the exclusivity provisions of 42 U.S.C. § 262(k)(7)(B) prohibit the FDA from even accepting a biosimilar application during the reference product's four-year exclusivity period. An application under this subsection may not be submitted to the secretary until the date that is four years after the date on which the reference product was first licensed under Subsection (a).

The subsequent eight years of market exclusivity prohibits the FDA from approving a biosimilar product until the date that is 12 years after the reference product was first licensed under the provision of a full biologics license application (Effective Date of Biosimilar Application

Table 3.4 Market Exclusivity of Major Biosimilar Possibilities Based on Composition or Method of Use Patent

Biologic	Brand Name	Approval Date	Data Exclusivity	Market Exclusivity	U.S. Patent Expiry
Adalimumab	Humira	Dec 2002	Dec 2006	Dec 2014	Dec 2016
Infliximab	Remicade	Aug 1998	Aug 2002	Aug 2010	Sep 2018
Rituximab	Rituxan	Nov 1997	Nov 2001	Nov 2009	Jul 2018
Etanercept	Enbrel	Nov 1998	Nov 2002	Nov 2010	Apr 2029
Bevacizumab	Avastin	Feb 2004	Feb 2008	Feb 2016	Mar 2019
Trastuzumab	Herceptin	Sep 1998	Sep 2002	Sep 2010	Jun 2019
Filgrastim	Neupogen	Feb 1991	Feb 1995	Feb 2003	Dec 2013
PEG-Filgrastim	Neulasta	Jan 2002	Jan 2006	Jan 2014	Oct 2015
Procrit/Epogen	Epoetin-α	June 1989	Jun 1993	Jun 2011	Aug 2013

Approval: Approval of an application under this subsection may not be made effective by the Secretary until the date that is 12 years after the date on which the reference product was first licensed under Subsection (a) [42 U.S.C. § 262(k)(7)(A)]). No additional exclusivity is available to reference product sponsors that file supplemental BLA applications, for example, to secure approval for the use of a biologic to treat a second or a subsequent indication. Furthermore, the BPCI Act expressly prohibits reference product sponsors (or their related entities) from using subsequent BLA filings to "evergreen" their period of regulatory exclusivity by filing a new application for a change that results in new indication, route of administration, dosing schedule, dosage form, delivery system, delivery device, or modification to the structure of the product that does not result in a change in the potency, the safety, or the purity of the reference product (42 U.S.C. § 262(k)(7)(C)). Table 3.4 provides the data exclusivity and the market exclusivity expiry dates for the top nine biologics in the United States This list is based on available expiry dates of composition or method of use; this may change over time as new patents appear, so the reader is advised to consult for its accuracy.

The regulatory exclusivities function to protect originator products from biosimilar entrants attempting to use the 351(k) pathway, but not from competitors who secure allowance pursuant to a 351(a) biologics license application. This explains why biopharmaceutical companies protect their products with a combination of regulatory, patent, and trade secret exclusivities. It also explains why biopharmaceutical companies are unlikely to rely solely on regulatory exclusivities to protect their products.

It should be noted that the statutory provisions do not prevent a biopharmaceutical company from filing a full BLA for the approval of a competitive product that has the same active ingredient as a branded biologic marketed in the United States. For example, the FDA approved tbo-filgrastim (short-acting recombinant GCSF) in August 2013, which has the same active ingredient as Amgen's Neupogen (filgrastim), based on Teva Pharmaceutical's biologics license application.

Teva's tbo-filgrastim is available in the United States under the brand name Granix® (Granix is approved to reduce the duration of severe neutropenia in patients with nonmyeloid malignancies receiving myelosuppressive anticancer drugs associated with a clinically significant incidence of febrile neutropenia [tbo-filgrastim prescribing information, issued 2013, Teva Pharmaceuticals, Inc.]). While Granix is a filgrastim, it is not "biosimilar" to Neupogen. Teva's application was filed under 351(a) and made no reference to, and did not rely on, Amgen's filgrastim data. Its approval was based on an independent demonstration of the safety and the efficacy of tbo-filgrastim. It should be noted that filgrastim has several indications for which tbo-filgrastim is not approved including severe chronic neutropenia, stem cell mobilization, acute myeloid leukemia, and bone marrow transplant (Filgrastim [Neupogen] Prescribing Information, revised September 2013, Amgen Inc.). While a 351(k) applicant can rely on the originator's safety and efficacy data to extrapolate all indications for the biosimilar based on the extensive comparative analytical similarity, a 351(a) applicant can rely only on actual clinical data from its own trials.

Teva Pharmaceutical filed for tbo-filgrastim approval before the enactment of the BPCI Act. Therefore, it did not have the option of using the abbreviated 351(k) pathway (tbo-filgrastim is licensed as a biosimilar in Europe). However, in the future, biopharmaceutical companies seeking approval for biologic therapies comprising the same active ingredient as a branded product will have the option of choosing between the two pathways. Filing a BLA allows an applicant to avoid the exclusivity time bars as well as other provisions and uncertainties that accompany the use of the 351(k) pathway. However, submitting a 351(a) application for a biosimilar requires submission of a complete analytical and clinical package as required for any new biologic.

Unlike a generic applicant who receives 180 days of market exclusivity for being the first approved generic, the only biosimilar exclusivity available to a drug licensed under the provisions of 351(k) is a period of market exclusivity for the first applicant to obtain approval for a biosimilar product deemed to be interchangeable with the reference product; the length of the market exclusivity is not defined in the statute and will depend on whether the first interchangeable applicant has been sued for patent infringement by the reference product sponsor, and whether the suit remains pending when the first interchangeable product application is approved. The *interchangeable exclusivity* originates from a statutory provision that prevents the FDA from approving an application for a second or a subsequent interchangeable biosimilar during the exclusivity period. However, the market exclusivity does not prevent the FDA from approving a second or a subsequent biosimilar application.

Therefore, the first interchangeable biosimilar product could conceivably find itself competing not only with the reference product but also with one or more biosimilar products, a scenario which might seem to significantly diminish the value of obtaining an interchangeable designation. However, because an interchangeable biosimilar product does not require notification of the prescribing physician, it would likely be prescribed over a competitive biosimilar product that does require notification.

The pediatric exclusivity available to biosimilar applicants under the 351(k) pathway provides an additional six-month period of exclusivity beyond the period provided for any other applicable regulatory exclusivity (e.g., data, market or orphan drug). It does not attach to the end of any patent exclusivity protecting the product.

3.10 The 505(b)(2) versus 351(k) choice

Prior to the passage of the BPCI Act and to this day, another regulatory pathway, the 505(b)(2) pathway, could be used to obtain approval of certain follow-on biologics. Like the 351(k) pathway, the 505(b)(2) pathway allows the applicant to rely on the safety and effectiveness data of a previously approved product. The 505(b)(2) pathway, while largely used to obtain approval of small-molecule drugs, has been used on several occasions to obtain approval of biologics that are similar to the reference product and marketed as biosimilars in Europe. A 505(b)(2) application is an application for the approval of different dosage forms, formulations, or combination products of already-approved drugs, but can also be available for the approval of biologics that are similar to, and rely on the information contained in, a previously approved NDA. The 505(b)(2) pathway is available for a relatively narrow category of biologics—specifically, those that had been approved under an NDA before the BPCI Act was signed into law on March 23, 2010—and it is only available for that narrow category of biologics until March 23, 2020 (§ 7002(e) of the Affordable Care Act [ACA]). But for the biologics that fit into this category, the 505(b)(2) pathway offers a pathway for marketing approval. Notably, any product approved under the 505(b)(2) pathway will be considered approved under the 351(k) pathway once the 10-year phase-in period is complete (ACA, § 7002(e)(4)). Fundamentally, the 351(k) pathway concerns products that are regulated as biologics under the BPCI Act, while the 505(b)(2) pathway concerns products that are regulated as drugs under the FDCA.

The 505(b)(2) pathway offers marketing approval for certain biosimilars—at least for the next five years. In addition to a more predictable regulatory pathway, the litigation pathway for 505(b)(2) products is more familiar and predictable as well. The pathways involve vastly different regulatory frameworks. Table 3.5 summarizes some of these differences.

Table 3.5 Comparison of 351(k) and 505(b)(2) Pathways

Approval under 351(k)	**Approval under 505(b)(2)**
Available for biosimilars	Available for drugs and certain biologics
Evaluation: Biosimilarity to a reference product (highly similar to reference product, no clinically meaningful differences)	Evaluation: Proof of safety and efficacy
Litigation: BPCIA ("patent dance")	Litigation: Hatch–Waxman (30-month stay)
Market exclusivity: Limited market exclusivity for the first interchangeable biosimilar against other interchangeable biosimilars	Market exclusivity: Likely not applicable for biosimilars, although five years of new chemical exclusivity has been awarded for recombinant versions of previously animal-derived products

A number of biologics have been approved under the 505(b)(2) pathway. Examples of five 505(b)(2) products, all produced by recombinant DNA technology, include the following:

- Basaglar® (Insulin glargine injection): In August 2014, the FDA granted tentative approval for Eli Lilly's Basaglar, a recombinantly produced insulin glargine for treating diabetes. As a 505(b)(2) product, the approval relied in part on clinical studies carried out for Sanofi's Lantus (insulin glargine). Basaglar does not have final approval due to the Hatch–Waxman litigation involving Sanofi's patents and the associated 30-month stay. Time to tentative approval was quick, however, coming to exactly 10 months. The same product was approved as a biosimilar, in 2014, in Europe.
- Omnitrope® (Somatropin for injection): In its 2006 decision to approve Sandoz's Omnitrope, a recombinant growth hormone replacement therapy, the FDA addressed and rejected citizen petitions from Pfizer, Biotechnology Industry Organization, and Genentech opposing Omintrope's approval. FDA's decision to approve Omnitrope set forth the required level of similarity between Omnitrope and the reference product, Pfizer's Genotropin, for approval under the 505(b)(2) pathway. Notably, Omnitrope was approved as a biosimilar in Europe in 2006.
- Hylenex® (Hyaluronidase human injection): In December 2005, less than nine months after submission of the 505(b)(2) application, the FDA approved Hylenex, a recombinant version of human hyaluronidase. Hylenex is marketed by Baxter and it facilitates subcutaneous fluid administration. At the time Hylenex was approved, ovine-derived hyaluronidase was marketed as Vitrase by ISTA Pharmaceuticals, Inc. Despite the fact that Vitrase was FDA approved, the FDA concluded that Hylenex was a new chemical entity compared to the prior versions of hyaluronidase and awarded Hylenex five years of market exclusivity.

- Fortical® (Calcitonin-salmon): The FDA approved Unigene's Fortical (recombinantly produced calcitonin-salmon) in August 2005 as a 505(b)(2) product. Unigene's application relied on the regulatory filings for Novartis's Miacalcin® (calcitonin-salmon synthetic), a treatment for osteoporosis. Novartis submitted a citizen petition, asking the FDA to deny Fortical approval because Unigene's 505(b)(2) application did not provide both (a) two years of bone mineral density data and (b) at least the minimal fracture data that the FDA required for Miacalcin. Highlighting the lesser regulatory burden for a 505(b)(2) application compared to an NDA, the FDA denied Novartis's petition, stating that these data were not necessary for the approval of Fortical.
- GlucaGen® (Glucagon injection): One of the first 505(b)(2) biologics, Novo Nordisk's GlucaGen was approved in June 1998. GlucaGen is a recombinant version of glucagon. Novo Nordisk relied on the NDA for Glucagon USP (derived from purified beef and pork pancreas) for GlucaGen's approval. Years after GlucaGen was approved, the FDA used GlucaGen as an example of how the 505(b)(2) route could be used to obtain approval of follow-on biologics. Novo Nordisk objected, saying that GlucaGen was a case of "extraordinary circumstances" and that ordinarily, the 505(b)(2) route should be used only for "chemically derived" drugs. The FDA rejected Novo Nordisk's position in its decision granting approval to Omnitrope.

3.11 The Purple Book

On September 9, 2014, the FDA published its first edition of the biologic equivalent of the Orange Book. While the *Purple Book* lists biological products, including any biosimilar and interchangeable biological products licensed by the FDA under the PHSA, it is more formally known as *Lists of Licensed Biological Products with Reference Product Exclusivity and Biosimilarity Interchangeability Evaluations*. However, unlike the Orange Book, it does not include patents relevant to the biological originator product; the lists include only the date a biological product was licensed under 351(a) of the PHSA and whether the FDA evaluated the biological product for reference product exclusivity under Section 351(k)(7) of the PHSA. The Purple Book also enables a user to see whether a biological product licensed under Section 351(k) of the PHSA has been determined by the FDA to be biosimilar to or interchangeable with a reference biological product (an already-licensed FDA biological product). Biosimilar and interchangeable biological products licensed under Section 351(k) of the PHSA will be listed under the reference product to which biosimilarity or interchangeability was demonstrated. Separate lists for those biological products regulated by the CDER and the CBER will be periodically updated.

These lists are designed to help enable a user to see whether a particular biological product has been determined by the FDA to be biosimilar to or interchangeable with a reference biological product. The lists cross-reference the names of biological products licensed under Section 351(a) of the PHSA with the names of biosimilar or interchangeable biological products licensed under Section 351(k) of the PHSA by the FDA (see Section 3.12 for an explanation of the Sections 351(a) and 351(k) of the PHSA). There will be separate lists for those biological products regulated by the CDER and the CBER.

For products licensed under Section 351(a) of the PHSA, the lists identify the date the biological product was licensed and whether the FDA evaluated the biological product for reference product exclusivity under Section 351(k)(7) of the PHSA. If the FDA has determined that a biological product is protected by a period of reference product exclusivity, the list will identify the date of first licensure and the date that the reference product exclusivity (including any attached pediatric exclusivity) will expire. The list will not identify periods of orphan exclusivity and their expiration dates for biological products as those dates are available at the searchable database for orphan-designated and/or approved products.

Biosimilar and interchangeable biological products licensed under Section 351(k) of the PHSA will be listed under the reference product to which biosimilarity or interchangeability was demonstrated.

Although the FDA has not made a determination of the date of the first licensure for all 351(a) biological products included on the lists, it does not mean that the biological products on the list are not, or were not, eligible for exclusivity. A determination of the date of the first licensure and of when any remaining reference product exclusivity will expire for a biological product submitted under Section 351(a) of the PHSA will be generally made for reasons of regulatory necessity and/or at the request of the 351(a) application license holder.

These lists will be updated when the FDA licenses a biological product under Section 351(a) or Section 351(k) of the PHSA and/or makes a determination regarding the date of the first licensure for a biological product licensed under Section 351(a) of the PHSA.

3.12 The FDA questions and answers

3.12.1 Background

The questions and answers (Q&As) are grouped in the following categories:

- Biosimilarity or Interchangeability
- Provisions Related to Requirement to Submit a BLA for a "Biological Product"
- Exclusivity

The Q&A format is intended to promote transparency and facilitate development programs for proposed biosimilar products by addressing questions that may arise in the early stages of development. In addition, these Q&As respond to questions the Agency has received from prospective BLA and NDA applicants regarding the appropriate statutory authority under which certain products will be regulated. The FDA intends to update this guidance to include additional Q&As as appropriate. Table 3.1 describes the status of the draft guidance Q&As provided in this guidance and the final guidance Q&As that are included in the guidance on *Biosimilars: Questions and Answers Regarding Implementation of the Biologics Price Competition and Innovation Act of 2009*. The FDA has maintained the original numbering of the Q&As used in the February 2012 draft guidance. Q&As that have been finalized appear in the final guidance, and the omission of these Q&As from this revised draft guidance is marked by several asterisks between nonconsecutively numbered Q&As.

3.12.2 Biosimilarity or interchangeability

Q. I.1: Whom should a sponsor contact with questions about its proposed biosimilar development program?

A. I.1: If the reference product for a proposed biosimilar product is regulated by the Center for Drug Evaluation and Research (CDER), contact the Therapeutic Biologics and Biosimilars Team (TBBT) in CDER's Office of New Drugs at 301-796-0700.

If the reference product for a proposed biosimilar product is regulated by the Center for Biologics Evaluation and Research (CBER), contact the Office of Communication, Outreach and Development (OCOD) at 800-835-4709 or 240-402-7800 or by email to ocod@fda.hhs.gov.

For general questions related to the FDA's implementation of the BPCI Act, contact Sandra Benton in CDER's Office of Medical Policy at 301-796-2500.

Q. I.2: When should a sponsor request a meeting with the FDA to discuss their proposed biosimilar development program, and what data and information should a sponsor provide to the FDA as background for this meeting?

A. I.2: Sponsors can request meetings at any time point in their development program. The FDA recommends that sponsors refer to the draft guidance for industry titled *Formal Meetings between the FDA and Biosimilar Biological Product Sponsors or Applicants* to determine the most appropriate meeting type to request. This draft guidance describes the different meeting types intended to facilitate biosimilar development programs in accordance with the Biosimilar User Fee Act of 2012 (BsUFA) and the criteria/data needed to support the request. The type of meeting granted will depend on the stage of product development and whether the information submitted in the meeting package meets the criteria for the kind of meeting.

See the FDA's draft guidance for industry on *Formal Meetings between the FDA and Biosimilar Biological Product Sponsors or Applicants*: http://www.fda.gov/downloads/Drugs/GuidanceComplianceRegulatoryInformation/Guidances/UCM345649.pdf.

See the FDA's BsUFA website: http://www.fda.gov/ForIndustry/UserFees/BiosimilarUserFeeActBsUFA/defaul.htm.

Q. I.3: Can a proposed biosimilar product have a different formulation than the reference product?

A. I.3: Yes, differences between the formulation of a proposed product and the reference product may be acceptable. A 351(k) application must contain information demonstrating that the biological product is highly similar to the reference product notwithstanding minor differences in clinically inactive components. In addition, an applicant would need to show that there are no clinically meaningful differences between the biological product and the reference product in terms of safety, purity, and potency. It may be possible, for example, for a proposed product formulated without human serum albumin to demonstrate biosimilarity to a reference product formulated with human serum albumin. For more information about FDA's current thinking on the interpretation of the statutory standard for biosimilarity, see the FDA's draft guidances for industry on *Quality Considerations in Demonstrating Biosimilarity of a Therapeutic Protein Product to a Reference Product* and *Scientific Considerations in Demonstrating Biosimilarity to a Reference Product*.

Q. I.4: Can a proposed biosimilar product have a delivery device or container closure system that is different from its reference product?

A. I.4: Yes, some design differences in the delivery device or container closure system used with the proposed biosimilar product may be acceptable. It may be possible, for example, for an applicant to obtain licensure of a proposed biosimilar product in a pre-filled syringe or in an auto-injector device (which are considered the same dosage form), even if the reference product is licensed in a vial presentation, provided that the proposed product meets the statutory standard for biosimilarity and adequate performance data for the delivery device or container closure system are provided. For a proposed biosimilar product in a different delivery device or container closure system, the presentation must be shown to be compatible for use with the final formulation of the biological product through appropriate studies, including, for example, extractable/leachable studies and stability studies. Also, for design differences in the delivery device or container closure system, performance testing, and a human factors study may be needed.

However, a prospective biosimilar applicant will not be able to obtain licensure under section 351(k) for its product when a design difference in the delivery device or container closure system results in any of the following:

- A clinically meaningful difference between the proposed product and the reference product in terms of safety, purity, and potency;
- A different route of administration or dosage form; or
- A condition of use (e.g., indication, dosing regimen) for which the reference product has not been previously approved; or otherwise does not meet the standard for biosimilarity.

Additional considerations apply for a proposed interchangeable product. For example, in reviewing an application for a proposed interchangeable product, the FDA may consider whether the differences from the reference product significantly alter critical design attributes, product performance, or operating principles, or would require additional instruction to healthcare providers or patients, for patients to be safely alternated or switched between the reference product and one or more interchangeable products without the intervention of the prescribing healthcare provider. Additional performance data about the delivery device may also be necessary.

A proposed biosimilar product in a delivery device will be considered a combination product and may, in some instances, require a separate application for the device.

Q. I.5: Can an applicant obtain licensure of a proposed biosimilar product for fewer than all routes of administration for which an injectable reference product is licensed?

A. I.5: Yes, an applicant may obtain licensure of a proposed biosimilar product for fewer than all routes of administration for which an injectable reference product is licensed. An applicant must demonstrate that there are no clinically meaningful differences between the proposed biosimilar product and the reference product in terms of safety, purity, and potency. In a limited number of circumstances, this may include providing information from one or more studies using a route of administration for which licensure is not requested (e.g., a study using subcutaneous administration may provide a more sensitive comparative assessment of immunogenicity of the reference product and a proposed biosimilar product, even though licensure of the proposed biosimilar product is requested only for the intravenous route of administration).

Q. I.6: Can an applicant obtain licensure of a proposed biosimilar product for fewer than all presentations (e.g., strengths or delivery device or container closure systems) for which a reference product is licensed?

A. I.6: Yes, an applicant is not required to obtain licensure for all presentations for which the reference product is licensed. However, if an applicant seeks licensure for a particular indication or other condition of use for which the reference product is licensed and that indication or condition of use corresponds to a certain presentation of the reference product, the applicant may need to seek licensure for that particular presentation (see also questions and answers I.4 and I.5).

Q. I.7: Can an applicant obtain licensure of a proposed biosimilar product for fewer than all conditions of use for which the reference product is licensed?

A. I.7: Yes, a biosimilar applicant generally may obtain licensure for fewer than all conditions of use for which the reference product is licensed. The 351(k) application must include information demonstrating that the condition or conditions of use prescribed, recommended, or suggested in the proposed labeling submitted for the proposed biosimilar product have been previously approved for the reference product (see section 351(k)(2)(A)(i)(III) of the PHS Act).

Q. I.8: Can a sponsor use comparative animal or clinical data with a non-U.S.-licensed product to support a demonstration that the proposed product is biosimilar to the reference product?

A. I.8: Yes, a sponsor may use a non-U.S.-licensed comparator product in certain studies to support a demonstration that the proposed biological product is biosimilar to the U.S.-licensed reference product. However, as a scientific matter, analytical studies and at least one clinical pharmacokinetic (PK) study and, if appropriate, at least one pharmacodynamic (PD) study, intended to support a demonstration of biosimilarity must include an adequate comparison of the proposed biosimilar product directly with the U.S.-licensed reference product unless it can be scientifically justified that such a study is not needed.

If a sponsor seeks to use data from an animal study or a clinical study comparing its proposed biosimilar product to a non-U.S.-licensed product to address, in part, the requirements under section 351(k)(2)(A) of the PHS Act, the sponsor should provide adequate data or information to scientifically justify the relevance of these comparative data to an assessment of biosimilarity and establish an acceptable bridge to the U.S.-licensed reference product. As a scientific matter, the type of bridging data needed will always include data from analytical studies (e.g., structural and functional data) that directly compare all three products (i.e., the proposed biosimilar product, the U.S.-licensed reference product, and the non-U.S.-licensed comparator product), and is likely to also include bridging clinical PK and/or PD study data for all three products. All three pairwise comparisons should meet the pre-specified acceptance criteria for analytical and PK and/or PD similarity. The acceptability of such approach will be evaluated on a case-by-case basis, and should be discussed in advance with the Agency. For certain complex biological products, a modified approach may be needed. A final determination about the adequacy of the scientific justification and bridge will be made during the review of the application.

Issues that a sponsor may need to address to use a non-U.S.-licensed comparator product in a biosimilar development program include, but are not limited to, the following:

- The relevance of the design of the clinical program to support a demonstration of biosimilarity to the U.S.-licensed reference product for the condition(s) of use and patient population(s) for which licensure is sought;
- The relationship between the license holder for the non-U.S.-licensed comparator product and BLA holder for the U.S.-licensed reference product;
- Whether the non-U.S.-licensed comparator product was manufactured in a facility(ies) licensed and inspected by a regulatory authority that has similar scientific and regulatory standards as the FDA (e.g., International Conference on Harmonisation [ICH] countries);
- Whether the non-U.S.-licensed comparator product was licensed by a regulatory authority that has similar scientific and regulatory standards as the FDA (e.g., ICH countries) and the duration and extent to which the product has been marketed; and
- The scientific bridge between the non-U.S.-licensed comparator product and the U.S.-licensed reference product, including comparative physicochemical characterization, biological assays/functional assays, degradation profiles under stressed conditions, and comparative clinical PK and, when appropriate, PD data, to address the impact of any differences in formulation or primary packaging on product performance.

A sponsor also should address any other factors that may affect the relevance of comparative data with the non-U.S.-licensed comparator product to an assessment of biosimilarity with the U.S.-licensed reference product.

A sponsor may submit publicly available information regarding the non-U.S.-licensed comparator product to justify the extent of comparative data needed to establish a bridge to the U.S.-licensed reference product. The complexity of the products, particularly with respect to higher order structure, post-translational modifications (e.g., glycosylation) and the degree of heterogeneity associated with the product may impact the considerations for the scientific justification regarding the extent of bridging data. Additional factors that the FDA may consider regarding the extent of bridging data include, but are not limited to, the following:

- Whether the formulation, dosage form, and strength of the U.S.-licensed reference product and non-U.S.-licensed comparator products are the same;
- The route of administration of the U.S.-licensed reference product and non-U.S.-licensed comparator products;
- The design of the physicochemical and biological/functional assessments and the use of multiple orthogonal methods with adequate sensitivity to detect differences among the products;
- The scientific justification for the selection of the non-U.S.-licensed comparator lots used to establish the scientific bridge and how the selected lots relate to the material used in the nonclinical and clinical studies. The scientific bridge should include a sufficient number of lots of non-U.S.-licensed comparator product to capture adequately the variability in product quality attributes. When possible, the non-U.S.-licensed comparator lots used in the nonclinical or clinical studies should be included in the assessment performed to establish the analytical bridge.

Sponsors are encouraged to discuss with the FDA during the development program the adequacy of the scientific justification and bridge to the U.S.-licensed reference product. A final decision about the adequacy of this scientific justification and bridge will be made by the FDA during the review of the 351(k) application.

At this time, as a scientific matter, it is unlikely that clinical comparisons with a non-U.S.-licensed product would be an adequate basis to support the additional criteria required for a determination of interchangeability with the U.S.-licensed reference product.

Q. I.9: Is a clinical study to assess the potential of the biological product to delay cardiac repolarization (a QT/QTc study) or a drug–drug interaction study generally needed for licensure of a proposed biosimilar product? [Revised]

A. I.9 (Revised Proposed Answer): In general, a proposed biosimilar product may rely upon the reference product's clinical evaluation of QT/QTc interval prolongation and proarrhythmic potential and drug–drug interactions. If such studies were not required for the reference product, then these data generally would not be needed for licensure of the proposed biosimilar product. However, if the BLA holder for the reference product has been required to conduct postmarket studies or clinical trials under section 505(o)(3) of the FD&C Act to assess or identify a certain risk related to a QT/QTC study or a drug–drug interaction study and those studies have not yet been completed, then the FDA may impose similar postmarket requirements on the biosimilar applicant in appropriate circumstances.

Q. I.10: How long and in what manner should sponsors retain reserve samples of the biological products used in comparative clinical PK and/or PD studies intended to support a 351(k) application? [Revised]

A. I.10 (Revised Proposed Answer): Reserve samples establish the identity of the products tested in the actual study, allow for confirmation of the validity and reliability of the results of the study, and facilitate investigation of further follow-up questions that arise after the studies are completed. The FDA recommends that the sponsor of a proposed biosimilar product retain reserve samples for at least five years following a comparative clinical PK and/or PD study of the reference product and the proposed biosimilar product (or other clinical study in which PK or PD samples are collected with the primary objective of assessing PK similarity) that is intended to support a submission under section 351(k) of the PHS Act. For a three-way PK similarity study, samples of both comparator products should be retained, in addition to samples of the proposed biosimilar product.

For most protein therapeutics, the FDA recommends that a sponsor retain the following quantities of product and dosage units, which are expected to be sufficient for evaluation by state of the art analytical methods:

- A minimum of 10 dosage units each of the proposed biosimilar, reference product and, if applicable, comparator product, depending on the amount of product within each unit. In general, this should provide for a total product mass of equal to or greater than 200 mg in a volume equal to or greater than 10 mL.
- For multi-site studies, three or more dosage units each of the proposed biosimilar, reference product, and, if

applicable, comparator product, at the site where the highest number of patients enrolled, and one or more dosage units from the next highest enrolling sites until the minimum recommended total number of retained samples is met.

The FDA recommends that the sponsor contact the review division to discuss the appropriate quantities of reserve samples in the following situations:

- A product mass of equal to or greater than 200 mg in a volume equal to or greater than 10 mL requires a large number of dosage units.
- Biologics other than protein therapeutics.
- A product intended for multi-dose administration.

Q. I.11: Can an applicant extrapolate clinical data intended to support a demonstration of biosimilarity in one condition of use to support licensure of the proposed biosimilar product in one or more additional conditions of use for which the reference product is licensed?

A. I.11: Yes. If the proposed product meets the statutory requirements for licensure as a biosimilar product under section 351(k) of the PHS Act based on, among other things, data derived from a clinical study or studies sufficient to demonstrate safety, purity, and potency in an appropriate condition of use, the applicant may seek licensure for one or more additional conditions of use for which the reference product is licensed. However, the applicant would need to provide sufficient scientific justification for extrapolating clinical data to support a determination of biosimilarity for each condition of use for which licensure is sought.

Such scientific justification for extrapolation should address, for example, the following issues for the tested and extrapolated conditions of use:

- The mechanism(s) of action in each condition of use for which licensure is sought; this may include:
  - The target/receptor(s) for each relevant activity/function of the product;
  - The binding, dose/concentration–response and pattern of molecular signaling upon engagement of target/receptor(s);
  - The relationships between product structure and target/receptor interactions;
  - The location and expression of the target/receptor(s);

- The PK and biodistribution of the product in different patient populations (relevant PD measures also may provide important information on the mechanism of action);
- The immunogenicity of the product in different patient populations;
- Differences in expected toxicities in each condition of use and patient population (including whether expected toxicities are related to the pharmacological activity of the product or to "off-target" activities); and
- Any other factor that may affect the safety or efficacy of the product in each condition of use and patient population for which licensure is sought.

Differences between conditions of use with respect to the factors described above do not necessarily preclude extrapolation. A scientific justification should address these differences in the context of the totality of the evidence supporting a demonstration of biosimilarity.

In choosing which condition of use to study that would permit subsequent extrapolation of clinical data to other conditions of use, the FDA recommends that a sponsor consider choosing a condition of use that would be adequately sensitive to detect clinically meaningful differences between the two products.

The sponsor of a proposed product may obtain licensure only for a condition of use that has been previously licensed as the reference product. If a reference product has a condition of use that was licensed under section 506(c) of the FD&C Act and 21 CFR part 601, subpart E (accelerated approval), and the reference product's clinical benefit in this condition of use has not yet been verified in postmarketing trials, the proposed product sponsor should consider studying another condition of use for which the reference product is licensed to avoid potential complications in the event that postmarketing trials fail to verify the clinical benefit of the reference product for the condition of use.

Q. I.12: How can an applicant demonstrate that its proposed injectable biosimilar product has the same "strength" as the reference product?

A. I.12: Under section 351(k)(2)(A)(i)(IV) of the PHS Act, an applicant must demonstrate that the "strength" of the proposed biosimilar product is the same as that of the reference product. As a scientific matter, there may be a need to take into account different factors and approaches in determining the "strength" of different types of biological products.

In general, we expect injectable biological products to have both the same total content of drug substance (in mass or units of activity in a container closure) and the same concentration of drug substance (in mass or units of activity per unit volume) as the reference product to have the same "strength" under section 351(k)(2)(A)(i)(IV) of the PHS Act. We note, however, that for certain complex biological products, a modified approach may be needed.

The total content of drug substance generally should be expressed using the same measure as the reference product. For example, if the strength of the reference product is expressed as milligrams (mg) per total volume in a container closure, for example, mg/five milliliters (mL), the proposed biosimilar product generally should also describe its strength in mg/five mL, rather than units per five mL. If the total content of drug substance is expressed in units of activity (e.g., international units [IU] or units per total volume in a container closure), the units of the proposed biosimilar product should be the same as the reference product.

The concentration of the drug substance (in mass or units of activity per unit volume) generally should be expressed using the same measure as the reference product. The extinction coefficient used to calculate the concentration of a protein drug substance should be determined experimentally, and justification for the experimental method should be provided. If the proposed biosimilar product is a dry solid (e.g., lyophilized) from which a constituted or reconstituted solution is prepared, then the 351(k) application should contain information demonstrating that the concentration of the proposed biosimilar product, when constituted or reconstituted, is the same as that of the reference product.

The requirement for a 351(k) application to contain information demonstrating that the proposed product and the reference product have the same "strength" applies to both biosimilar products and interchangeable products.

Q. I.13: What constitutes "publicly-available information" regarding FDA's previous determination that the reference product is safe, pure, and potent to include in a 351(k) application?

A. I.13 (Proposed Answer): "Publicly-available information" in this context generally includes the types of information found in the "action package" for a BLA (see section 505(l)(2)(C) of the FD&C Act). However, the FDA notes that submission of publicly available information composed of less than the action package for the reference product BLA will generally not be considered a bar to submission or approval of an acceptable 351(k) application.

The FDA intends to post on the Agency's Web site publicly available information regarding FDA's previous determination that certain biological products are safe, pure, and potent in order to facilitate biosimilar development programs and submission of 351(k) applications. We note, however, that the publicly available information posted by the FDA in this context does not necessarily include all of the information that would otherwise be disclosable in response to a Freedom of Information Act request.

Q. I.14: Can an applicant obtain a determination of interchangeability between its proposed product and the reference product in an original 351(k) application?

A. I.14 (Proposed Answer): Yes. Under the BPCI Act, the FDA can make a determination of interchangeability in a 351(k) application or any supplement to a 351(k) application. An interchangeable product must be shown to be biosimilar to the reference product and meet the other standards described in section 351(k)(4) of the PHS Act. At this time, it would be difficult as a scientific matter for a prospective biosimilar applicant to establish interchangeability in an original 351(k) application given the statutory standard for interchangeability and the sequential nature of that assessment. The FDA is continuing to consider the type of information sufficient to enable the FDA to determine that a biological product is interchangeable with the reference product.

Q. I.15: Is a pediatric assessment under the Pediatric Research Equity Act (PREA) required for a proposed biosimilar product?

A. I.15: Under the Pediatric Research Equity Act (PREA) (section 505B of the FD&C Act), all applications for new active ingredients, new indications, new dosage forms, new dosing regimens, or new routes of administration are required to contain a pediatric assessment to support dosing, safety, and effectiveness of the product for the claimed indication unless this requirement is waived, deferred, or inapplicable.

Section 505B(n) of the FD&C Act, added by section 7002(d)(2) of the Affordable Care Act, provides that a biosimilar product that has not been determined to be interchangeable with the reference product is considered to have a "new active ingredient" for purposes of PREA, and pediatric assessment is required unless waived or deferred. Under the statute, an interchangeable product is not considered to have a "new active ingredient" for purposes of PREA. Therefore, if a biological product is determined to be interchangeable with the reference product, PREA would not be triggered, and a pediatric assessment of the interchangeable product would not be required. However, if an applicant first seeks licensure of its proposed product as a non-interchangeable biosimilar product and intends to seek subsequently licensure of the product as interchangeable, the applicant still must address

PREA requirements when it seeks initial licensure as a non-interchangeable biosimilar product.

The FDA encourages prospective biosimilar applicants to submit plans for pediatric studies as early as practicable during product development. If there is no active IND for the proposed product, and the sponsor intends to conduct a comparative clinical study as part of its development program, the initial pediatric study plan (PSP) should be submitted as a pre-IND submission. In this scenario, the FDA encourages the sponsor to meet with the FDA before submission of the initial PSP to discuss the details of the planned development program. It is expected that the sponsor will submit the initial PSP before initiating any comparative clinical study in its biosimilar development program. For more information see the draft question and answer I.17 in FDA's draft guidance for industry (revision 1) on *Biosimilars: Additional Questions and Answers Regarding Implementation of the Biologics Price Competition and Innovation Act of 2009*, which, when finalized, will represent the Agency's current thinking on this topic. See also the draft guidance for industry *Pediatric Study Plans: Content of and Process for Submitting Initial Pediatric Study Plans and Amended Pediatric Study Plans* (http://www.fda.gov/downloads/drugs/guidancecompliance regulatoryinformation/guidances/ucm360507.pdf).

Q. I.16: How can a proposed biosimilar product applicant fulfill the requirement for pediatric assessments under the Pediatric Research Equity Act (PREA)? [New]

A. I.16 (Proposed Answer): Applicants for proposed biosimilar products should address PREA requirements based on the nature and extent of pediatric information in the reference product labeling.

As a preliminary matter, we note that there are differences in the use of the term "extrapolation" in the context of a proposed biosimilar product under the BPCI Act and in the context of PREA. Under the BPCI Act, if a biosimilar applicant fulfills the requirements for demonstrating its product is biosimilar to a reference product in one condition of use for which the reference product is licensed (e.g., an indication for an adult population), information regarding the safety, purity, and potency of the reference product in one or more additional conditions of use for which the reference product is licensed (e.g., the same indication in the pediatric population) may be extrapolated to the proposed biosimilar product if sufficient scientific justification for extrapolation is provided by the applicant (see question and answer I.11 in FDA's guidance for industry on *Biosimilars: Questions and Answers Regarding Implementation of the Biologics Price*

Competition and Innovation Act of 2009). In this context, extrapolation occurs across drug products (i.e., from the reference product to the proposed biosimilar product).

Under PREA, a single sponsor with a single drug or biological product or drug or biological product line may conduct studies in an indication in one population (e.g., adults or older pediatric populations) and extrapolate efficacy findings to satisfy, in part, PREA requirements regarding use of that same product or product line in additional populations (e.g., younger pediatric populations). In this context, "extrapolation" occurs in a single product or product line without relying on studies comparing the product to an approved product and without conducting a full complement of additional studies in those additional populations. Under PREA, extrapolation of efficacy (but not safety or dosing) from adult populations to pediatric populations in a single drug or biological product or drug or biological product line may be permitted if the adult and pediatric indications are the same indication and the course of the disease and the effects of the drug are sufficiently similar in adult and pediatric patients. Extrapolation from one pediatric age group to another pediatric age group for a single drug or biological product or drug or biological product line also may be appropriate to fulfill a PREA requirement under these circumstances. However, under PREA, extrapolation of dosing or safety from adult populations to pediatric populations in a single drug or biological product or drug or biological product line generally is not permitted and will not satisfy a PREA requirement.

In the discussion that follows, the term "extrapolation" generally refers to extrapolation from the reference product to the proposed biosimilar product under the BPCI Act, not to extrapolation from adults or older pediatric populations to younger pediatric populations within a single product or product line under PREA.

- Adequate pediatric information in reference product is labeling
  - If the labeling for the reference product contains adequate pediatric information (information reflecting an adequate pediatric assessment) with respect to an indication for which a biosimilar applicant seeks licensure in adults, the biosimilar applicant may fulfill PREA requirements by satisfying the statutory requirements for showing biosimilarity and providing an adequate scientific justification under the BPCI Act for extrapolating the pediatric information from the reference product to the proposed biosimilar product. See question and answer I.11 in the FDA's

guidance for industry on Biosimilars: Questions and Answers Regarding Implementation of the Biologics Price Competition and Innovation Act of 2009 for additional information on extrapolation under the BPCI Act. If the submitted scientific justification for extrapolation under the BPCI Act is inadequate, a biosimilar applicant must submit appropriate data to fulfill applicable PREA requirements.

- Lack of adequate pediatric information in reference product labeling
  - If the labeling for the reference product does not contain adequate pediatric information for one or more indications for which a biosimilar applicant seeks licensure in adults, and applicable PREA requirements were deferred for the reference product for those indications, a biosimilar applicant should request a deferral of PREA requirements for those indications.

If PREA requirements were waived for the reference product sponsor for those indications, and if the biosimilar applicant believes that its proposed product meets the requirements for a full or partial waiver of PREA requirements under section 505B(a)(4) of the FD&C Act, the biosimilar applicant should request a full or partial waiver for those indications.

If a biosimilar applicant believes that none of the situations described above applies to its proposed product, the applicant should contact the FDA for further information.

Q. I.17: When should a proposed biosimilar product applicant submit an initial pediatric study plan (PSP)? [New]

A. I.17 (Proposed Answer): Section 505B(e) of the Federal Food, Drug, and Cosmetic Act (FD&C Act), as amended by Section 506 of the Food and Drug Administration Safety and Innovation Act (FDA SIA), requires applicants subject to the Pediatric Research Equity Act (PREA) to submit an initial pediatric study plan (PSP) no later than 60 calendar days after the date of an end-of-Phase 2 (EOP2) meeting, or at another time agreed upon by the FDA and the applicant. This provision of FDA SIA has an effective date of January 5, 2013. The FDA has issued draft guidance on the PSP process, including the timing of PSP submission, as required by section 505B(e)(7) of the FD&C Act.

Sections 505B(e)(2)(C) and 505B(e)(3) of the FD&C Act set forth a process for reaching an agreement between an applicant and the FDA on an initial PSP that lasts up to 210 days. Given the potential length of this process, and in the absence of an EOP2 meeting for a proposed biosimilar product, the FDA recommends that if a sponsor has not already initiated a comparative clinical study intended to address the requirements under section 351(k)(2)(A)(i)(I)(cc) of the Public Health Service (PHS) Act, the sponsor should submit an initial PSP as soon as feasible, but no later than 210 days before initiating such a study. This is intended to provide adequate time to reach an agreement with the FDA on the initial PSP before the study is initiated. Depending on the details of the clinical program, it may be appropriate to submit an initial PSP earlier in development. The FDA encourages the sponsor to meet with the FDA to discuss the details of the planned development program before submission of the initial PSP.

The initial PSP must include an outline of the pediatric study or studies that a sponsor plans to conduct (including, to the extent practicable, study objectives and design, age groups, relevant endpoints, and statistical approach); any request for a deferral, partial waiver, or full waiver, if applicable, along with any supporting documentation; and should also include any previously negotiated pediatric plans with other regulatory authorities. For additional guidance on submission of the PSP, including a PSP Template, please refer to http://www.fda.gov/Drugs/DevelopmentApprovalProcess/DevelopmentResources/ucm049867.htm. After the initial PSP is submitted, a sponsor must work with the FDA to reach timely agreement on the plan, as required by section 505B(e)(2)–(3) of the FD&C Act. It should be noted that requested deferrals or waivers in the initial PSP will not be formally granted or denied until the product is licensed.

Q. I.18: For biological products intended to be injected, how can an applicant demonstrate that its proposed biosimilar product has the same "dosage form" as the reference product? [New]

A. I.18 (Proposed Answer): Under section 351(k)(2)(A)(i)(IV) of the PHS Act, an applicant must demonstrate that the dosage form of the proposed biosimilar or interchangeable product is the same as that of the reference product. For purposes of implementing this statutory provision, the FDA considers the dosage form to be the physical manifestation containing the active and inactive ingredients that deliver a dose of the drug product. In the context of proposed biosimilar products intended to be injected, the FDA considers, for example, "injection" (e.g., a solution) to be a different dosage form from "for injection" (e.g., lyophilized powder). Thus, if the reference product is an "injection," an applicant could not obtain licensure of a proposed biosimilar "for injection" even if the applicant demonstrated that the proposed biosimilar product, when constituted or reconstituted, could meet the other requirements for an application for a proposed biosimilar product.

For purposes of section 351(k)(2)(A)(i)(IV) of the PHS Act, the FDA also considers emulsions and suspensions of products intended to be injected to be distinct dosage forms. Liposomes, lipid complexes, and products with extended-release characteristics present special scenarios due to their unique composition, and prospective applicants seeking further information should contact the FDA.

It should be noted, however, that this interpretation regarding the same dosage form is for purposes of section 351(k)(2)(A)(i)(IV) of the PHS Act only. For example, this interpretation should not be cited by applicants seeking approval of a new drug application under section 505(c) of the FD&C Act or licensure of a BLA under section 351(a) of the PHS Act for purposes of determining whether separate applications should be submitted and assessed separate fees for different dosage forms. For more information about the prescription drug user fee bundling policy, see the FDA's guidance for industry on *Submitting Separate Marketing Applications and Clinical Data for Purposes of Assessing User Fees*, available at http://www.fda.gov/downloads/Drugs/GuidanceComplianceRegulatoryInformation/Guidances/UCM079320.pdf.

Q. I.19: If a non-U.S.-licensed product is proposed for importation and use in the U.S. in a clinical investigation intended to support a proposed biosimilar development program (e.g., a bridging clinical PK and/or PD study), is a separate IND required for the non-U.S.-licensed product? [New]

A. I.19 (Proposed Answer): No, a sponsor may submit a single IND for its proposed biosimilar development program, and may submit information supporting the proposed clinical investigation with the non-U.S.-licensed comparator product under the same IND. This scenario may occur, for example, if a sponsor seeks to use data from a clinical study comparing its proposed biosimilar product to a non-U.S.-licensed product to address, in part, the requirements under section 351(k)(2)(A) of the PHS Act, and proposes to conduct a clinical PK and/or PD study in the U.S. with all three products (i.e., the proposed biosimilar product, the U.S.-licensed reference product, and the non-U.S.-licensed product) to support establishment of a bridge to the U.S.-licensed reference product and scientific justification for the relevance of these comparative data to an assessment of biosimilarity.

A non-U.S.-licensed comparator product is considered an investigational new drug in the United States, and thus would require an IND for importation and use in the United States (see 21 CFR 312.110(a)). If a sponsor intends to conduct a clinical investigation in the United States using a non-U.S.-licensed comparator product, the IND requirements in 21 CFR part 312 also would apply to this product (see, e.g., 21 CFR 312.2).

With respect to chemistry, manufacturing, and controls (CMC) information, a sponsor should submit to the IND as much of the CMC information required by 21 CFR 312.23(a)(7) as is available. However, the FDA recognizes that a sponsor may not be able to obtain all of the CMC information required by 21 CFR 312.23(a)(7) for a non-U.S.-licensed comparator product for which it is not the manufacturer. In these circumstances, the sponsor can request that the FDA waive the requirement for complete CMC information on the non-U.S.-licensed comparator product (21 CFR 312.10). The IND must include, as part of the waiver request, at least one of the following:

- A sufficient explanation why compliance with the complete requirements of 21 CFR 312.23(a)(7) is unnecessary or cannot be achieved,
- Information that will satisfy the purpose of the requirement by helping to ensure that the investigational drug will have the proper identity, strength, quality, and purity, or
- Other information justifying a waiver.

Information that is relevant to whether the investigational drug will have the proper identity, strength, quality, and purity may include, for example, information indicating whether the investigational drug has been licensed by a regulatory authority that has similar scientific and regulatory standards as the FDA (e.g., International Conference on Harmonisation [ICH] countries). This should include, to the extent possible, summary approval information and current product labeling made public by the foreign regulatory authority. In addition, a sponsor should also provide information on the conditions and containers that will be used to transport the drug product to the U.S. clinical site(s) and information on the relabeling and repackaging operations that will be used to relabel the drug product vials for investigational use. (This should include information on how exposure of the product to light and temperature conditions outside of the recommended storage conditions will be prevented. A risk assessment on the impact the relabeling operations may have on drug product stability should also be included.)

The sponsor should consult with the appropriate the FDA review division regarding the CMC information necessary to support the proposed clinical trial.

As applicable to all investigational drugs, the FDA reminds sponsors that the investigator brochure (IB) for studies to be conducted under the IND should be carefully prepared to ensure that it is not misleading, erroneous, or materially incomplete, which can be a basis for a clinical hold (see 21 CFR 312.42(b)

(1)(iii) and (b)(2)(i)). For example, the term *reference product* should be used in the IB only to refer to the single biological product licensed under section 351(a) of the Public Health Service Act against which the proposed biosimilar product is evaluated for purposes of submitting a 351(k) application. The IB and study protocol(s) should use consistent nomenclature that clearly differentiates the proposed biosimilar product from the reference product. The IB and study protocol(s) also should clearly describe whether the comparator used in each study is the U.S.-licensed reference product or a non-U.S.-licensed comparator product, and use consistent nomenclature that clearly differentiates these products. If a non-U.S.-licensed comparator product is being used in a study conducted in the United States, the IB and study protocol(s) should clearly convey that the product is not FDA-approved and is considered an investigational new drug in the United States. The IB and study protocol(s) also should avoid conclusory statements regarding regulatory determinations (e.g., "comparable," "biosimilar," "highly similar") that have not been made.

3.12.3 Provisions related to requirement to submit a BLA for a "biological product"

Q. II.1: How does the FDA interpret the category of "protein (except any chemically synthesized polypeptide)" in the amended definition of "biological product" in section 351(i)(1) of the PHS Act?

A. II.1: The BPCI Act amends the definition of "biological product" in section 351(i) of the PHS Act to include a "protein (except any chemically synthesized polypeptide)" and provides that an application for a biological product must be submitted under section 351 of the PHS Act, subject to certain exceptions during the 10-year transition period ending on March 23, 2020, described in section 7002(e) of the Affordable Care Act.

The FDA has developed the following regulatory definitions of "protein" and "chemically synthesized polypeptide" to implement the amended definition of "biological product" and provide clarity to prospective applicants regarding the statutory authority under which products will be regulated.

Protein—The term "protein" means any alpha amino acid polymer with a specific defined sequence that is greater than 40 amino acids in size.

For purposes of this definition, the size of the molecule is based on the total number of amino acids and is not limited to the number of amino acids in a contiguous sequence. However, compounds greater than 40 amino acids in size will be scrutinized to determine whether they are related to a natural peptide of shorter length and, if so, whether the additional amino acids raise any concerns about the risk/benefits profile of the product.

Chemically synthesized polypeptide—The term "chemically synthesized polypeptide" means any alpha amino acid polymer that (1) is made entirely by chemical synthesis; and (2) is less than 100 amino acids in size.

A chemically synthesized polypeptide, as defined, is not a "biological product" and will be regulated as a drug under the FD&C Act unless the polypeptide otherwise meets the statutory definition of a "biological product."

For purposes of this definition, the size of the molecule is based on the total number of amino acids and is not limited to the number of amino acids in a contiguous sequence. However, chemically synthesized compounds greater than 99 amino acids in size will be scrutinized to determine whether they are related to a natural peptide of shorter length and, if so, whether the additional amino acids raise any concerns about the risk/benefits profile of the product.

The FDA's interpretation of these statutory terms is informed by several factors, including the following. The scientific literature describes a "protein" as a defined sequence of alpha amino acid polymers linked by peptide bonds, and generally excludes "peptides" from the category of "protein." A "peptide" generally refers to polymers that are smaller, perform fewer functions, contain less three-dimensional structure, are less likely to be post-translationally modified, and thus are characterized more easily than proteins.

Consistent with the scientific literature, the FDA has decided that the term "protein" in the statutory definition of the biological product does not include peptides. To enhance regulatory clarity and minimize administrative complexity, the FDA has decided to distinguish proteins from peptides based solely on size (i.e., the number of amino acids).

In the absence of clear scientific consensus on the criteria that distinguish proteins from peptides, including the exact size at which a chain(s) of amino acids becomes a protein, the FDA reviewed the pertinent literature and concluded that a threshold of 40 amino acids is appropriate for defining the upper size boundary of a peptide. Accordingly, the FDA considers any polymer composed of 40 or fewer amino acids to be a peptide and not a protein. Therefore, unless a peptide otherwise meets the statutory definition of a "biological product" (e.g., a peptide vaccine), it will be regulated as a drug under the FD&C Act.

The statutory category of "protein" parenthetically excludes "any chemically synthesized polypeptide." There are several definitions of "polypeptide" in the scientific literature. Some are broad (e.g., polypeptide means any amino acid polymer) while others are more narrow (e.g., polypeptide means any amino acid polymer composed of fewer than 100 amino acids). The FDA believes that a narrow definition of the polypeptide is most appropriate in this context because, among other reasons, this avoids describing an exception to the category of protein using a term that relates to a larger class of molecules. Therefore, the FDA interprets the statutory exclusion for "chemically synthesized polypeptide" to mean any molecule that is made entirely by chemical synthesis and that is composed of up to 99 amino acids. Such molecules will be regulated as drugs under the FD&C Act unless the chemically synthesized polypeptide otherwise meets the statutory definition of a "biological product."

There may be additional considerations for proposed products that are combination products or meet the statutory definition of both a "device" and a "biological product." We encourage prospective sponsors to contact the FDA for further information on a product-specific basis.

Q. II.2: How is "product class" defined for purposes of determining whether an application for a biological product may be submitted under section 505 of the FD&C Act during the transition period?

A. II.2: For purposes of section 7002(e)(2) of the Affordable Care Act, a proposed biological product will be considered to be in the same "product class" as a protein product previously approved under section 505 of the FD&C Act on or before March 23, 2010, if both products are homologous to the same gene-coded sequence (e.g., the INS gene for insulin and insulin glargine) with allowance for additional novel flanking sequences (including sequences from other genes). Products with discrete changes in gene-coded sequence or discrete changes in post-translational modifications may be in the same product class as the previously approved product even if the result may be a change in product pharmacokinetics.

For naturally derived protein products that do not have identified sequences linked to specific genes and that were approved under section 505 of the FD&C Act on or before March 23, 2010, a proposed biological product is in the same product class as the naturally derived protein product if both products share a primary biological activity (e.g., the four-number Enzyme Commission code for enzyme activity).

However, for any protein product (whether naturally derived or otherwise), if the difference between the proposed product and the protein product previously approved under section 505 of the FD&C Act alters a biological target or effect, the products are not in the same product class for purposes of section 7002(e)(2) of the Affordable Care Act.

Q. II.3: What type of marketing application should be submitted for a proposed antibody–drug conjugate? [New]

A. II.3 (Proposed Answer): As described in further detail below, a BLA should be submitted for a proposed monoclonal antibody that is linked to a drug (antibody–drug conjugate). The FDA considers an antibody–drug conjugate to be a combination product composed of a biological product constituent part and a drug constituent part (see 21 CFR 3.2(e)(1); 70 FR 49848, 49857–49858; August 25, 2005).

CDER is the FDA center assigned to regulate antibody–drug conjugates, irrespective of whether the biological product constituent part or the drug constituent part is determined to have the primary mode of action (see section 503(g) of the FD&C Act; see, e.g., Transfer of Therapeutic Biological Products to the Center for Drug Evaluation and Research [June 30, 2003], available at http://www.fda.gov/CombinationProducts/JurisdictionalInformation/ucm136265.htm; Intercenter Agreement between the Center for Drug Evaluation and Research and the Center for Biologics Evaluation and Research [October 31, 1991], available at http://www.fda.gov/CombinationProducts/JurisdictionalInformation/ucm121179.htm).

To enhance regulatory clarity and promote consistency, CDER considered several factors to determine the appropriate marketing application type for antibody–drug conjugates, including the relative significance of the safety and effectiveness questions raised by the constituent parts, particularly the highly specific molecular targeting by the antibody to a cell type, cellular compartment, or other marker at the site of action (as distinguished from mere alteration of systemic pharmacokinetics).

In light of such factors, CDER considers submission of a BLA under section 351 of the PHS Act to provide the more appropriate application type for antibody–drug conjugates.

Sponsors seeking to submit a BLA for a proposed antibody–drug conjugate should contact CDER's Office of New Drugs at 301-796-0700 for further information.

3.12.4 Exclusivity

Q. III.1: Can an applicant include in its 351(a) BLA submission a request for reference product exclusivity under section 351(k)(7) of the PHS Act?

A. III.1 (Proposed Answer): Yes. The FDA is continuing to review the reference product exclusivity provisions of section 351(k)(7) of the PHS Act and has published a draft guidance addressing certain exclusivity issues (see FDA's draft guidance for industry on *Reference Product Exclusivity for Biological Products Filed under Section 351(a) of the PHS Act*, available at http://www.fda.gov/downloads/drugs/guidancecomplianceregulatoryinformation/guidances/ucm407844.pdf). An applicant may include in its BLA submission a request for reference product exclusivity under section 351(k)(7) of the PHS Act, and the FDA will consider the applicant's assertions regarding the eligibility of its proposed product for exclusivity. The draft guidance describes the types of information that reference product sponsors should provide to facilitate FDA's determination of the date of the first licensure for their products.

Q. III.2: How can a prospective biosimilar applicant determine whether there is unexpired orphan exclusivity for an indication for which the reference product is licensed?

A. III.2: A searchable database for Orphan Designated and/or Approved Products and indications is available on FDA's Web site and is updated on a monthly basis (see http://www.accessdata.fda.gov/scripts/opdlisting/oopd/index.cfm). The FDA will not approve a subsequent application for the "same drug" for the same indication during the seven-year period of orphan exclusivity, except as otherwise provided in the FD&C Act and 21 CFR part 316.

3.13 FDA's explicit views on development of biosimilars

While there is a longer history of approvals of biosimilar products in Europe and certainly in the developing countries, the FDA has taken a more calculated, more conservative view. Surprisingly, the first biosimilar-like products were approved by the FDA long before EMA began a formal biosimilar product program, but this was done under the statutory authority that the FDA enjoys. Now the challenges that the FDA faces are more regulatory. A keen understanding of the thinking of the FDA will greatly contribute to the biosimilar product developers because the United States still represents about 50% of the world market and still securing the FDA approval is the standard that most biosimilar product companies would like to earn.

Recently, Dr. Steven Kozlowski, director of Biotechnology Products in the Center for Drug Evaluation and Research at the FDA, testified before a congressional committee and shared the thinking of the FDA regarding the development of biosimilar products. This testimony that focused on therapeutic proteins reveals many interesting and subtle directions in developing biosimilar products that are important for a biosimilar product developer to understand, more particularly, as this pertains to how the development of measurement science, standards, and related technologies might make it easier to characterize FDA-regulated biological products. Dr. Kozlowski recognized three specific properties of biological products that cannot be sufficiently measured, but are critical for understanding the behavior of biological protein products and suggested that better analytical methods that can measure these three properties would be extremely helpful in determining the similarity of similar biological protein products.

In approving biosimilar products, the FDA wants to understand the characterization and composition of these products, more specifically, what materials they are made up of, and how the materials are arranged (i.e., the structure) at a molecular level. For some products, particularly the nonbiological products, the characterization is relatively straightforward since adequate analytical technology currently exists that is capable of fully understanding the structural nuances of these products. However, in the era of molecular biology where many new therapies are manufactured by inserting novel genes into living cells so as to produce therapeutic proteins by biologic processes, a new challenge has come about that raises the bar on the technology of analytical testing.

3.13.1 Size and complexity of biological drugs: Protein therapeutics

Compared to assessing the structure of small-molecule drugs, which have generally fewer than 100 atoms, assessing the structure of biological drugs is a formidable task. Therapeutic proteins are much larger than typical small-molecule drugs. Using molecular weight as a measure of size, human growth hormone is more than 150 times larger than aspirin, and a mAb is more than five times larger still than human growth hormone. Therapeutic proteins are also much more complex than typical small-molecule drugs.

The manufacture of biological drugs is also quite complex. Most biological drugs are composed of many thousands of atoms linked together in a precise arrangement (called the primary structure). This organization of atoms is further organized into a 3D HOS by the folding of the linked atoms into a specific pattern that is held together by relatively unstable connections. A protein molecule consists of a long chain of building blocks called amino acids, of which there are 20 types—a single protein chain can be made up of hundreds of amino acids. The sequential order of these building blocks in the chain can be critical for medicinal activity. Protein chains with the same sequence of amino acids can fold in different ways—much like a single piece of rope can be tied to a variety of different knots. The specific folding of these chains is also very important in carrying out their therapeutic functions.

In addition, many of the linked amino acids can have modifications attached. These attachments can be small (only a few atoms) or very large (similar in size to the rest of the protein). One commonly observed attachment is the addition of complex groups of sugar molecules, called oligosaccharides. Attachments occur at very specific locations on the protein and, like folding, can have a great impact on the therapeutic function of the protein. A protein can thus be represented as a long chain with 20 different types of links with different possible attachments on the links.

To further complicate matters, biological drugs are not composed of structurally identical units. Instead, they are a mixture of products with slightly different features. This is referred to as microheterogeneity and can be represented as a mixture of very similar chains that differ in a few links or in a few of the attachments. The protein chains themselves can then be linked or aggregated (i.e., clumped). It is a challenge to analyze and characterize the composition of such a mixture. Even with currently available analytical technologies, some uncertainty regarding the actual structure of a biologic usually remains. Simple measurements of biological activity, such as enzyme activity, may provide additional information about a product. But there is currently no way to, a priori, understand how the product will perform in patients (e.g., distribution in the body, immune responses against the product). As a result, nonclinical or clinical studies are necessary to assess the safety and the effectiveness of the product.

3.13.2 Potential benefits of improved analytical methods

Advances in analytical tests during the last two decades have driven progress in biopharmaceutical manufacturing, but there is still room for significant improvement. New or enhanced analytical technologies and measurement systems and standards that can more accurately and precisely assess the HOS and the attachments of biological drugs would provide additional assurance of the quality of biological drugs in at least three specific ways:

- Improved analytical methods would enable quicker and more confident assessments of the potential effects of changes in the manufacturing process, the equipment, or the raw materials.
- At present, the manufacturers and the FDA are hampered by the inability to measure fully structural differences that could be caused by changes in the manufacturing process. Since these unknown structural differences could change the properties of the product, the FDA might only approve a manufacturing change after seeing the results of studies of the product in animals or humans. This can significantly slow the implementation of innovative process improvements and impede the

manufacturer's ability to react to changes in raw material supplies, which could reduce the availability of the drug to patients who need it. Improved analytical methods could reduce the requirements for the animal and/or human studies for evaluation of manufacturing changes. In addition, for products that have abbreviated pathways for approval, improved analytical methods could facilitate comparison of products and detection of differences between manufacturers.
- The development of analytical methods that can evaluate the quality of the biologic throughout the manufacturing process would provide a superior system for ensuring product quality. This would enable increased productivity and improved quality control during the manufacturing process. Improved analytical methods would increase general knowledge in the field of biopharmaceuticals.

The FDA intends to heavily rest its regulatory decisions based on the knowledge of improved analytical methods; this poses a direct challenge to the industry to come up with novel methodologies that will be robust and more reassuring of the structural variability. The FDA has proven this resolve several times by approving complex products, both biological- and nonbiological based on analytical similarity demonstration, allowing the sponsors to launch these products without any testing in patients. The FDA has been legally challenged but won the argument and has frequently stated that a robust analytical similarity demonstration is more useful that targeted clinical trials. This philosophy and this resolve of the FDA are critical to understand.

A good example of how the increased knowledge can inform both regulatory decision making and product design is that of therapeutic proteins like mAbs that affect a patient's immune system to kill tumor cells, and some that do not. One reason for this difference was discovered only after the development of an analytical technique that enabled scientists to characterize the structure of the sugar chains attached to the antibodies. It was discovered that antibodies with certain sugar chains were more consistently able to direct an immune system to kill tumor cells than antibodies with different sugar chains. The FDA initially used this knowledge to require monitoring and control of these sugar chains to ensure consistent clinical benefit to patients. But this knowledge has also enabled the industry to design new mAb products with enhanced tumor-killing activity. These discoveries have led to a great emphasis on the glycan patterns of mAbs and an appreciation why a biosimilar product must emulate all binding and activity characteristics of the reference product, regardless of the specific relevance of the mode of action. For example, the ADCC activity, although not directly related to drugs like TNF blockers, is required to be matched to obtain the FDA approval of the extrapolation of multiple indications. These topics are discussed in detail in later chapters.

3.13.3 Potential benefits of new measurement standards

With the development of new analytical methods comes the need for new standards to evaluate them. The term *standard* can apply to measurements or to processes, and although process standards are valuable in ensuring effective manufacturing process operation and validation, the measurement standards need to be revisited. A measurement standard can be standardized test materials used to evaluate the performance of a measurement method, or it can be a particular analytical procedure used to take a measurement. Standardized test materials can be used to assess the precision and the accuracy of many different analytical technologies and are, thus, more likely to foster competition and development of new and improved analytical methods by industry and academia. Standard test materials could be used to verify the ability of an analytical method to detect differences between product batches from a single manufacturer or products from different manufacturers. For example, if a method is being developed to assess the sugars attached to a protein, the analytical method could be used to test a set of related standard test materials in order to determine the precision and the accuracy of the method. In this way, a given technology can be optimized, or a variety of different technologies can be compared for their ability to accurately and quantitatively assess the quality of a product. The development of such measurement standards would also be extremely valuable for ensuring that current and future analytical methods are properly working and are providing consistent results from assay to assay and from lab to lab.

3.13.4 Three specific properties needing improved measurement

The FDA has identified three properties of therapeutic proteins that cannot be sufficiently measured at this time, but are very important for understanding the behavior of protein drugs. Improved analytical methods to measure these three properties would be particularly useful in determining the extent of similarity of biological protein products intended to be similar.

3.13.4.1 Posttranslation modifications As previously indicated, proteins contain added structural features, such as attached sugar chains, that may be critical for their clinical activity. These attached modifications can be complex and heterogeneous, and we currently lack standardized analytical methods to qualitatively and quantitatively assess the structure as it relates to the intact protein and understand the relationship of the modifications to potency and clinical performance. We are particularly interested in better methods for analyzing the sugars (glycosylation) and other modifications known to affect the medicinal activity of these products.

3.13.4.2 3D structure As previously described, proteins must be folded into a 3D structure to become functional (sometimes a 3D structure can be misfolded). The proteins within a biologic will have one major 3D structure along with a distribution of other variants differing in a 3D structure. Our current ability to predict the potency of biological drugs would be enhanced if we had improved ability to measure and quantify the correct (major) 3D structure, the aberrant 3D structures (misfolding), and the distribution of different 3D structures.

3.13.4.3 Protein aggregation Some biological products can stick to one another. When many protein molecules stick together, they are referred to as aggregates and have the potential to cause adverse immune responses in patients. There are many forms and sizes of aggregates, and many current methodologies have gaps in their ability to detect different types of aggregates. Our ability to minimize adverse immune reactions would be enhanced if we had improved ability to measure and quantify various types of aggregates.

The field of biopharmaceuticals is rapidly advancing—in many ways more quickly than analytical technologies. New measurement tools and standards would be of value in all areas, particularly, reliable and discriminating material standards that can enhance the use of current methodologies and encourage new technologies to fill current gaps. Moreover, as the field of biopharmaceuticals continues to advance, there is the potential for greater research and development in the evolving area of biosimilar products, which stand to save consumers billions of dollars over time.

3.14 The comparative EMA and FDA mind-set

An analysis of the differences between the FDA and the EMA forms a good basis to understand the complexity of developing biosimilars. While the emphasis in this book is on understanding what the FDA considers to be essential elements of biosimilarity, it is to be expected that companies filing for the FDA approval would also want to secure the EU markets, requiring a planning that will cover the expectations of both agencies. Given in the following is a cursory overview of the mind-sets of the two agencies.

Both the EMA and FDA are continuously evolving their approach to approving biosimilars; the changes in the approval standards will come as a result of the experience of approving these products, their safety market confidence, and also to a better understanding of the science involved in assessing the safety and the effectiveness of these products. It is for this reason that I am calling this *current* mind-set.

- The guiding principle of a biosimilar development program is to establish similarity between the biosimilar and the reference product by the *best possible means*, ensuring that the previously proven safety and efficacy of the reference medicinal product also apply to the biosimilar. [Best possible ways are more clearly identified in the FDA expectations—analytical and functional similarity.]

- A biosimilar should be *highly similar* [exactly what the FDA lists as the minimum level of acceptance; however, EMA fails to provide a tiered approach as the FDA does] to the reference medicinal product in physicochemical and biological terms. Any observed differences have to be duly justified with regard to their potential impact on safety and efficacy. [The FDA calls it "no clinically meaningful difference."]
- A stepwise approach is normally recommended throughout the development program, starting with a comprehensive physicochemical and biological characterization. The extent and nature of the nonclinical in vivo studies and clinical studies to be performed depend on the level of evidence obtained in the previous step(s) including the robustness of the physicochemical, biological, and nonclinical in vitro data [exactly as the FDA recommends].
- Generally, the aim of clinical data is to address slight differences shown at previous steps and to confirm the comparable clinical performance of the biosimilar and the reference product. Clinical data cannot be used to justify substantial differences in quality attributes. [EMA now admits that the role of clinical studies is to address "slight differences" and does not allow the use of clinical studies to overcome the lack of similarity—for the FDA guidance that would require the sponsor to follow the 351(a) route instead.]
- If the biosimilar comparability exercise indicates that there are relevant differences between the intended biosimilar and the reference medicinal product making it unlikely that biosimilarity will eventually be established, a stand-alone development to support a full Marketing Authorization Application should be considered instead [same as FDA, where a 351(a) route is recommended].
- The ultimate goal of the biosimilar comparability exercise is to exclude any relevant differences between the biosimilar and the reference medicinal product. Therefore, studies should be sensitive enough with regard to design, conduct, end points, and/or population to detect such differences. [The FDA uses "no clinically meaningful difference." However, this is a debatable point; for example, while the ADCC may not be relevant to demonstrating similarity, the FDA will still require the biosimilar product to match that, within acceptable limits.]
- In specific circumstances, a confirmatory clinical trial may not be necessary. This requires that similar efficacy and safety can clearly be deduced from the similarity of physicochemical

characteristics, biological activity/potency, and PK and/or PD profiles of the biosimilar and the reference product. In addition, it requires that the impurity profile and the nature of excipients of the biosimilar itself do not give rise to concern. [This is a significant change in the mind-set of EMA and fully matches the FDA expectations. The fact that a limited clinical trial may not provide all attributes required to allow extrapolation makes the clinical trials less useful.]

- The standard generic approach (demonstration of bioequivalence with a reference medicinal product by appropriate bioavailability studies) which is applicable to most chemically-derived medicinal products is in principle not sufficient to demonstrate the similarity of biological/biotechnology-derived products due to their complexity. The biosimilar approach, based on a comprehensive comparability exercise, will then have to be followed. [This is what the FDA requires as well, except that the FDA does not use "comparability," since that is reserved for postapproval changes as provided in the ICH guidance; many writers and agencies make this mistake.]
- The scientific principles of such a biosimilar comparability exercise are based on those applied for evaluation of the impact of changes in the manufacturing process of a biological medicinal product (as outlined in ICH Q5E). [The concept of identifying critical quality attributes (CQAs) is common between the FDA and the EMA; one of the CQAs for these drugs is the protein content; for most generics, the content is not a CQA since it is easily conformed to because of the release range allowance.]
- Whether the biosimilar approach would be applicable to a certain biological medicinal product depends on the state of the art of analytical methods, the manufacturing processes employed, as well as the availability of clinical models to evaluate comparability. [This is an exclusion criterion; however, given the progress made in analytical chemistry of proteins and other complex molecules, this barrier is falling fast; the most significant example is the recent approval of glatiramer acetate (Copaxone equivalent) by FDA, a product that was claimed to be extremely complex and unpredictable and manufactured using a proprietary process.]
- The biosimilar approach is more likely to be successfully applied to products that are highly purified and can be thoroughly characterized (such as many biotechnology-derived medicinal products). The biosimilar approach is more difficult to apply to other types of biological medicinal products, which by their nature are more difficult to characterize, such as biological substances arising from extraction from biological sources and/or those for which little clinical and regulatory experience has been gained. [This remains an issue, and indeed

both agencies refer to highly purified products since they are easier to characterize; however, there is a move through guidance from the FDA on *Complementary and Alternative Medicine Products* that can resolve these uncertainties.]

- The active substance of a biosimilar must be similar, in molecular and biological terms, to the active substance of the reference medicinal product. For example, for an active substance that is a protein, the amino acid sequence is expected to be the same. [This is similar to the FDA's expectation; however, for products like small–molecular weight heparin, EMA may allow similar active pharmaceutical ingredient (API), not necessarily identical, and to support that, EMA will require a clinical trial.]
- The posology and route of administration of the biosimilar must be the same as those of the reference medicinal product. [While this is also a statutory description in the BPCI Act, this restrictions can be challenging to the development of biosimilar products as the originators have begun abusing the IP to protect dosing and indications as well, although many of them will be knocked off through IP rights, yet they create a dilemma that the agencies need to address.]
- Deviations from the reference product as regards strength, pharmaceutical form, formulation, excipients or presentation require justification. If needed, additional data should be provided. Any difference should not compromise safety. [This is not contradictory to the recommendation earlier as it does not affect posology, just the presentation; however, it will likely be challenging, both scientifically as well as in commercial operations, to develop a different product. Sandoz used a different buffer in its product, and this remains a criticism of their GCSF product.]
- Intended changes to improve efficacy (e.g., glycol optimization) are not compatible with the biosimilarity approach. However, differences that could have an advantage as regards safety (for instance lower levels of impurities or lower immunogenicity) should be addressed, but may not preclude biosimilarity. [This position of EMA is confusing as on the one hand, it considers modifications such as PEGylation to be a different product, yet if it improves safety, which PEGylation does, then it leaves room for biosimilar considerations; the FDA is very clear on this—these will be considered a different product, regardless of the impact on safety.]
- The biosimilar shall, with regard to the quality data, fulfill all requirements for Module 3 as defined in Annex I to Directive 2001/83/EC, as amended and satisfy the technical requirements of the European Pharmacopoeia and any additional requirements, such as defined in relevant CHMP [Committee for Medicinal Products for Human Use] and ICH guidelines.

[The FDA does not require compliance with any pharmacopeia and while adherence to ICH guidelines is expected, the FDA generally takes a view that all guidelines are guidance and not a requirement and the filer is allowed to challenge or improve upon them.]

- Comparable safety and efficacy of a biosimilar to its reference product has to be demonstrated or otherwise justified in accordance with the data requirements laid down in Directive 2001/83/EC, as amended. General technical and product-class specific provisions for biosimilars are addressed in EMA/CHMP guidelines. For situations where product-class specific guidance is not available, applicants are encouraged to seek scientific advice from Regulatory Authorities. [The FDA differentiates efficacy from effectiveness; the FDA also does not need any compliance with product-specific guidance as provided by EMA; these are helpful, yet not binding, for U.S. filing.]
- If biosimilarity has been demonstrated in one indication, extrapolation to other indications of the reference product could be acceptable with appropriate scientific justification. [The FDA is more liberal and allows extrapolation without extraordinary justification.]
- There is no regulatory requirement to repeat the demonstration of biosimilarity against the reference product, e.g., in the context of a change in the manufacturing process, once the Marketing Authorization has been granted. [The FDA follows the same process under the Comparability Protocol.]
- In order to support pharmacovigilance monitoring and in accordance with Article 102(e) of Directive 2001/83/EC, as amended, all appropriate measures should be taken to identify clearly any biological medicinal product which is the subject of a suspected adverse reaction report, with due regard to its brand name and batch number. [The FDA follows a similar path.]
- The reference medicinal product must be a medicinal product authorized in the EEA, on the basis of a complete dossier in accordance with the provisions of Article 8 of Directive 2001/83/EC, as amended. [The requirement of complete dossier, meaning full set of clinical trials, will exclude a biosimilar product to emulate another biosimilar product.]
  - A single reference medicinal product, defined on the basis of its marketing authorization in the EEA [European Economic Area], should be used as the comparator throughout the comparability program for quality, safety and efficacy studies during the development of a biosimilar in order to allow the generation of coherent data and conclusions.
- However, with the aim of facilitating the global development of biosimilars and to avoid unnecessary repetition of clinical

trials, it may be possible for an Applicant to compare the biosimilar in certain clinical studies and in in vivo non-clinical studies (where needed) with a non-EEA authorized comparator (i.e., a non-EEA authorized version of the reference medicinal product) which will need to be allowed by a regulatory authority with similar scientific and regulatory standards as EMA (e.g., ICH countries). In addition, it will be the Applicant's responsibility to demonstrate that the comparator authorized outside the EEA is representative of the reference product authorized in the EEA. [This opens the door to use a U.S. product for clinical and in vivo nonclinical studies only—however, all other in vitro similarity testing must still be conducted with an EU-authorized product and if a non-EU reference product is used for clinical trials, then there must be bridging in vitro studies with that product as well. A reciprocal concession is not available in the FDA guidance. See below for specific details.]

- For a demonstration of biosimilar comparability at the quality level, side-by-side analysis of the biosimilar product (from the commercial scale and site) with EEA authorized reference product must be conducted. However, combined use of non-EEA authorized comparator and EEA authorized reference product is acceptable for the development of the Quality Target Product Profile of the biosimilar product.
- If certain clinical and in vivo nonclinical studies of the development program are performed with the non-EEA authorized comparator, the Applicant should provide adequate data or information to justify scientifically the relevance of these comparative data and establish an acceptable bridge to the EEA-authorized reference product. As a scientific matter, the type of bridging data needed will always include data from analytical studies (e.g., structural and functional data) that compare all three products (the proposed biosimilar, the EEA-authorized reference product and the non-EEA-authorized comparator), and may also include data from clinical PK and/or PD bridging studies for all three products. The overall acceptability of such an approach and the type of bridging data needed will be a case-by-case/product-type decision, and is recommended to be discussed upfront with the Regulatory Authorities. However, the final determination of the adequacy of the scientific justification and bridge will only be made during the assessment of the application. [It is noteworthy that in the recent approval of Zarxio, Sandoz provided a bridging comparison of the EU Neupogen versus the U.S. Neupogen; however, the requirement of using the U.S. reference-listed drug was not waived.]

3.15 Pharmacovigilance

Postauthorization pharmacovigilance is considered essential to guarantee the product's safety and efficacy over time; as part of a comprehensive risk management program, this includes regular testing for consistent manufacturing of the drug. The most critical safety concern relating to biopharmaceuticals (including biosimilars) is immunogenicity. Pharmacovigilance is important in the biosimilar market because of the limited ability to predict clinical consequences of seemingly innocuous changes in the manufacturing process and the scientific information gap—an understanding that arose from the example of Eprex, where an otherwise innocuous change in the packaging design resulted in several deaths from pure red cell aplasia. As a consequence, the CHMP guidelines emphasize the need for particular attention to pharmacovigilance, especially to detect rare but serious side effects. Pharmacovigilance systems should differentiate between licensed reference product and biosimilar products so that effects of biosimilars are not lost in the background of reports on licensed reference products. Further, the risk management plans for biosimilars should focus on increasing pharmacovigilance measures, identifying immunogenicity risk, and implementing special postmarketing surveillance.

Biologicals carry specific risks. Safety problems, for example, infliximab and the risk for tuberculosis, have been identified via spontaneous reports of suspected adverse drug reactions (ADRs). Data obtained from the ADR database (VigiBase), maintained by the WHO Collaborating Centre for International Drug Monitoring, indicated that biologicals have a different safety profile compared with all other drugs in the database and, within the group of biological products, differences exist between mechanistic classes. In addition, because not all adverse reactions can be predicted or detected during development, spontaneous reporting remains an important tool for the early detection of signals. Further, pharmacovigilance plans developed and implemented by manufacturers are frequently part of the postapproval commitments to regulatory agencies to provide follow-up safety assessments.

Bibliography

FDA—Guidance for Industry: Assay Development for Immunogenicity Testing of Therapeutic Proteins. http://www.fda.gov/downloads/Drugs/GuidanceComplianceRegulatoryInformation/Guidances/UCM192750.pdf.

FDA—Guidance for Industry: Clinical Pharmacology Data to Support a Demonstration of Biosimilarity to a Reference Product (Draft Guidance). http://www.fda.gov/downloads/Drugs/GuidanceComplianceRegulatoryInformation/Guidances/UCM397017.pdf.

FDA—Guidance for Industry: Comparability Protocols—Chemistry, Manufacturing, and Controls Information. http://www.fda.gov/ucm/groups/fdagov-public/@fdagov-drugs-gen/documents/document/ucm070545.pdf.

FDA—Guidance for Industry: Comparability Protocols Protein Drug Products and Biological Products—Chemistry, Manufacturing, and Controls Information. http://www.fda.gov/ucm/groups/fdagov-public/@fdagov-drugs-gen/documents/document/ucm070262.pdf.

FDA—Guidance for Industry: Cooperative Manufacturing Arrangements for Licensed Biologics. http://www.fda.gov/BiologicsBloodVaccines/GuidanceComplianceRegulatoryInformation/Guidances/General/ucm069883.htm.

FDA—Guidance for Industry for the Submission of Chemistry, Manufacturing, and Controls Information for a Therapeutic Recombinant DNA–Derived Product or a Monoclonal Antibody Product for In Vivo Use. http://www.fda.gov/downloads/BiologicsBloodVaccines/GuidanceComplianceRegulatoryInformation/Guidances/General/UCM173477.pdf.

FDA—Guidance for Industry: Formal Meetings between the FDA and Biosimilar Biological Product Sponsors or Applicants (Draft Guidance). http://www.fda.gov/downloads/Drugs/GuidanceComplianceRegulatoryInformation/Guidances/UCM345649.pdf.

FDA—Guidance for Industry: Non-inferiority Clinical Trials. http://www.fda.gov/downloads/Drugs/GuidanceComplianceRegulatoryInformation/Guidances/UCM202140.pdf.

FDA—Guidance for Industry: Quality Considerations in Demonstrating Biosimilarity to a Reference Protein Product (Draft Guidance). http://www.fda.gov/downloads/Drugs/GuidanceComplianceRegulatoryInformation/Guidances/UCM291134.pdf.

FDA—Biosimilars: Questions and Answers regarding Implementation of the Biologics Price Competition and Innovation Act of 2009 Guidance for Industry. http://www.fda.gov/downloads/Drugs/GuidanceComplianceRegulatoryInformation/Guidances/UCM444661.pdf.

FDA—Guidance for Industry: Reference Product Exclusivity for Biological Products Filed under Section 351(a) of the PHS Act (Draft Guidance). http://www.fda.gov/downloads/Drugs/GuidanceComplianceRegulatoryInformation/Guidances/UCM407844.pdf.

FDA—Guidance for Industry: Scientific Considerations in Demonstrating Biosimilarity to a Reference Product (Draft Guidance). http://www.fda.gov/downloads/Drugs/GuidanceComplianceRegulatoryInformation/Guidances/UCM291128.pdf.

FDA—Points to Consider in the Manufacture and Testing of Monoclonal Antibody Products for Human Use. http://www.gpo.gov/fdsys/granule/FR-1997-02-28/97-5006.

ICH Guidance for Industry M4Q: The CTD—Quality (ICH M4Q) http://www.ich.org/fileadmin/Public_Web_Site/ICH_Products/CTD/M4_R1_Quality/M4Q__R1_.pdf.

ICH Guidance for Industry Q1A(R2): Stability Testing of New Drug Substances and Products (ICH Q1A(R2)). http://www.ich.org/products/guidelines/quality/quality-single/article/stability-testing-of-new-drug-substances-and-products.html.

ICH Guidance for Industry Q2(R1): Validation of Analytical Procedures: Text and Methodology (ICH Q2(R1)). http://www.ich.org/fileadmin/Public_Web_Site/ICH_Products/Guidelines/Quality/Q2_R1/Step4/Q2_R1__Guideline.pdf.

ICH Guidance for Industry Q2B: Validation of Analytical Procedures: Methodology (ICH Q2B). http://www.ich.org/fileadmin/Public_Web_Site/ICH_Products/Guidelines/Quality/Q2_R1/Step4/Q2_R1__Guideline.pdf.

ICH Guidance for Industry Q3A: Impurities in New Drug Substances (ICH Q3A). http://www.ich.org/products/guidelines/quality/quality-single/article/impurities-in-new-drug-substances.html.

ICH Guidance for Industry Q5A: Viral Safety Evaluation of Biotechnology Products Derived from Cell Lines of Human or Animal Origin (ICH Q5A). http://www.ich.org/products/guidelines/quality/quality-single/article/viral-safety-evaluation-of-biotechnology-products-derived-from-cell-lines-of-human-or-animal-origin.html.

ICH Guidance for Industry Q5B: Quality of Biotechnological Products: Analysis of the Expression Construct in Cells Used for Production of r-DNA Derived Protein Products (ICH Q5B). http://www.ich.org/products/guidelines/quality/quality-single/article/analysis-of-the-expression-construct-in-cells-used-for-production-of-r-dna-derived-protein-products.html.

ICH Guidance for Industry Q5C: Quality of Biotechnological Products: Stability Testing of Biotechnological/Biological Products (ICH Q5C). http://www.ich.org/products/guidelines/quality/quality-single/article/stability-testing-of-biotechnologicalbiological-products.html.

ICH Guidance for Industry Q5D: Quality of Biotechnological/Biological Products: Derivation and Characterization of Cell Substrates Used for Production of Biotechnological/Biological Products (ICH Q5D). http://www.ich.org/products/guidelines/quality/quality-single/article/derivation-and-characterisation-of-cell-substrates-used-for-production-of-biotechnologicalbiologica.html.

ICH Guidance for Industry Q5E: Comparability of Biotechnological/Biological Products Subject to Changes in Their Manufacturing Process (ICH Q5E). http://www.ich.org/products/guidelines/quality/quality-single/article/comparability-of-biotechnologicalbiological-products-subject-to-changes-in-their-manufacturing-proc.html.

ICH Guidance for Industry Q6B Specifications: Test Procedures and Acceptance Criteria for Biotechnological/Biological Products (ICH Q6B). http://www.ich.org/products/guidelines/quality/quality-single/article/specifications-test-procedures-and-acceptance-criteria-for-biotechnologicalbiological-products.html.

ICH Guidance for Industry Q7(A): Good Manufacturing Practice Guidance for Active Pharmaceutical Ingredients (ICH Q7A). http://www.ich.org/products/guidelines/quality/article/quality-guidelines.html.

ICH Guidance for Industry Q8(R2): Pharmaceutical Development (ICH Q8(R2)). http://www.ich.org/products/guidelines/quality/quality-single/article/pharmaceutical-development.html.

ICH Guidance for Industry Q9: Quality Risk Management (ICH Q9). http://www.ich.org/products/guidelines/quality/quality-single/article/quality-risk-management.html.

ICH Guidance for Industry Q10: Pharmaceutical Quality System (ICH Q10). http://www.ich.org/products/guidelines/quality/quality-single/article/pharmaceutical-quality-system.html.

ICH Guidance for Industry Q11: Development and Manufacture of Drug Substances (ICH Q11). http://www.ich.org/products/guidelines/quality/quality-single/article/development-and-manufacture-of-drug-substances.html.

ICH Guidance for Industry S6(R1): Preclinical Safety Evaluation of Biotechnology-Derived Pharmaceuticals (ICH S6(R1)). http://www.ich.org/products/guidelines/safety/safety-single/article/preclinical-safety-evaluation-of-biotechnology-derived-pharmaceuticals.html.

Chapter 4 Understanding biosimilarity

Love is the power to see the similarity in the dissimilar.

Theodor Adorno

4.1 Background

The main intent of the BPCI Act is to reduce the cost of development of biosimilar products; the highest-cost line item is clinical trials in patients; as a result, if the "safety, purity, and potency" of a biosimilar candidate can be established without testing it in patients, then there is no need for clinical trials—this is position that the FDA takes.

While Europe has been approving biosimilars for several years, the approach taken to approve these products has been more conservative and less structured; now that the FDA has approved its first biosimilar product, there is some clarity; still this is a beginning of a long road of difficulties in understanding what is meant by biosimilarity. How similar is similar? And does one predict the requirements that the FDA might impose on demonstrating biosimilarity?

This chapter deals with developing an understanding about biosimilarity as expressed by the FDA in its publications, guidances, and regulatory documents that the FDA shared with the public. In addition, this understanding is further based on face-to-face meetings that the author has held with the FDA in seeking clarification about this topic.

4.1.1 Definitions

A biosimilar product is defined by regulatory agencies as the following:

- FDA: The product is highly similar to the reference product notwithstanding minor differences in clinically inactive components, and there are no clinically meaningful differences between the biological product and the reference product in terms of safety, purity, and potency of the product.
- EMA: A biosimilar medicine is a biological medicine that is developed to be similar to an existing biological medicine (the *reference medicine*). Like the reference medicine, the biosimilar has a degree of natural variability. When approved, its

variability and any differences between it and its reference medicine will have been shown not to affect safety or effectiveness.
- WHO: A biotherapeutic product, which is similar in terms of quality, safety, and efficacy to an already-licensed reference biotherapeutic product.

Both WHO and EMA require a product to be *similar*, while the FDA requires them to be at least *highly similar* to qualify as a biosimilar. Regarding the variability, the FDA states "no clinically meaningful difference ... in terms of safety, purity and potency," and the EMA states "its variability ... not to affect safety or effectiveness." The WHO emphasizes "quality, safety and efficacy," and makes the description more confounding than what is suggested by the FDA and the EMA. These subtle differences are important in understanding the mind-set of these agencies. Both the FDA and the EMA shun from using *quality*, which is a broad and perhaps an assumptive term. The FDA stays away from *effectiveness* or *efficacy*, while both the EMA and WHO emphasize it, although differently. It should be noted that the correct description is effectiveness that is demonstrated by comparison, whereas efficacy is a controlled clinical trial outcome against a placebo. Effectiveness can be shown by many methods including patient trials; efficacy is generally proven in patients only. This subtle difference is missed out in the WHO definition and in the guidelines of several other countries.

Recent draft guidance issued by the EMA (October 2014) brings the EMA closer to the thinking of the FDA to allow as many approvals without clinical trials in patients when justified. The rhetoric of the originators that extensive clinical trials are the only way to establish safety and efficacy (effectiveness) of biosimilar products is being set aside by the regulatory agencies. However, the onus of proving that a clinical trial is not needed, or only minimal trials are sufficient, lies on the sponsor of the biosimilar product, and it is, for this reason, the understanding of the science and the art involved in establishing evidence of biosimilarity is crucial for success.

4.2 The FDA mind-set

The BPCI Act of 2009 was passed as part of health reform (ACA) that President Obama signed into law on March 23, 2010. The BPCI Act creates an abbreviated licensure pathway for biological products shown to be biosimilar to or interchangeable with an FDA-licensed reference product. A biological product that is demonstrated to be highly similar to an FDA-licensed biological product (the reference product) may rely on licensure, among other things, publicly available information regarding the FDA's previous determination that the reference product is safe, pure, and potent. This licensure pathway permits a biosimilar biological product to be licensed under 351(k) of the PHSA based on less than a full complement of product-specific preclinical and clinical data.

4.2.1 The FDA defines biosimilars or biosimilarity

- The biological product is highly similar to the reference product notwithstanding minor differences in clinically inactive components.
- There are no clinically meaningful differences between the biological product and the reference product in terms of safety, purity, and potency of the product.

4.2.2 What reference product means

- The single biological product, licensed under Section 351(a) of the PHSA, against which a biological product is evaluated in an application submitted under Section 351(k) of the PHSA.

Note: A biological product, in a 351(k) application, may not be evaluated against more than one reference product.

4.2.3 What interchangeable or interchangeability means

- The biological product is biosimilar to the reference product.
- It can be expected to produce the same clinical result as the reference product in any given patient.
- For a product that is administered more than once to an individual, the risk in terms of safety or diminished efficacy of alternating or switching between use of the product and its reference product is not greater than the risk of using the reference product without such alternation or switch.

Note: The interchangeable product may be substituted for the reference product without the intervention of the healthcare provider who prescribed the reference product.

4.2.4 351(k) application content

A 351(k) application must include information demonstrating the following:

- The biological product is biosimilar to a reference product.
- The biological product utilizes the same MOAs for the proposed conditions of use—but only to the extent that the mechanisms are known for the reference product.
- The biological product's conditions of use proposed in labeling have been previously approved for the reference product.

- The biological product has the same route of administration, dosage form, and strength as the reference product.
- The biological product is manufactured, processed, packed, or held in a facility that meets standards designed to assure that the biological product continues to be safe, pure, and potent.

4.2.5 351(k) information on biosimilarity

The PHSA requires that a 351(k) application include, among other things, information demonstrating biosimilarity based on data derived from the following:

- Analytical studies demonstrating that the biological product is highly similar to the reference product notwithstanding minor differences in clinically inactive components
- Animal studies (including the assessment of toxicity)
- A clinical study or studies (including the assessment of immunogenicity and PK or PD) that are sufficient to demonstrate safety, purity, and potency in one or more appropriate conditions of use for which the reference product is licensed and for which licensure is sought for the biosimilar product

Note: The FDA may determine, in its discretion, that an element described above is unnecessary in a 351(k) application.

4.2.6 Licensure

The FDA shall license the biological product under Section 351(k) of the PHSA if the FDA determines that the information submitted in the application (or supplement) is sufficient to show that

- The biological product is biosimilar to the reference product; or
- The biological product meets the standards described in 351(k)(4) and is, therefore, interchangeable with the reference product; and
- The applicant (or another appropriate person) consents to the inspection of the facility, in accordance with Section 351(c).

Note: The BPCI Act does not require that the FDA promulgate guidance or regulation before reviewing or approving a 351(k) application.

4.2.7 Reference product

The PHSA defines the *reference product* for a 351(k) application as the "single biological product licensed under section 351(a) against which a biological product is evaluated."

- Data from animal studies and certain clinical studies comparing a proposed biosimilar product with a non-U.S.-licensed product may be used to support a demonstration of biosimilarity to a U.S.-licensed reference product.

- The sponsor should provide adequate data or information to scientifically justify the relevance of these comparative data to an assessment of biosimilarity and to establish an acceptable bridge to the U.S.-licensed reference product.

4.2.8 Nonlicensed product

The support for the use of non-U.S.-licensed comparator requires bridging data that would include the following:

- Direct physicochemical comparison of all three products (proposed biosimilar to U.S.-licensed reference product; proposed biosimilar to non-U.S.-licensed comparator product; U.S.-licensed reference product to non-U.S.-licensed comparator product)
- Likely three-way bridging clinical PK and/or PD study
- All three pairwise comparisons meeting prespecified acceptance criteria for analytical and PK and/or PD similarities

4.2.9 The FDA guidance

- The FDA guidance focuses on therapeutic protein products.
- The FDA guidance discusses general scientific principles.
- The FDA guidance outlines a stepwise approach to generating data and the evaluation of residual uncertainty at each step.
- The FDA guidance introduces the totality-of-the-evidence approach.

4.2.10 The key development concepts

The goals of stand-alone and biosimilar developments are different.

- The goal of stand-alone development is to demonstrate that the proposed product is safe and efficacious.
- Drug development starts with preclinical research, moves to phases 1 and 2, and culminates in phase 3 pivotal trials to show safety and efficacy.
- The goal is to demonstrate biosimilarity between the proposed product and a reference product.
- The goal is not to independently establish safety and effectiveness of the proposed product.

4.2.11 Stepwise approach

The FDA has outlined a stepwise approach to generating data in support of a demonstration of biosimilarity:

- Evaluation of residual uncertainty at each step
- Totality-of-the-evidence approaches in evaluating biosimilarity
- Establishing that there is no one pivotal study that demonstrates biosimilarity

- Application of a stepwise approach to data generation and the evaluation of residual uncertainty
- Evaluation and understanding of the question being answered when considering designing a study:
  - What is the residual uncertainty?
  - What differences have been observed and how to best evaluate the potential impact?
  - What will the data tell you? Will it answer the question?

4.2.12 Totality of the evidence

- No "one-size-fits-all" assessment
- The FDA scientists will evaluate the applicant's integration of various types of information to provide an overall assessment that a biological product is a biosimilar to a U.S.-licensed reference product

4.2.13 Analytical similarity data

- The foundation of a biosimilar development program
- Extensive structural and functional characterization, which is necessary
- Understanding the molecule and function
- Identifying critical quality attributes (CQAs) and clinically active components
- Understanding the relationship between the quality attributes and the clinical safety and efficacy profiles to determine if any residual uncertainty about biosimilarity remains; this allows prediction of clinical similarity from the quality data

4.2.14 Generating analytical similarity data

- Characterize reference product variability and product quality characteristics
- Characterize proposed biosimilar product quality characteristics
- Identify and evaluate the impact of differences
  - The potential effect of the differences in safety, purity, and potency should be addressed and supported by appropriate data
  - The biological products must be highly similar and have no clinically meaningful differences

4.2.15 Assessing analytical similarity

Critical factors for consideration in assessing analytical similarity include the following:

- Expression system
- Manufacturing process

- Assessment of physicochemical properties
- Functional activities
- Receptor-binding and immunochemical properties
- Impurities
- Reference product and reference standards
- Finished drug product
- Stability

4.2.16 Choice of analytics

It is expected that appropriate analytical test methods will be selected based on the following:

- The nature of the protein being characterized
- The knowledge regarding the structure
- The heterogeneity of the reference product and the proposed biosimilar product including the following:
  - Known and potential impurities
  - Characteristics that are critical to product performance

4.2.17 Analytical tools

A variety of tools is available to characterize proteins, more particularly testing biosimilars side by side as suggested by the FDA (Figure 4.1).

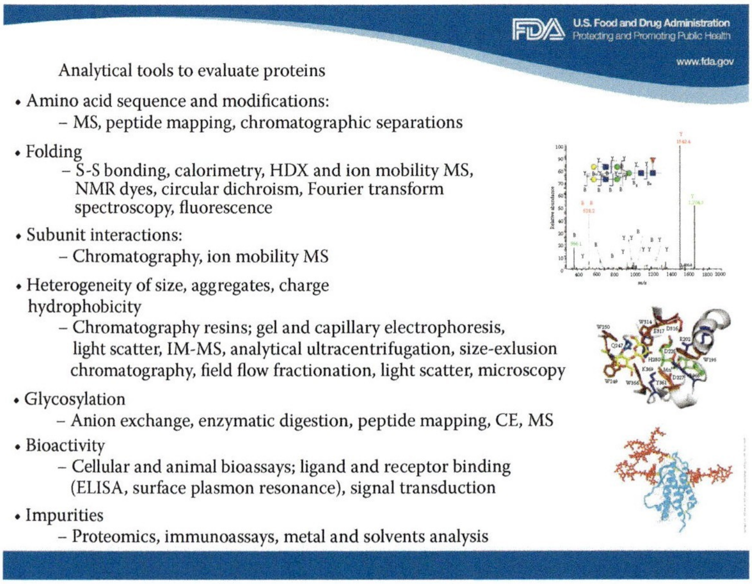

Figure 4.1 Analytical tools to support biosimilarity. (Courtesy of FDA, Silver Spring, MD.)

4.2.18 Animal data

Animal toxicity data are useful when uncertainties remain about the safety of the proposed product prior to initiating clinical studies.

- The scope and the extent of animal toxicity studies will depend on publicly available information and/or data submitted in the biosimilar application regarding the reference product and the proposed biosimilar product, and the extent of known similarities or differences between the two.
- A comparison of PK/PD in an animal model may be useful.

4.2.19 Clinical studies

The nature and the scope of clinical studies will depend on the extent of residual uncertainty about the biosimilarity of the two products after conducting extensive structural and functional characterizations and, where relevant, animal studies.

4.2.20 Type of clinical data

- As a scientific matter, the FDA expects an adequate clinical PK, and PD if relevant, comparison between the proposed biosimilar product and the reference product.
- As a scientific matter, at least one clinical study that includes a comparison of the immunogenicity of the proposed and reference products will be generally expected.
- As a scientific matter, a comparative clinical study will be necessary to support a demonstration of biosimilarity if there are residual uncertainties about whether there are clinically meaningful differences between the proposed and reference products based on structural and functional characterizations, animal testing, human PK and PD data, and clinical immunogenicity assessment.

4.2.21 Comparative human PK and PD data

- Demonstrate PK (and PD) similarity.
- Assess clinically meaningful differences between the proposed biosimilar and the reference products.
- PK and/or PD is generally considered the most sensitive clinical study/assay in which to assess for differences, should they exist.
- Support a demonstration of biosimilarity with the assumption that similar exposure (and PD response) provides similar efficacy and safety (i.e., an exposure–response relationship exists).
- Clinical PK data generally will be expected; PD data are desirable (case-by-case consideration).

4.2.22 Human PK and PD study considerations

- Study design
  - Study population: Study population is an adequately sensitive population to detect any differences, should they exist
  - PD end point: PD end point reflects the biological effects of the drug, they may (or may not) be on mechanistic path of MOA or disease process
  - Route of administration: All routes versus a single route
- Data analysis plan
  - Acceptance range: 80%–125% (90% confidence interval [CI] for PK and PD), scientifically justify use of other ranges
  - Choice of primary end points (e.g., PK—AUC, C_{max}; PD—area under the effect curve [AUEC])
- Others
  - Incidence of immunogenicity

4.2.23 Comparative clinical study considerations

- A comparative clinical study of a biosimilar development program should be designed to investigate whether there are clinically meaningful differences between the proposed product and the reference product.
- Consider the adequacy of the population, sample size, and study duration to detect differences, should they exist.
- The goal of the study is to support a demonstration of no clinically meaningful differences.
- Typically, an equivalence design with symmetric inferiority and superiority margins would be used, but other designs may be justified depending on product-specific and program-specific considerations.

4.2.24 Totality of the evidence

Based on the definition of the BPCI Act, biosimilarity requires that there are no clinically meaningful differences in terms of safety, purity, and potency. Safety could include PK and PD, safety and tolerability, and immunogenicity studies. Purity includes all CQAs during manufacturing process. Potency is referred to as efficacy studies. In the 2015 FDA draft guidance on scientific considerations, the FDA recommends that a stepwise approach be considered for providing the totality of the evidence to demonstrating biosimilarity of a proposed biosimilar product as compared to a reference product.

The stepwise approach starts with analytical studies for structural and functional characterizations (Figure 4.2). The stepwise approach continues with animal studies for toxicity and clinical pharmacology studies

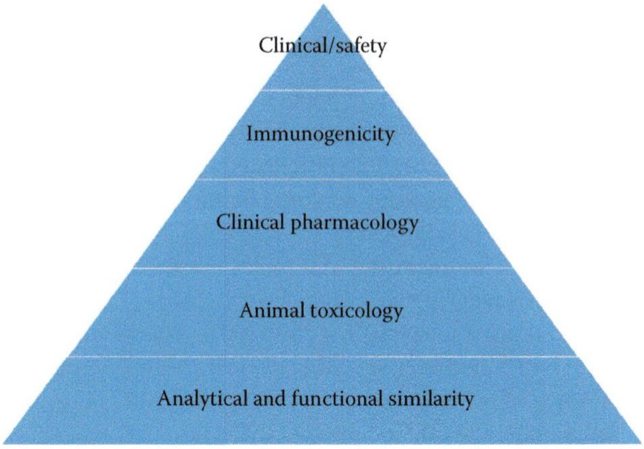

Figure 4.2 Totality of the evidence to demonstrate biosimilarity. Highly similar analytical and PK/PD data assume lower risk of clinical differences.

such as PK/PD studies, followed by investigations of immunogenicity, and clinical studies for safety/tolerability and efficacy.

The sponsors are encouraged to consult with medical/statistical reviewers of the FDA with the proposed plan or strategy of the stepwise approach to a regulatory agreement and acceptance. This is to make sure that the information provided is sufficient to fulfill the FDA's requirement for providing the totality of the evidence for the demonstration of biosimilarity of the proposed biosimilar product as compared to the reference product. As an example, more precisely, the analytical studies are to assess the similarity in CQAs at various stages of the manufacturing process of the biosimilar product as compared to those of the reference product. To assist the sponsors to fulfill the regulatory requirement for providing the totality of the evidence of analytical similarity, the FDA suggests several approaches depending on the criticality of the identified quality attributes relevant to the clinical outcomes.

4.2.25 Extrapolation

- The potential exists for a biosimilar product to be approved for one or more conditions of use for which the U.S.-licensed reference product is licensed based on extrapolation of data intended to demonstrate biosimilarity in one condition of use.
- Sufficient scientific justification for extrapolating data is necessary.

4.2.26 Extrapolation considerations

The FDA guidance outlines factors/issues that should be considered when providing scientific justification for extrapolation including, for example (as a subset of the issued described in the FDA guidance document),

- The MOA(s) in each condition of use for which licensure is sought;
- The PK and the biodistribution of the product in different patient populations;
- The immunogenicity of the product in various patient populations; and
- Differences in expected toxicities in each condition of use and patient population.
- Differences between conditions of use do not necessarily preclude extrapolation.

4.2.27 Summary of key concepts

- Demonstrating biosimilarity is different from stand-alone product development.
  - A stand-alone-like program will not demonstrate biosimilarity.
  - The approach and the development program should and will be different based on the intended outcome to demonstrate biosimilarity.
- Analytical similarity data are the foundation for biosimilar development.
  - Understanding the relationship between the quality attributes and the clinical safety and efficacy profiles helps in enhancing the ability to determine residual uncertainty about biosimilarity and to predict expected clinical similarity from the quality data.
- The nature and the scope of clinical studies will depend on the extent of residual uncertainty about the biosimilarity of the two products after conducting an extensive analytical similarity assessment.
- Comparative clinical studies will be necessary to support a demonstration of biosimilarity if there are residual uncertainties about whether there are clinically meaningful differences between the proposed biosimilar and reference products.
- Scientific justification must be provided to support extrapolation to other conditions of use.
- The content of a biosimilar development program is based on stepwise development, and approvability is based on the totality of the evidence submitted by the sponsor.

4.3 Similarity concept

Drugs for human and animal use can be generally divided into two broad categories: fixed structure ingredients (FSIs) or variable structure entities (VSEs). The former category mainly includes synthesized drugs with a unitary structure; the latter category mainly includes biological and complex synthetic drugs such as cytokines, mAbs, short-chain heparin, and glatiramer acetate as examples. However, the regulatory approval of new biological drugs goes through a BLA process, even though some have been approved under NDA. All FSIs have been approved under NDA.

The NDA classification is further divided into three categories. Section 505 of the act describes three types of NDAs: (a) an application that contains full reports of investigations of safety and effectiveness (Section 505(b)(1)); (b) an application that contains full reports of investigations of safety and effectiveness but where at least some of the information required for approval comes from studies not conducted by or for the applicant and for which the applicant has not obtained a right of reference (Section 505(b)(2)); and (c) an application that contains information to show that the proposed product is identical in active ingredient, dosage form, strength, route of administration, labeling, quality, performance characteristics, and intended use, among other things, to a previously approved product (Section 505(j)). A supplement to an application is an NDA.

The drugs approved under BLA are classified into two categories: (a) 351(a), which is a full application compared to Section 505(b)(1), and (b) 351(k), which is a comparable hybrid of 505(b)(2) and 505(j). Both NDA and BLA are handled by CDER but only for following the biologic drugs. Only therapeutic biological products are filed with CDER; others go to CBER:

- mAbs for in vivo use
- Cytokines, growth factors, enzymes, immunomodulators, and thrombolytic
- Proteins intended for therapeutic use that are extracted from animals or microorganisms, including recombinant versions of these products (except clotting factors)
- Other nonvaccine therapeutic immunotherapies

Table 4.1 provides a broader comparison of biological drugs versus chemical drugs for a demonstration of equivalence.

Since the manufacturing of biological drugs involves a living entity, the expression of these molecules always results in a VSE, not an FSI. It is for this reason that they may not be called identical, only similar. Biosimilarity, demonstration of similarity in clinical and safety response, is not analogous to *bioequivalence*, a term that has long been in use to describe generic FSIs; bioequivalence assumes the same availability of drug at the site of action (the statutory definition) and, therefore, the same action (a physiological presumption). Biosimilarity, on the other hand, assumes sufficient similarity in structure, function, PK and PD properties, immunogenicity, side effects, and, where necessary, clinical effectiveness to declare biosimilarity.

Table 4.1 Comparison of Biological Drugs and Chemical Drugs for Regulatory Equivalence Determination Criteria under the FDA Approvals

Equivalence Attribute	Chemical Drugs—505(j)	Biological Products—351(k)
Chemical equivalence	Yes	No; variations similar to originator molecule allowed
Pharmaceutical equivalence	Yes; Q/Q compliance required	No; different formulations allowed
PK equivalence of 80%–125%	Yes, unless waived for certain class of drugs and parenteral dosage forms	Yes, regardless of the delivery mode
PD equivalence in healthy subjects	No	Yes, unless a suitable model is not available such as for mAbs
MoA-based evaluation	No	Yes; risk factors are determined based on MoA
Head-to-head testing with a reference product for analytical similarity, stability, nonclinical attributes	No, except for release attributes where compendia standards are not available	Yes
Tier-based statistical analysis of CQAs	No	Yes; CQAs may not show a difference of more than ($\sigma R/8$); CQA determined based on risk factors
Immunogenicity evaluation	No	Yes, both at the nonclinical stage, if conducted, and at the clinical pharmacology level; healthy subjects are better suited for this testing unless disease state impacts PK/PD
Finished product safety attributes	No, unless product packaging affects safety	Yes; alternate formulations and devices are allowed, and their impact on safety should be determined
Nonclinical	Yes, unless classified as *generally recognized as safe* or waived	Yes, only if a suitable model is available; generally, it is not suitable for mAbs unless residual uncertainty remains in analytical similarity
Clinical effectiveness	No; in some limited cases for complex molecular mixtures	No, unless PD evaluation based on MoA does not remove any residual uncertainty; varies widely among agencies
Biosimilarity tiers	No	Yes
Bioequivalence	Yes	No

A significant understanding of the FDA expectation comes from what the Agency expects to be demonstrated at the IND and the subsequent stages. Figure 4.3 shows the expectations of the FDA for new biological drugs and Figure 4.4 displays the expectations for proposed biosimilars.

It is noteworthy that the structural characterization requirement is less robust for new entities; the same goes for the use of qualified or validated test methods to establish the stability of the product for biosimilars. The characterization and the demonstration of analytical similarity go on until the 351(k) application is filed.

4.4 Stages of analytical similarity

"Analytical studies provide the foundation for an assessment of the proposed protein product for submission ..." and include "analytical studies

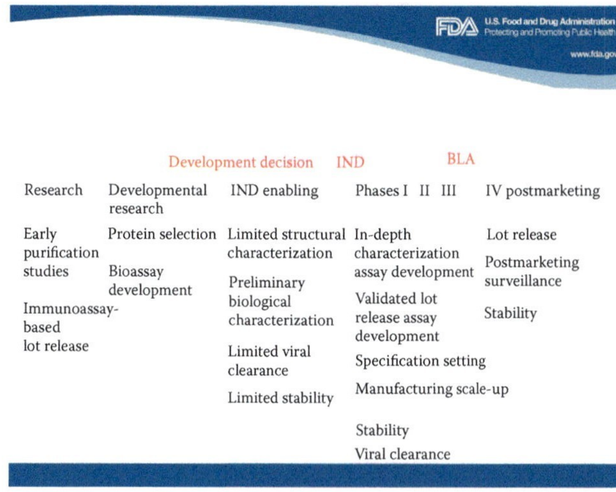

Figure 4.3 The FDA expectations of data required for IND filing and subsequent phases for a new biological entity. (From FDA—Biosimilars: An Update—Focused on Quality Considerations, http://www.fda.gov/downloads/AdvisoryCommittees/CommitteesMeetingMaterials/Drugs/AdvisoryCommitteeforPharmaceuticalScienceandClinicalPharmacology/UCM315764.pdf.)

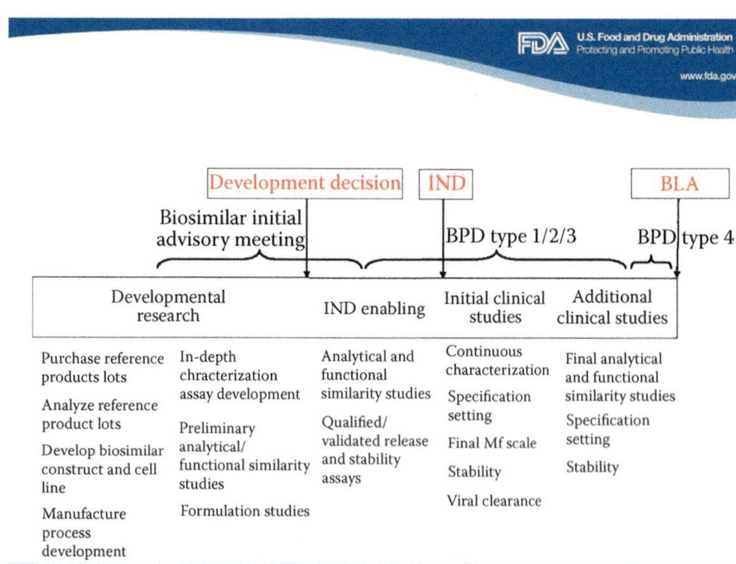

Figure 4.4 The FDA expectations of data required for IND filing and subsequent phases for a new biosimilar candidate. (From FDA—Biosimilars: An Update—Focused on Quality Considerations, http://www.fda.gov/downloads/AdvisoryCommittees/CommitteesMeetingMaterials/Drugs/AdvisoryCommitteeforPharmaceuticalScienceandClinicalPharmacology/UCM315764.pdf.)

that demonstrate that the biological product is highly similar to the reference product notwithstanding minor differences in clinically inactive components" (*FDA Guidance for Industry Quality Considerations in Demonstrating Biosimilarity to Reference Protein Product*, 2012).

A 351(k) application in the United States and similar applications in Europe and other developed countries must contain, among other things, information demonstrating that the proposed product is biosimilar to a reference product based on data derived from analytical studies, animal studies, and a clinical study or studies, unless the FDA determines, in its discretion, that certain studies are unnecessary in a 351(k) application. The goal of a biosimilar development program is thus to demonstrate that the proposed product is biosimilar to the reference product. The overall plan for developing a case of biosimilarity involves the following:

- Stage 1: Analytical and functional similarity: A large number of tests are currently available, and many more are appearing in the literature that can be used to demonstrate the level of similarity. The goal of the biosimilar product development is to create a battery of orthogonal tests that qualifies the product for the category fingerprint-like similarity, wherein the need for any additional testing such as trials in patients is obviated.
- Stage 2: Preclinical or nonclinical safety: Once an acceptable level of analytical and functional similarity has been established, the sponsor should consult with the agencies on the need for this testing and the extent of testing. There is a new consensus developing in the regulatory agencies that purports to avoid any animal testing unless it provides any useful safety information. The nonclinical study must be conducted in species that show safety signals similar or proportional to humans; therefore, it is possible that for some drugs like mAbs, no animal species may be suitable. When a new drug is developed, several animal species are used as the MOA and the safety profile is not known, but for biosimilar products, the comparison with reference product requires species capable of showing an adverse response. This distinction is important to avoid initiating studies similar to what the originator had conducted. The species must be meaningful, and this requires a discussion with regulatory agencies before starting these studies. For example, while rats constitute an excellent species to demonstrate the safety of filgrastim, for adalimumab, only PK studies in a couple of monkeys may be required if the biosimilar product is not structurally and functionally highly similar.
- Stage 3: Clinical pharmacology: The routine PK/PD studies in healthy subjects or where necessary, in patients, is required by all agencies. There is, however, sufficient room for negotiating the size of these trials that may include selecting only the doses within a linear range, avoiding multiple-dose studies and using

creative statistical models to design trials to reduce the number of the subject required. The clinical pharmacology studies also serve the purpose of evaluating safety and immunogenicity; the adverse events recorded in these studies are of high value in establishing biosimilarity. Monitoring antibodies in these studies further supports immunogenicity comparisons.

- Stage 4: Clinical trials in patients: These may be required in two instances, first, when the regulatory agencies are not convinced of the similarity of the product, leaving sufficient residual uncertainty, and second, where PD studies are not meaningful in healthy subjects and these are linked to the safety of the product. Even when conducted, these clinical studies in patients are limited to a single indication and in the easiest population to recruit, reducing the burden of cost and time for the biosimilar product developer; however, it requires a lot of scientific finesse on the part of the sponsor to secure concessions from the regulatory agencies on their clinical trial protocols.
- Stage 5: Postmarket surveillance: Postmarket surveillance is required in EU, but the FDA is flexible, and it may not be necessary; under risk evaluation and mitigation strategies, the FDA will declare what, if any, surveillance studies are needed. The developer may, however, want to conduct open-label studies postapproval to support its marketing plans. Once it is approved, the biosimilar product need not revert to the reference product for any similarity studies, except where it is desired for marketing purposes.

4.5 Levels of similarity

Until the FDA took a giant step in 2014 to define various levels of similarity leading to biosimilarity, the standard of biosimilarity needed for approval was somewhat vague. Figure 4.5 shows a tier-based definition

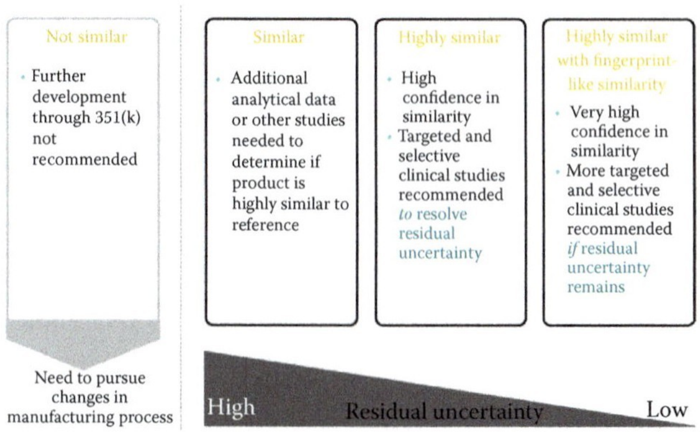

Figure 4.5 Confidence-based levels of biosimilarity.

of biosimilarity as suggested by the FDA. The specific language used to describe each tier is pivotal in understanding the regulatory consequences.

4.5.1 Level 1: Not similar

At Level 1, the functional similarity is not in line with the reference product. This includes bioassays, in vitro binding tests, glycan patterns, and immunogenicity profile for products for which immunogenicity is a concern. The determination by the Agency whether a product is not similar can be challenged by the sponsor, but it will require extensive toxicology studies and other nonclinical evaluations, many of which may be difficult to plan in the absence of an understood MOA. For example, mAbs are difficult to evaluate at the nonclinical testing level because of lack of a suitable toxicology model in common species used for such studies. The developer needs to evaluate the cost of challenging this tier status vis-à-vis the cost of a 351(a) filing.

4.5.2 Level 2: Not highly similar

This tier stipulates "additional analytical or other data needed to determine if the product is not highly similar to the reference." This discussion with the Agency will likely take place in a Type 2 meeting where the sponsor presents an orthogonal evaluation of the biosimilar candidate comparing it with the reference product. Whereas it is not the expectation that all orthogonal tests will provide an equal level of similarity, the purpose of this classification is to encourage the sponsor to move to the highly similar tier, the minimum tier required to be classified as a biosimilar product.

The developer would be required to present a detailed plan of testing that is expected to provide confidence that the product can be classified as Level 3, and any differences that are observed are not clinically meaningful. This judgment is subject to interpretation and highly determined by the anticipated clinical responses. In those instances where the product is administered on a chronic basis, the residual uncertainty can be reduced by conducting protocols that require switching between the reference and the test products, particularly in animal models, to demonstrate that any functional dissimilarity is not clinically meaningful.

Generally, the product must meet most of the primary, secondary, and tertiary structural similarities and most of the functional similarity. The additional studies as recommended are intended to support the assertion that the observed variability is not exacerbating any toxic or immunogenic response and that repeated use will not result in a noticeable inferior clinical response.

In all instances, these additional tests will depend on the type of product, such as cytokine versus mAb, and will incur the substantial additional expense to prove similarity.

If the differences identified are related to the process such as the variability in the size-exclusion chromatography or the analytical centrifugation, these can be corrected with appropriate formulation changes; it is noteworthy that the Agency does not require the Q1-/Q2-type similarity of formulation common for small-molecule drugs. Realizing that the formulations of biological drugs may be under IP protection, the Agency welcomes alternate formulations as long as these do not require changing the dose or the indication. For example, an alternate route, for example, subcutaneous dosing in place of intravenous, will be a major change and does not fall within the category or similarity evaluation. The first biosimilar approved by FDA, Zarxio, has a different buffer formulation than its reference product, Neupogen.

4.5.3 Level 3: Highly similar

Level 3 is the minimal level that the Agency requires for a biosimilar candidate. At this point, there is high confidence in similarity in both the analytical and the functional level and further development requires securing the approval for targeted and selective clinical studies to resolve residual uncertainty. It is this residual uncertainty that needs to be understood. The uncertainty begins with first not being able to understand the source of dissimilarity. For example, if there are process-related impurities that are indigenous to any acceptable process changes, these must be fully characterized and proven to be clinically not meaningful.

In those instances where the functionality profile is not identical to in vitro bioassays or other binding assays, the Agency may require an abbreviated study to show that these differences are not impacting the efficacy or the toxicity. It is understood at this stage that any clinical studies suggested will be abbreviated, and this may not require patient participation or even efficacy trials. If suitable PD profiles are available in healthy subjects, these should be evaluated first.

In some instance, such as in the case of mAbs, the nonclinical profiling is highly species dependent, reducing the value of animal testing to reduce uncertainty. However, where robust models are available to resolve the uncertainty issues with animal studies, these should be suggested.

4.5.4 Level 4: Highly similar with fingerprint-like similarity

When proven to qualify for a Level 4 classification, the sponsor has already proven it to be biosimilar by the first part of the level description: "highly similar." Now if the data presented across an orthogonally planned evaluation that all parameter studies are fully reproducible in the biosimilar candidate, more targeted studies may be required, "if residual uncertainty" remains. The last part of the definition is crucial to developing biosimilar products. What this classification means is that if the product is similar to fingerprint-like comparisons, no further studies may be required if the similarity data removes residual uncertainty.

It is important, therefore, to understand what constitutes residual uncertainty. As discussed earlier, any uncertain or unexpected observation about the product creates a residual or remaining uncertainty. Note that it is not the uncertainty or the unexpected observations but that these remain uncertain is the focus of description. For example, if the biosimilar candidate shows extra chromatography peaks that are fully identified and are established to not impact the structure of the protein at any level, then these do not remain residually uncertain.

4.6 Fingerprint similarity

The regulatory guidance provided by the FDA has always been evolutionary and in some instances revolutionary—in the case of biosimilars, it is the latter; the concept of biosimilarity is based on the scientific rationale that has evolved, yet still questioned by many. A good example of how the FDA, unlike any other regulatory agency in the world, takes a bold step is exemplified by the example of the approval of low–molecular weight heparin (LMWH). The product was approved without any phase 3 clinical trials, despite the hue and cry by the originator of the product (meaning several citizens' petitions, extensive press coverage to clinicians to confuse the science, and commercial efforts to protect a multibillion dollar franchise).

The FDA stated that

> the EMA has set guidelines for LMWH products such as enoxaparin that only require the products to contain a similar (as opposed to the same) active ingredient to that contained in another already marketed LMWH product. Because the proposed LMWH product in Europe will contain an active ingredient that is similar to (as opposed to the same as) the brand name product, there might be uncertainties as to whether the two products are the same with regard to safety and effectiveness. Thus, sponsors of a similar enoxaparin product under the EMA framework are expected to provide clinical studies showing comparable effectiveness to the proposed similar LMWH product as well as clinical data showing comparable safety (including with respect to Heparin Induced Thrombocytopenia).
>
> In contrast, the FDA requires a generic enoxaparin product to contain the same active ingredient as Lovenox. Based on the FDA's scientific experience and expertise, and relevant scientific information, the FDA has concluded that the five criteria (see response to Q#8) are sufficient to ensure that the generic enoxaparin product has the same active ingredient as Lovenox. The FDA also evaluates impurities in the generic enoxaparin product, particularly with respect to their effect on immunogenicity. With the FDA approach, there is no scientific need to perform additional clinical studies to demonstrate equivalence of clinical effectiveness and

> safety of generic enoxaparin to Lovenox. Although the EMA Guideline requires clinical studies to demonstrate comparable effectiveness to a similar LMWH, the FDA notes that its approach (i.e., the five criteria) is more sensitive to differences between two enoxaparin products than the clinical studies recommended in the EMA guideline.
>
> Thus, sponsors of a similar enoxaparin product under the EMA framework are expected to provide clinical studies showing comparable effectiveness to the proposed similar LMWH product as well as clinical data showing comparable safety (including with respect to Heparin Induced Thrombocytopenia).

Figure 4.6 shows the five criteria used in the approval of enoxaparin to show its fingerprint-like similarity.

The reason why I provided the example of enoxaparin, which is not a protein, is because this product is at least as equally complex as proteins, perhaps more, when we look at the simple proteins as filgrastim and growth hormone.

No other regulatory agency in the world allows two levels of approval of biosimilars—biosimilars and interchangeable biosimilars. A significant market advantage can be gained if a product is approved as interchangeable. In most cases, the sponsor reaching this level of similarity will be able to request a waiver of any further clinical trials in patients and in most cases in healthy subjects. This has long been the goal of many regulatory agencies and, in its true expression, holds the promise to reduce

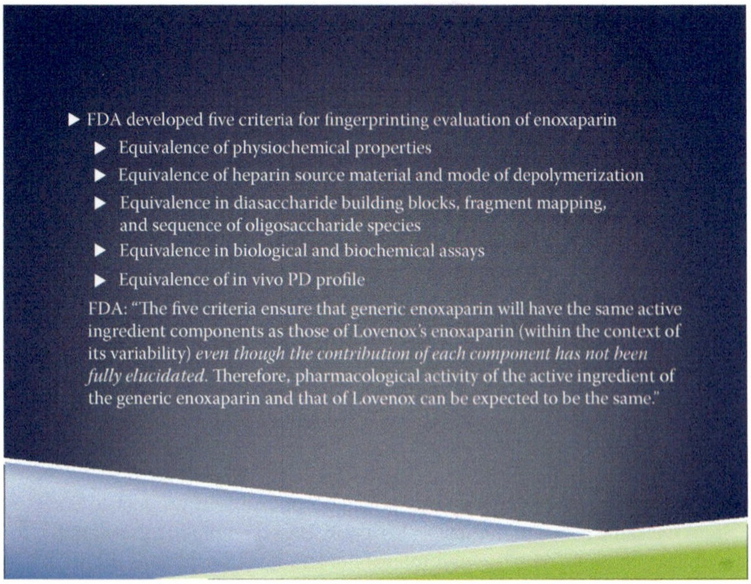

Figure 4.6 Fingerprinting and enoxaparin: The FDA perspective. (From FDA—Biosimilars: An Update—Focused on Quality Considerations, http://www.fda.gov/downloads/AdvisoryCommittees/CommitteesMeetingMaterials/Drugs/AdvisoryCommitteeforPharmaceuticalScienceandClinicalPharmacology/UCM315764.pdf.)

the cost of biosimilar drugs. The FDA had taken a lead when it approved several complex and biological products without any clinical studies in patients and in all likelihood wanted to expand this practice based on the science of understanding the molecules.

The use of fingerprint-like similarity to obviate clinical trials is not new to the FDA. One of the better recent examples is the approval of enoxaparin. In approving enoxaparin, an LMWH, the FDA developed five criteria for fingerprinting evaluation of enoxaparin:

- Equivalence of physicochemical properties
- Equivalence of heparin source material and mode of depolymerization
- Equivalence in disaccharide building blocks, fragment mapping, and sequence of oligosaccharide species
- Equivalence in biological and biochemical assays
- Equivalence of in vivo PD profile

In approving enoxaparin, the FDA stated that

> the five criteria ensure that generic enoxaparin will have the same active ingredient components as those of Lovenox's enoxaparin (within the context of its variability) even though the contribution of each component has not been fully elucidated. Therefore, pharmacological activity of the active ingredient of the generic enoxaparin and that of Lovenox can be expected to be the same.

While enoxaparin is not a protein, its complexity is perhaps more comparable to those some simpler proteins. For biosimilar products, the FDA lists fingerprint-like similarity requirements as shown in Figure 4.7.

The attributes that are significant to establish fingerprint-like similarity are shown in Figures 4.8 and 4.9.

4.7 Comparability versus similarity

It should be noted that biosimilarity is the outcome of various similarity exercises. We do not demonstrate structural and functional biosimilarities; it is merely analytical similarity. We also do not demonstrate structural or functional comparability; we demonstrate similarity. There is a difference between these two terms as *comparability* refers to postapproval changes requiring a comparison between the products before and after the changes are made. Generally, the term *comparability* is used in conjunction with *protocol* to define this exercise. We can use *comparison* but not *comparability* if we do not want to confuse the agencies about the intent of the exercise.

In light of the confusion created in the literature, in the regulatory guidance worldwide and by developers, it is important to understand the

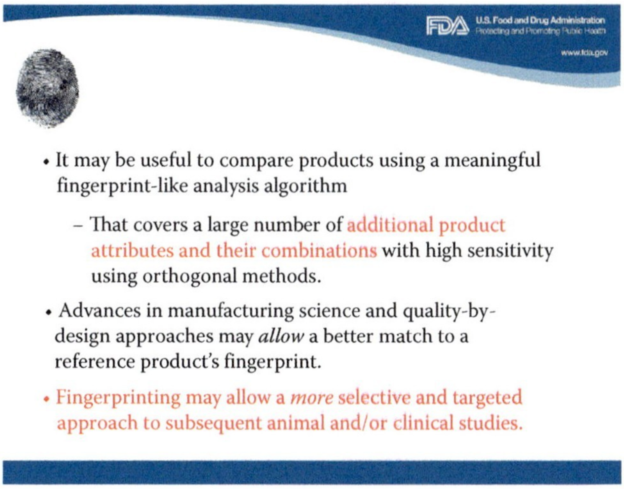

Figure 4.7 How the FDA defines fingerprinting. (From FDA—Biosimilars: An Update—Focused on Quality Considerations, http://www.fda.gov/downloads/AdvisoryCommittees/CommitteesMeetingMaterials/Drugs/AdvisoryCommitteeforPharmaceuticalScienceandClinicalPharmacology/UCM315764.pdf.)

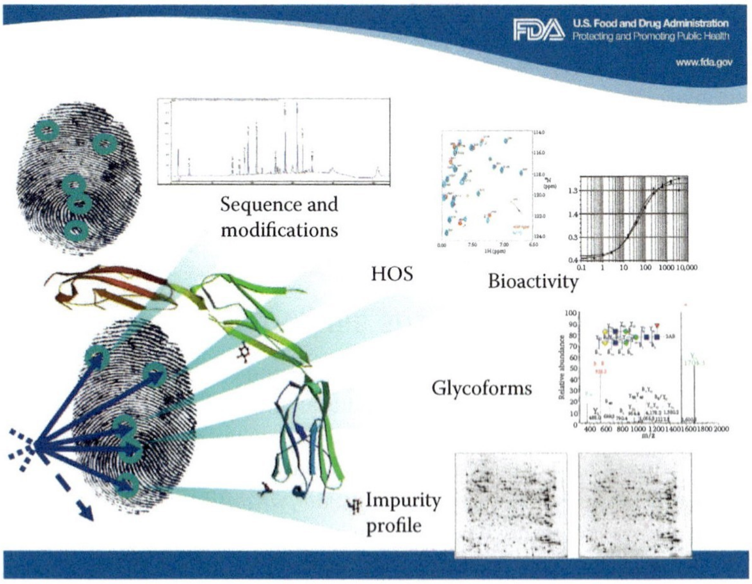

Figure 4.8 Fingerprinting attributes in general. (From FDA—Biosimilars: An Update—Focused on Quality Considerations, http://www.fda.gov/downloads/AdvisoryCommittees/CommitteesMeetingMaterials/Drugs/AdvisoryCommitteeforPharmaceuticalScienceandClinicalPharmacology/UCM315764.pdf.)

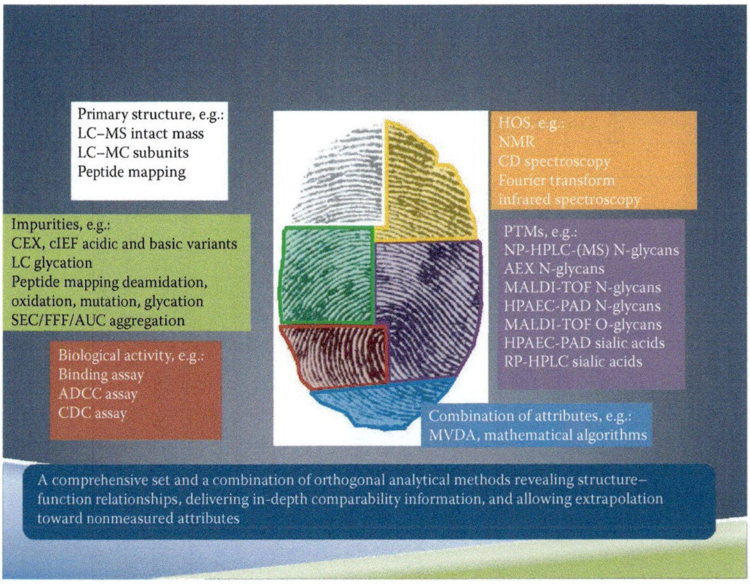

Figure 4.9 Fingerprinting attributes of mAbs and fusion proteins. (From FDA—Biosimilars: An Update—Focused on Quality Considerations, http://www.fda.gov/downloads/AdvisoryCommittees/CommitteesMeetingMaterials/Drugs/AdvisoryCommitteefor PharmaceuticalScienceandClinicalPharmacology/UCM315764.pdf.)

difference between comparability testing and similarity testing, as well the terms like *comparator product* and *reference product.*

Comparability protocol refers to a protocol suggested by regulatory agencies (http://www.fda.gov/downloads/drugs/guidancecomplianceregulatory information/guidances/ucm070262.pdf) with specific indications on validating changes made the CMC section of protein drugs after these products are approved and in commerce. This falls in the class of changes such as CBE0 and CBE30. Comparability usually comprises the process change by the same sponsor where historical data are available (e.g., development, process qualification, and control), and the acceptance criteria are relatively easy to set. On the other hand, similarity testing involves attribute comparisons between a biosimilar candidate and a reference product or where there is a change in manufacturer where limited (or no historical) data are available and, therefore, involves more rigorous analytical and statistical evaluations.

A good example is that of a study of the comparability protocols for Aranesp, Rituxan, and Enbrel. In this study, samples of multiple lots before and after changes in the comparability protocols were collected and analyzed between 2007 and 2010. Figure 4.10 shows the changes observed before and after the comparability protocols were completed. These appear to be significant changes, yet the agencies allowed these changes.

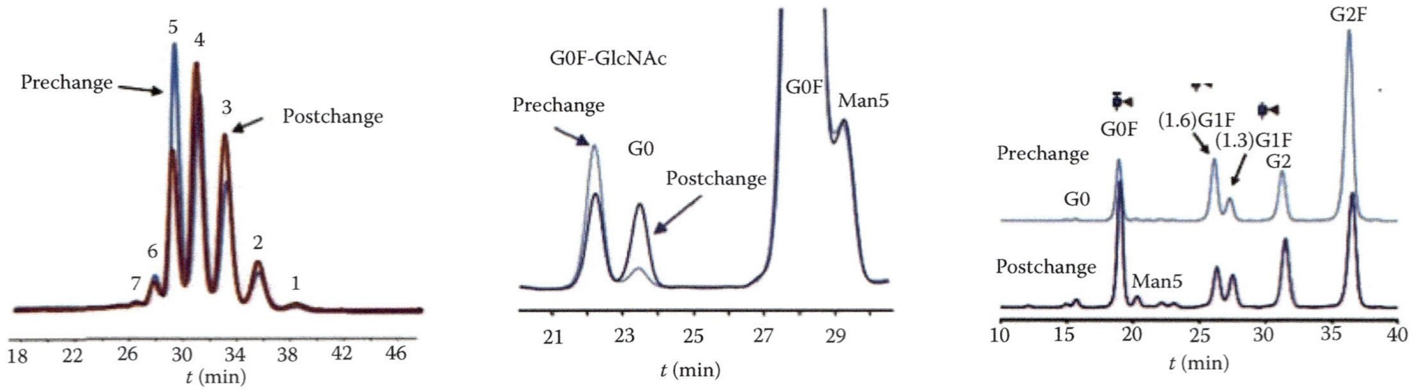

Figure 4.10 Changes in quality attributes of glycosylated biopharmaceuticals under comparability protocol. *Left to right:* Aranesp, Rituxan, and Enbrel. (Reprinted by permission from Macmillan Publishers Ltd., *Nature Biotechnology*, Schiestl, M., Stangler, T., Torella, C., Čepeljnik, T., Toll, H., and Grau, R. Acceptable changes in quality attributes of glycosylated biopharmaceuticals, 29, 310–312, copyright 2011).

The changes made by the originator in the comparability protocol exercises are generally available in regulatory documents, and these documents along with establishment inspection reports (EIRs) of the facilities where the originator product is made are excellent sources of information for the biosimilar product developer. The EIRs are available under the Freedom of Information Act. It is noteworthy that these reports provide great insight into what is considered a critical attribute and how it is controlled in a risk-based evaluation of the development plan of the biosimilar product developer.

The use of *comparability* has specific meaning for postapproval changes and should be discouraged when compiling documents for the FDA filing. Figure 4.10 shows an example of variability in the comparability protocol presentation to FDA; differences arising out of changes are acceptable as long as they do not have any clinically meaningful difference. The reason why the regulatory agencies let a manufacturer make changes without necessarily having to demonstrate clinical similarity is that the manufacturer knows its molecule well and is able to satisfy the regulatory agencies that these changes are not critical to the safety and the efficacy of the product.

Much of published literature, however, ignores this differentiation. However, this should not be confused with the use of *comparison*, which is an evaluation of two products at any stage. *Compare to* is used to liken two things or to put them in the same category. *Compare to* is a proper choice when you intend to simply assert that two things are alike. *Compare with* is used to place two things side by side for the purpose of examining their similarities or differences as is the case in biosimilarity testing; so use *compared with* instead of *compared to* and never *comparability*. An example of an improper choice is "Physicochemical and functional comparability between the proposed biosimilar rituximab GP2013 and originator rituximab" (Visser et al. 2013).

4.8 Biosimilarity tetrahedron

Realizing that there is a significant difference in the development of biological drugs and a biosimilar, there is a need to add a fourth classification of attributes, identity, to the existing list of safety, purity, and potency that the FDA prescribes for biological drugs. And this allows us to create a tetrahedron, wherein each of these categories of attributes is equally important, and must be checked off for similarity to demonstrate overall biosimilarity to qualify approval under the 351(k) statute. Figure 4.11 shows the tetrahedron of biosimilarity.

A keen understanding of each of the four pillars of this tetrahedron and its three components is required to execute a successful biosimilarity demonstration program.

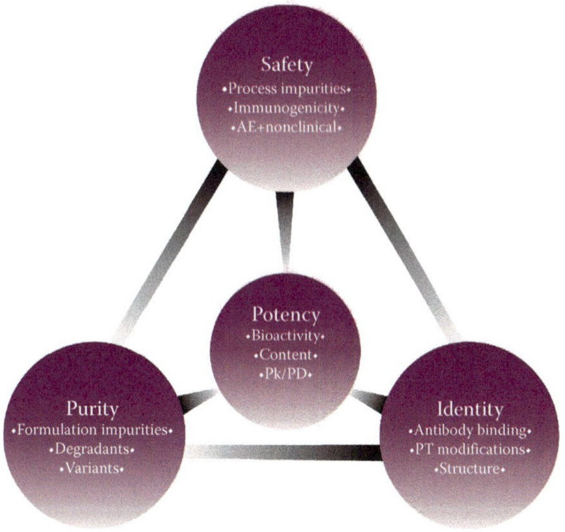

Figure 4.11 Biosimilarity tetrahedron.

The four pillars of establishing biosimilarity are equally important just as the molecular tetrahedron, wherein the angle between the groups is exactly 109.5°, but a stepwise approach requires establishing similarity at the most fundamental level first. The biosimilar product developer will start with characterizing the originator product and, having done so, study its own candidate in this order: identity, potency, purity, and safety. The reason for this order lies in the risk-based management of attributes. If it is determined that it is the correct product and has the effectiveness, its purity and safety can be managed since the contributors of the last two characterizations are possible to modulate with formulation change, process change, and several techniques but it must first have the right structure and activity.

4.9 Quality attributes

A large number of quality attributes are associated with the development of biosimilars (Table 4.2), making it difficult to provide a high level of certainty of similarity between molecules. However, the recent guidelines of the ICH Q8 on pharmaceutical development and the rollout of the Quality by Design and Process Analytical Technology initiatives from the FDA have improved understanding of the impact of manufacturing processes and their starting materials on product quality.

The greatest challenge to a biosimilar developer comes in choosing a correct battery of tests that are significant to all classifications of attributes shown in the depiction of the biosimilarity tetrahedron in Figure 4.11;

Table 4.2 Methods for Quality Safety and Efficacy Assessment of Biosimilars

Attribute	Method
Primary sequence (peptide map and amino acid sequence analysis), immunogenicity (immunoassay), other identity indicators	IE, HPLC, gel electrophoresis
Potency	Cell-based bioassay, expression gene bioassay, ADCC, CDC
Conformation	Near/far-ultraviolet circular dichroism spectroscopy, Fourier transform infrared spectroscopy, x-ray crystallography, and differential scanning calorimetry
Glycosylation	Monosaccharide composition analysis, oligosaccharide profile, CE, LC-MS, MS/MS, ESI, MALDI-TOF
Phosphorylation	Peptide mapping with MS
Truncation	SE-HPLC, gel electrophoresis, AUC, peptide mapping with MS, RP-HPLC
Glycation	Peptide mapping with (MS, HPLC), methylation, isomerization (RP-HPLC)
PEGylation	HPLC, CE
Aggregation	SE-HPLC, gel electrophoresis, light scattering, and AUC
Oxidation	Peptide mapping with MS
Deamidation	Capillary IEF, peptide mapping with MS, and CEX-HPLC, C-terminal lysine
	(Capillary IEF, peptide mapping with MS, and CEX-HPLC), misfolds (RP-HPLC)
Host cell proteins	ELISA, DNA, endotoxin (limulus amebocyte lysate assay)
Binding	Cell assays, spectroscopy, ELISA
Biological activity	Cell assays, animal models

Note: ADCC, antibody-dependent cell-mediated cytotoxicity; AUC, analytical ultracentrifugation; CDC, complement-dependent cytotoxicity; CE, capillary electrophoresis; CEX, cation exchange; ELISA, enzyme-linked immunosorbent assay; ESI, electrospray ionization; HPLC, high-performance liquid chromatography; IE, ion exchange; IEF, isoelectric focusing; LC-MS, liquid chromatography–mass spectroscopy; MALDI-TOF, matrix-assisted laser desorption/ionization time of flight mass spectrometry; MS/MS, tandem mass spectrometry; RP-HPLC, reverse phase HPLC; SE, size exclusion.

while more tests are more desirable, the choice of tests to demonstrate biosimilarity must be based on an evaluation of safety, purity, and potency. And that depends a great deal on the mode of action (MoA). For example, when developing simpler molecules like filgrastim, a set of CQAs is easy to select as shown in Table 4.3.

The primary structure must be identical, while secondary and tertiary structures must be highly similar, just like purity and stability profiles as well as the receptor binding and biological activity.

Table 4.3 Selected CQAs for Analytical and Functional Similarity Demonstration for Filgrastim

		Clinical Relevance			
Criticality	**Attribute**	**Effectiveness**	**Safety**	**Immunogenicity**	**Methodology**
Very high	Amino acid sequence	✓	✓	✓	Peptide mapping
	Potency	✓	✓		Bioassay
	Target binding	✓	✓		Antibody binding
	Protein concentration	✓	✓		UVAS (ultraviolet absorption spectrometry)
High	Subvisible particles		✓	✓	Light obscuration
	Oxidized variants	✓			RP-HPLC
	HOS	✓		✓	Circular dichroism
	High–molecular weight variants/aggregates			✓	SE chromatography
Low	Truncated variants				RP-HPLC
Very low	Deamidation				CE chromatography

The success of biosimilar product development greatly depends on the expertise in analytical sciences. Whereas it is relatively easy to assert the similarity of fixed-structure small molecules, demonstrating the similarity of proteins is a more difficult task. Proteins have a variable structure and to determine what attribute variability is critical for safety, purity, and potency requires a deeper understanding of the MOA, the side effects, and the immunogenic profile.

Advances in analytical instrumentation have made it possible for us to better understand the differences in the structures and also to identify what constitutes a significant difference that will be meaningful to clinical effectiveness. However, this requires that the sponsors of biosimilar products be fully prepared to bring in all modern tools of analysis, both physicochemical and functional, and where possible create new testing models to prove that there are no structural differences between the biosimilar product and the reference product that will have any clinically meaningful difference. It would not be inaccurate to state that the biosimilar product developer needs to know the science even better than the originator since the challenge for the biosimilar developer is to convince the regulatory agencies of the similarity in comparison to another product, not placebo, as done by the originator.

Comprehensive analytical similarity assessment reduces the degree of uncertainty. Analytical similarity assessment is a repetitive and iterative operation conducted throughout biosimilar product development, with the goal to increase knowledge and confidence in analytical similarity: assess quality attributes important to similar safety, purity, and potency of the selection of host cells, pools, and clones to drug substance/drug product process to nonclinical development and finally the clinical production.

The establishment of an analytical similarity program begins with making available the state-of-the-art analytical characterization and functional assays to assess any structural difference. These methods are relevant to known MOAs, biological functions, safety, and immunogenicity profiles, and are further derived from the knowledge of the conserved attributes for the same class of molecules; e.g., IgG1 exhibits effector functions.

It is noteworthy that over the past two decades, the science of protein analytics has significantly changed, and the regulatory agencies expect the biosimilar developer to use the most advanced and novel methods. The electronic revolution presents us with methodologies that are millions of times more sensitive, such as mass spectrometry and nuclear magnetic resonance. This can be challenging for some developers since the cost of establishing this analytic apparatus can be onerous, not just in the equipment but also in the qualified personnel to perform and conduct these analyses. Whereas some developers may find it less capital intensive to outsource their testing, and there are several very good choices available, an in-house analytical testing program cannot be obviated given the speed and the frequency of testing required in the development programs.

The analytical similarity exercise begins with securing both the lots of reference product as well as the reference standards where available; the U.S. Pharmacopoeial Convention has recently added several monographs of recombinant protein products and reference standards have become available. However, the difference between the two should be clearly understood. Similarity should be assessed against criteria established based on the reference product and not against the standard. Monograph standards may or may not have any relationship with the reference originator product and may or may not capture all attributes of clinical relevance. The similarity is assessed against the reference product, while specification normally centers on the standard. This can create a situation that when the standard is close to the mean of reference product range, the specification also centers on reference product range, but when the standard is close to the edge of reference product range, specification no longer centers on reference product range. This should be clearly demonstrated in regulatory submissions as a justification for establishing specification. The standards used to measure biosimilar activity should represent the reference product, with attention to strength and biological and functional properties.

The sample age at the time of testing should be factored in when comparing stability-induced attributes. One way to satisfy this requirement is to collect, where possible, reference product lots of different ages and develop a range of attributes over the course of the expiry of the product; this will allow overlapping the biosimilar product analytical results over an appropriate course of the plot. This may apply to some testing more than others. For example, purity and product-related impurities are prime testings. This includes potency, aggregates, and impurities.

Similarity assessments are performed on drug product lots manufactured from unique drug substance lots using the to-be-commercial process that will support marketing applications. The last requirement may be unique to biosimilar development requirement since scale change can significantly alter the product characteristics. The 505(j) or 505(b)(2) applicants may choose a smaller scale for the development, and this choice is not available to biosimilar developers, notwithstanding any justified scaling that is fully justifiable. To comply with this requirement, the to-be-commercial process should lot at representative scale and will have same unit operations and critical raw materials used for toxicology, clinical, and commercial lots; the site of manufacturing should be the same as used for the clinical lots, and analytical data are accumulated for similarity assessment over development life cycle.

Much vagueness exists in the literature regarding the method of demonstrating analytical similarity; it is not a one-time side-by-side testing of the reference product and the biosimilar product using a limited number of obvious tests. It involves accumulating knowledge of reference products of different ages on the market to understand the range and the variability of the originator manufacturing process. Knowledge about any comparability protocols conducted by the originator is very useful in understanding the nature of these processes. Know that the FDA and the EMA allow manufacturers to change their process including change of host cells, change of manufacturing sites, and change in specification and purity profiles over the life of the product. In the United States, this is called, *comparability protocol*. This is allowed because the manufacturer has an in-depth and keen understanding of the product and the process, an experience that the biosimilar product developer is missing.

The specification of what constitutes similarity is established ahead of the analytical testing exercise. Results for each attribute are evaluated against its predefined similarity assessment criteria, and the predefined similarity evaluation criteria are established based on two general approaches:

- Nonstatistically derived similarity evaluation criteria: Similarity is met when all test lots meet the predefined evaluation criteria established based on knowledge of reference products and instrument and assay capabilities.
- Statistically derived similarity assessment criteria: Similarity is assessed using statistical equivalence testing when the data are deemed best evaluated by comparing differences in the means between the two products.

Any attribute failing the similarity criteria should be subjected to impact assessment using a risk-based approach. Confidence in analytical similarity can be built upon increasing rigor and objectivity that may lead to following outcomes:

- Extensive analytical testing shows that CQAs fail to meet similarity criteria and are likely to impact safety and efficacy. In such case, apply impact assessment for all analytical differences based on the magnitude of the difference and the

potential biological relevance; this product may not qualify as a biosimilar product.
- Ensuring high similarity with no analytical difference between all CQAs which could impact efficacy, immunogenicity, and safety.
- Ensuring high similarity with no analytical differences for all CQAs and a statistically rigorous pattern match for all other quantitative attributes relative to that of the reference product lots.

The factors that can potentially impact the ability to demonstrate that the biosimilar product is highly similar to the reference product may include, for example, the ages of the biosimilar product and reference product lots tested; optimizing assays and prespecifying the criteria under which wider similarity acceptance criteria for a particular assay would be considered appropriate.

As more advanced and reproducible methods become available to characterize molecules, new possibilities have arisen to make the orthogonal testing an excellent tool to remove any residual uncertainty. Since these testings may require novel methods, the regulatory agencies do not need the test procedures used for analytical and functional similarities to be fully validated, just proven suitable. However, any method used to release the product must be validated as is required for all testing.

4.10 Purity

This element of the biosimilarity tetrahedron includes impurities that are related to the product, as well as the process; for example, a genetic mutation producing an excess of the acetylated product beyond the accepted purity profile will be a significant event. These variations are related to the structure of the recombinant cell line and are very difficult to modulate. However, some binding characteristics and glycan patterns are dependent on process conditions and where possible need to be optimized.

More specifically, the impurities may come from the following:

- The majority molecular form and its variants and isoforms, each carrying an intrinsic biological activity close to the majority molecular form's biological activity (for instance, erythropoietin [EPO] and its isoforms and three distinct forms present in etanercept)
- The impurities that are linked to the product but which practically carry no biological activity; these may come from degradation as well
- The impurities linked to the production process or to the purification scheme

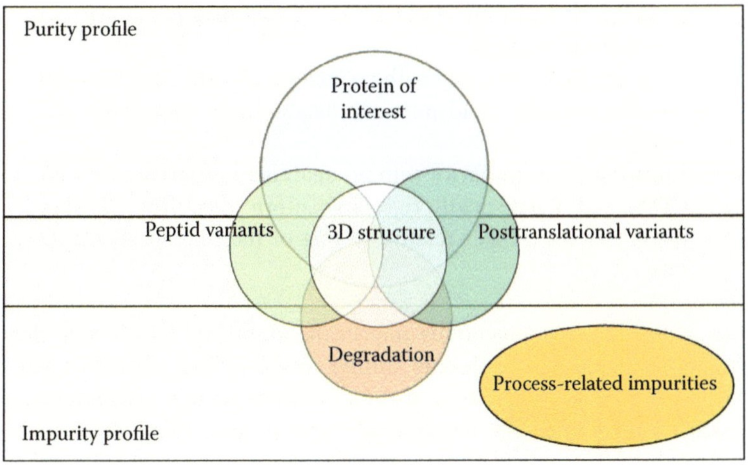

Figure 4.12 Contributors to impurities in biosimilar products.

The variants may be inherent to the product, produced as a result of the manufacturing process, or derived from degradation. The testing may include evaluation over the shelf life of the product. While the activity and the safety of biosimilar products are mainly determined by their structural variants, the impurity profile has a significant impact on all aspects of the product characteristics, from activity to immunogenicity.

The fundamental point of start is to examine the impurities that can appear in the product (Figure 4.12). The purity can be due to variations in the protein structure, the degradants, and the process-related impurities; all of these must be identified. Common tests used for this detection include SE-HPLC, CEX-HPLC, reduced CE-SDS, nonreduced CE-SDS. Product-related variants should be characterized by separation methods. Size variants include truncation, dimers, and multimers; charge and hydrophobic variants include N-terminal modification, C-terminal modification, deamidation, and oxidation. Regulatory agencies have specific allowances for impurities, generally not more than 3% at expiry and no single impurity more than 1%. All impurities must be identified. However, some differences such as in the levels of C-terminal lysine may have no impact on safety and efficacy and can be justified. Good examples of this are the variants reported for adalimumab, lysine-0, lysine-1, and lysine-2; all lysine groups are removed once the antibody enters the body and are not related to the activity of the antibody. However, the sponsors of biosimilars to adalimumab may face the challenge of assuring that each lot has the same lysine variants; AbbVie has filed a patent on how to control these variants, even though they are not relevant.

4.10.1 Product-related impurities

Product-related impurities are basically types of protein modification such as deamidation or oxidation. Characterizing product-related impurities is a major task and requires analyzing those using highly sensitive and accurate methods. While the goal is to have the lowest possible number of process-related modifications, these are often inevitable as a result of sample handling process, for example, in proteins that have been stored for some time during a stability study. They are unintentional and a source of structural heterogeneity in protein. These changes are known as PTMs and may be undesirable. Mass spectrometry can be used to detect even the smallest modifications, which are usually analyzed using a combination of electrophoretic, HPLC, and peptide mapping methods. Normally, mass spectrometry data are qualitative rather than quantitative. However, a quantitative approach can be taken to evaluate the degree of modification taking place. Several types of analyses are possible including the study of deamidation, oxidation, glycosylation, phosphorylation, N- and C-terminal truncation, acetylation, and pyroglutamate formation. All of these can be analyzed using a combination of two-dimensional (2D) gel electrophoresis, HPLC, and peptide mapping.

Deamidation is commonly observed as a PTM of the amino acid asparagine, which turns into a mixture of isoaspartate and aspartate via a succinimide intermediate. The rate of modification is influenced by factors such as the presence and interaction of surrounding amino acids and the pH and temperature buffers. Deamidation of glutamine also occurs, but much less frequently. It will be desirable to find out whether the protein has undergone deamidation because it leads to a change in pI and, therefore, the presence of charge heterogeneity. This can be reliably observed by one-dimensional IEF or IEX-HPLC. These variants can affect the effectiveness and even immunogenicity.

Oxidation of proteins is usually observed in methionine residues and to a lesser extent in tryptophan or tyrosine. As the name suggests, it is promoted by a form of oxygen, such as peroxide, but is also influenced by light, pH, temperature, buffers, and other factors. In many proteins, methionines in certain positions of an amino acid are especially prone to oxidation, presumably due to differences in solvent accessibility. The relative impact of oxidized products is less severe than that of deamidated variants.

Proteases are an enzyme class showing very diverse specificities and characteristics. Some have one specific substrate in vivo, while some are much more promiscuous. This makes it very difficult to detect unknown protease contaminations, which are a major problem in production and storage of protein- or peptide-based pharmaceuticals and diagnostic assays. Highly specific fluorescence resonance energy transfer (FRET) substrates (the sequence either directly deriving from drug substance or adapted to assay issues) can be used to detect proteolytic enzymes for the in-process control of the upstream and the downstream production of therapeutic proteins. Peptidic FRET substrates contain a donor (a fluorophore) and an acceptor (quencher) which absorbs at the emission

Table 4.4 Product-Related Impurities of Filgrastim

Impurity	Method of Testing
Oxidized species	RP-HPLC; LC–MS
Covalent dimers	LC–MS
Partially reduced species	LC–MS
Sequence variants: His → Gln, Asp → Glu, and Thr → Asp	LC–MS
fMet1 species	LC–MS
Succinimide species	LC–MS
Phosphoglucunoylation	LC–MS
Acetylated species	LC–MS
N-terminal truncated species	LC–MS

wavelength of the fluorophore. The quencher absorbs the energy emitted by the fluorophore only as long as they are in close proximity, connected by the peptide chain. Enzymatic hydrolysis causes an increase of fluorescence irrespective of the cleavage position, provided that donor and acceptor are disconnected.

Table 4.4 lists some of the product-related impurities listed for filgrastim products.

4.10.2 Process-related impurities

The category of process-related impurities creates a large challenge for a biosimilar product developer since these impurities might have a significant impact on all of the three concerns: purity, potency, and safety of the product. Some impurities come from the host cells and others from the downstream process; the final packaging may itself add to these impurities such as tungsten or silicon. Common tests used include host cell protein (HCP) using 2D SDS–polyacrylamide gel electrophoresis (PAGE), Protein A, DNA, 2D SDS-PAGE, and HCP using LC/MS/MS. However, the FDA does not expect the process-related impurities (such as HCPs) present in the biosimilar product to match those observed in the reference product. However, process-related impurities in biosimilar product should be assessed side by side with the reference product. The FDA recommends performing a risk-based assessment regarding any differences in process-related impurities identified between the biosimilar product and the reference product. If the manufacturing process used to produce biosimilar product introduces impurities different from or levels of impurities higher than those present in the reference product, additional pharmacological/toxicological or other studies may be necessary to evaluate the potential risk of any differences, and any differences should be justified. The adequacy of the risk-based assessment will be a review issue.

Regarding the HCP assay, the sponsor must provide a summary description of the source (in-house or commercial) of the antiserum used for the detection of HCP impurities. The FDA recommends developing a cell line–specific HCP detection reagent. For licensure, the anti-HCP antiserum needs to be qualified to detect potential HCP impurities. The data need to include 2D SDS-PAGE gels of the range of HCPs detected by a sensitive protein stain, such as silver stain, compared to the range detected by western blot analysis (or another similarly sensitive assay) using the antiserum employed in the assay. It is the FDA's experience that the analysis of HCP coverage by a one-dimensional SDS-PAGE gel method is not sufficiently sensitive for this purpose.

Process-related impurities, such as HCPs, can be detected using ELISA, 2D gel electrophoresis, western blotting, or mass spectrometry. Examples of process-induced modifications, which may be introduced during sample preparation, downstream processing, or other steps involving the use of chemicals, heat, or light are methylation or acetylation of side chains, fragmentation, and glycation. Biologically induced modifications, which may be introduced into the cell or supernatant by the complex biological system itself, are often crucial to the correct biological function of the protein. Examples include phosphorylation, sulfation, and formylglycine. Investigations for these modifications require the use of RP-HPLC, intact mass determination or peptide mapping.

An ELISA, which is useful when looking at quality control features such as drug purification, lot release, and stability testing, can be applied to detect and quantify specific analytes by applying antibodies to a complex matrix. The major aim is to demonstrate the specificity of the antibodies used in developing the assay. For process-related protein impurities, such as HCPs or column leakage (Protein A), quantitative and qualitative ELISAs are performed in a microtiter plate format using an enzyme-linked detection system with an absorbance or fluorescence readout.

Other significant process-related impurities for biosimilars include tungsten level, leachables and extractables, and visible and invisible particles. While some of these impurities may have a lesser impact on the formulation of small-molecule drugs, these can have a significant effect on the formulation of proteins. The most widely quoted role of process-related impurities is the case of EPO. The incidence of pure red cell aplasia in chronic kidney disease patients treated with epoetins substantially increased in 1998, was shown to be antibody mediated, and was predominantly associated with subcutaneous administration of Eprex®. A technical investigation identified organic compounds that leached from uncoated rubber stoppers in prefilled syringes containing polysorbate 80 as the most probable cause of the increased immunogenicity. The rubber stoppers were switched without conducting the impact on the formulation assuming they have no effect.

4.11 Potency

The potency of the biosimilar products is compared with that of the originator reference product as a definite measure of biosimilarity based on two considerations: protein content and functional response of the protein. Affecting both of these attributes are the formulation elements, such as inactive ingredients and other attributes like osmolality, pH, appearance, color, clarity, and surfactant or stabilizer concentration. It should be noted that the regulatory agencies allow the use of alternate inactive ingredients as long as they introduce any "clinically meaningful difference." In some cases, this may be difficult to prove and, therefore, the biosimilar product developer is left with fewer choices of excipients. However, the grade of excipients used can be significant. Lately, many higher-quality common components used in these products have become available, higher quality meaning fewer impurities and higher consistency of the specification. The biosimilar product developer is encouraged to acquire the best-quality excipients, even if the originator is not using these grades; the reason why the originator may not be using these grades is to avoid conducting comparability exercise. However, changing the specification of excipients with just cause is also not recommended. When developing a 505(j) product, the goal of the sponsor is to create a quarter-over-quarter (Q/Q) formula; this is not only required, but it also creates needs for more studies since many of the quality attributes that may have little effect on 505(j) products can be significant for 351(k) products. Attributes like pH is necessary for stability, and the osmolality for the comfort of administration and aggregation (immunogenic potential); and the use of surfactants can introduce stability issues because of the traces of peroxides in them.

Potency testing includes three major components: the bioactivity in a bioassay, a receptor-binding study, and also the content of protein, which will then determine the overall potency that may be content dependent; finally, to be potent, the product must demonstrate equivalent PK (what the body does to the molecule) as well as PD (what drug does to the body).

4.11.1 Protein content

One of the most important attributes to meet is the protein concentration, a simple as it might sound. This may appear rather redundant but using methods like A280 can often be misleading, and the biosimilar product developer is strongly urged to adopt orthogonal methods like RP-HPLC for protein concentration. While many other attributes may be described with acceptable or justified ranges, the concentration or the strength must be met. The biosimilar product developer may face a dilemma when a sufficiently large number of reference lots are not available as this might affect the statistical robustness of testing.

4.11.2 Bioactivity

Relevant functional assays are the best possible predictors of clinical bioactivity; these tests help demonstrate the structure–function relationships and are therefore placed in the category of tests that must be evaluated using an equivalence statistical model. These assay types include the following:

- Target binding (soluble- and membrane-bound)
- Receptor binding (including neonatal FC–receptor [FcRn] for mAbs)
- Affinity: On/off rates
- Effector function (mAbs, ADCC, CDC, etc.)
- Enzyme kinetics (complex physiological substrates versus low–molecular weight analogs, K_m, k_{cat}, etc.)
- Cellular uptake by target cells (e.g., for replacement enzymes)
- Bioactivity (cell proliferation, cytotoxicity, apoptosis, signal transduction, etc.)

4.11.3 Cell-based assays

These assays are used to determine the potency of a biological product and to monitor specific biological activity. Specific enzyme activity assays, which determine the functionality of enzymes. Cell-based assays are commonly designed around a specific biological drug and its particular MoA. Several assay responses are possible, including cell proliferation, cell killing (cytotoxicity), differentiation, cytokine/mediator secretion (receptor activation), or enzyme activation. These can be used to determine the specific activity of proteins like mAbs, cytokines, hormones, and growth factors. By using cell lines that respond to the specific MoA, cell-based assays can determine the relative potency of a biological product in relation to a standard reference material. Potency assays provide assurance of the quality and the consistency of the product. Note that biological activity (receptor–ligand interactions) can also be determined by an ELISA. Furthermore, cell-based assays can be coupled with an ELISA as the readout. The data comparing a test and a reference drug can be analyzed using software such as PLA3.0 to fulfill the statistical evaluation requirements (http://www.bioassay.de).

4.11.4 Receptor-binding assays

Regardless of the nature of the initiating signal, the cellular responses are determined by the presence of receptors that specifically bind the signaling molecules. The binding of signal molecules causes a conformational change in the receptor, which then triggers the subsequent signaling cascade. Given that chemical signals can act either at the plasma membrane or within the cytoplasm (or nucleus) of the target cell, it is not surprising that receptors are found on both sides of the plasma membrane. The receptors for impermeant signal molecules are membrane-spanning proteins that include components both outside and on the cell surface. The extracellular domain of such receptors includes the binding site for the signal, while the intracellular domain activates intracellular signaling cascades after the signal binds. A large number of these receptors have been identified and are grouped into three families defined by the mechanism used to transduce signal binding into a cellular response:

- Membrane-impermeant signaling molecules can bind to and activate either (a) channel-linked receptors, (b) enzyme-linked receptors, or (c) G-protein–coupled receptors. Membrane-permeant signaling molecules activate intracellularly.
- Channel-linked receptors (also called ligand-gated ion channels) have the receptor and transducing functions as part of the same protein molecule. Interaction of the chemical signal with the binding site of the receptor causes the opening or the closing of an ion channel pore in another part of the same molecule. The resulting ion flux changes the membrane potential of the target cell and, in some cases, can also lead to the entry of Ca^{2+} ions that serve as a second messenger signal within the cell.
- Enzyme-linked receptors also have an extracellular binding site for chemical signals. The intracellular domain of such receptors is an enzyme whose catalytic activity is regulated by the binding of an extracellular signal. A great majority of these receptors are protein kinases, often tyrosine kinases, that target phosphorylate intracellular proteins, thereby changing the physiological function of the target cells. Noteworthy members of this group of receptors include the Trk family of neurotrophin receptors and other receptors for growth factors.
- G-protein–coupled receptors regulate intracellular reactions by an indirect mechanism involving an intermediate transducing molecule, called the GTP-binding proteins (or G-proteins). Because these receptors all share the structural feature of crossing the plasma membrane seven times, they are also referred to as 7-transmembrane receptors.

Intracellular receptors are activated by cell-permeant or lipophilic signaling molecules. Many of these receptors lead to the activation of signaling cascades that produce new mRNA and protein within the target cell. Often such receptors comprise a receptor protein bound to an inhibitory protein complex. When the signaling molecule binds to the receptor, the inhibitory complex dissociates to expose a DNA-binding domain on the receptor. This activated form of the receptor can then move into the nucleus and directly interact with nuclear DNA, resulting in altered transcription. Some intracellular receptors are primarily located in the cytoplasm, while others are in the nucleus. In either case, once these receptors are activated, they can affect gene expression by altering the DNA transcription.

For products like GCSF, interferon, and granulocyte macrophage colony–stimulating factor, proliferation assays are used; for mAbs, the assay will depend on the MOA (Table 4.5).

Table 4.5 Representative Functional Assay Types of mAbs

Antibody	Target	Assay
Infliximab	Inhibition of TNF-alpha signaling	Proliferation assay
Adalimumab	Inhibition of TNF-alpha signaling	Proliferation assay
Rituximab	CD20	Binding assay (cytometry), ADCC assay, CDC assay
Bevacizumab	Vascular endothelial growth factor	CDC assay
Trastuzumab	HER2, ErbB2	Proliferation assay, ADCC assay
Cetuximab	Epidermal growth factor receptor	Proliferation assay
Natalizumab	Alpha4-integrin	Binding assay (cytometry)

In a stepwise approach, once the structure of the product is established to be at least highly similar, its evaluation begins for the potency of the product. Matching the reference product profiles is done with a greater emphasis on matching all biological functions that include biological and functional activities, receptor binding, and immunochemical properties. Common tests used to demonstrate these include potency assay, effector functions (ADCC/CDC), Fc receptor family–binding activities, antigen binding, FcRN, and other MOAs. The test methods must be sensitive and resolving, and their importance well understood; for example, if ADCC is not matching, then optimization is required. However, all assays reported here have limitations that should also be understood, and it is for this reason that the regulatory agencies require orthogonal testing to confirm similarity.

In the recent approval of a biosimilar product for filgrastim, a cell proliferation assay using murine myelogenous leukemia cells (NFS-60 cell line) was used to evaluate the biological product. This cell line carries the GCSF receptor, and it is commonly used to assess the biological activity of this growth factor. The bioactivity data were reported as a percentage relative to the applicant's in-house reference standard calibrated against an international GCSF reference standard. These data were subjected to statistical analysis using equivalence testing where 2xSD (two times standard deviation) of the reference product was taken as the equivalence range.

4.12 Clinical similarity

There are three types of clinical studies conducted to establish biosimilarity:

- The clinical pharmacology study to measure PK and, where available, PD parameters; there is no waiver of these trials.
- The clinical response (meaning effectiveness and safety) in patients when no suitable PD model exists or where an appropriate animal model is not available to study the safety of the product; the FDA has made it abundantly clear that it is the

level of analytical and functional similarity that determines the need for these additional studies—if there remains any residual uncertainty about the similarity of the biosimilar product to the originator product.

- The clinical trials to study effectiveness and safety when an interchangeability claim is sought by the sponsor; there is no waiver of these trials.

4.12.1 Clinical study challenges

Any clinical trial of a biosimilar product for effectiveness and safety purpose is encumbered with practicality issues—practicality of managing a reasonable size of the trial. The difference between the trials between the originator product and the biosimilar product compared to the trials originally conducted when the originator product was approved under 351(a) approval is the comparison between two products or the comparison between a product and a placebo. This situation raises the bar on statistical considerations that the biosimilar product developer must face.

The goal of biosimilar development is to leverage as much information as possible in a stepwise fashion starting with the analytical characterization of the biosimilar product compared to the reference product. Following this "fingerprint" analysis (the FDA vocabulary), cell-based assays, preclinical evaluation, and human PK comparability data are added as evidence to demonstrate biosimilarity. Should there remain any residual uncertainty, a clinical study may be required that is likely the costliest exercise; therefore, to reduce this cost, the sponsor must evaluate novel protocols and statistical models.

4.12.2 Statistical understanding

The demonstration of the effectiveness is always performed side by side with a reference product. Such experimental designs can be tough to statistically manage since the purpose of these trials is to demonstrate equivalence and in some instance noninferiority (NI). The first licensed product development was not hampered by these considerations, and mostly a placebo was sufficient to show efficacy. It is for this reason that it is often not feasible in demonstrating differences between products where variability is high that may lead to a large number of patients to provide sufficient power to a study.

Using traditional statistical methods advocated by regulatory guidelines for originator products; for example, in order to appropriately calculate a clinical margin, the lower bound of the 95% CI of the treatment difference between the reference product and the placebo must first be calculated. Significant covariates in computing this lower bound are the sample size from the reference trial (meaning the smaller the sample size in the reference trial, the higher the variability on the lower end of the margin, which results in smaller margins for the biosimilar trial). This method is accepted by regulators, but it proves feasible only when the treatment margin and the sample size in the reference clinical trial are large. If the sample size in the reference trial is small, the lower bound of this 95% CI will be much lower than the treatment margin. This will result in large and potentially impractical sample sizes and their astronomical costs. There are several possibilities to reduce these sample sizes:

- When leveraging information at multiple time points from the clinical trial by using the repeated measures analysis, the sample size can be reduced, but only modestly (depending on the correlation between the two time points: the lower the correlation between time points, the larger the sample size reduction). The clinical margin has the greatest impact on sample size. The most efficient method is to choose the largest clinical margin possible that is deemed not clinically meaningful.
- The repeated measures analysis assesses data longitudinally, which enhances the data set and generally results in smaller sample sizes. This method is useful for incorporating a data point occurring early in treatment with data occurring at a later point in time, which enables an early look at the clinical activity. By using this statistical methodology, more data are leveraged. Often, the end point itself can affect sample size. Using a continuous variable will provide more information than a binary end point. Additionally, longitudinal end points can provide more information than a single time point as demonstrated in our repeated measures methodology case studies.
- In the batch-to-batch reference similarity, design biosimilarity is established if the difference between the biosimilar and the reference product is not significantly larger than the difference between the reference product and itself (from batch to batch). This method is a more intuitive process of defining biosimilarity compared to the traditional method. However, as a non-traditional method, this incurs regulatory risk if considering utilizing this design in a global biosimilar program. An additional hurdle is the lack of availability of published clinical data using different batches. A potential use of this method is where the "constancy assumption" no longer applies due to a shift in the standard of care from the time the data from the reference product was published to the present day. One such example is the doxorubicin and docetaxel background chemotherapy used in the originator filgrastim trials, while cyclophosphamide or TAC is now the standard. When this occurs, the margin can no longer be calculated and, therefore, this batch-to-batch method may be an option. Using this technique, it is possible to reduce the sample size compared to the traditional method, especially when it can be demonstrated that the reference product has small

within-batch variability but significant between-batch variability on the end point of interest. In effect, this approach shows that the biosimilar is as similar as the reference is to itself.

- When leveraging both preclinical data and historical data from the reference product, using an informative prior when using Bayesian methodology can lead to significant sample size savings. The rationale is that before the clinical trial is conducted, a volume of data already published on the reference product is available. While there is great potential, there also is a regulatory risk, if Type I error is not adequately controlled. The Bayesian method may be the most appropriate method to incorporate the totality of the evidence that is accumulated throughout the biosimilar development program.
- In considering the prior distribution, the sample size is highly sensitive to the prior distribution chosen for the trial. The justification of the chosen prior is critical for regulatory acceptance of this novel methodology as is extensive modeling.
- The use of Bayesian hierarchical model by borrowing of strength across indications assumes identical Type I error rate and power.

4.13 Bioanalytical considerations

The FDA guidance for the development of biosimilar products has one nonnegotiable requirement—a clinical pharmacology study to compare the PK profile and where appropriate, the PD profile. The comparison then goes beyond to evaluate the similarity of antibody levels to assess immunogenicity. All of these testings require the analysis of body fluids, more particularly blood, and given the nature of the product, it creates a significant consideration to validate the methods used to analyze blood samples. While blood and plasma concentration estimations are common, there are several differences in the approach when dealing with biosimilar products.

4.13.1 Disposition kinetics profiling assay

The plasma level profiles of small-molecule drugs are readily established using methods like chromatography, often combined with mass spectrometry; these methods are readily validated and qualified. However, the measurement of biological entities is frequently based on ligand-binding assays such as ELISA employing several technologies for detection. These assays can be competitive, wherein one binding reagent is used or two in the case of sandwich assays. The selectivity and the specificity of these methods often require substantial work to establish validation since there can be a high variability in the interaction of the binding reagents used. While the critical reagents will be selected to provide optimal sensitivity, selectivity, and specificity for both the originator and the biosimilar products, the format and the reagents that will most utilize the epitopes of closest similarity, if not identical, between the originator and the biosimilar, will be preferred; this is needed to reduce the variability in the assay and, therefore, providing a better comparison of the PK parameters determined. Since a common point of comparison is required, several considerations become important.

In the case of fusion proteins, as shown in Figure 4.13, the molecules are composed of two copies of an endogenous protein and the Fc region of human IgG1. The assay format can be selected to provide the most

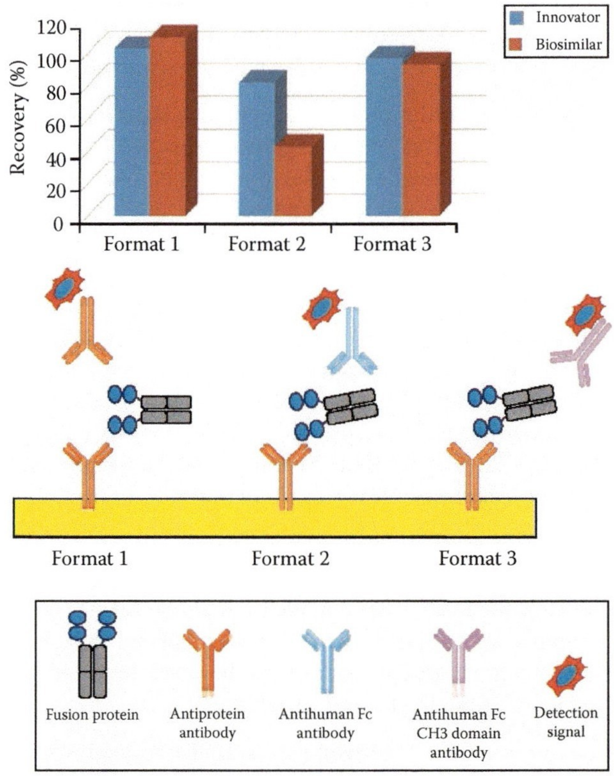

Figure 4.13 Assay format and its impact on the measurement of drug (originator and biosimilar). Format 1: Both the capture antibody and the detection antibody used are targeted against the endogenous protein. This format will not be specific for the intact drug, and endogenous proteins will cause cross-reactivity. Format 2: The capture antibody is directed against the endogenous protein, and the polyclonal detection antibody is targeted against the entire antihuman Fc region. This format is able to detect the intact drug but shows high variability in quantitating the originator and the biosimilar. This format will display nonparallelism between the originator and the biosimilar. Format 3: The capture antibody is directed against the endogenous protein, and the monoclonal detection antibody is targeted to the CH3 domain of the Fc region. This format is able to measure the intact drug and is able to similarly quantitate the originator and the biosimilar. (From Islam, R., *Bioanalysis*, 6, 349–356, 2014. With permission.)

suitable measurement of both the originator and the biosimilar product. Other factors that can modulate the results include the level of the endogenous counterpart, the free versus total analyte, and the mechanisms of therapeutic protein's absorption and disposition.

4.13.2 Potency

While establishing the PK assay development, the potency is defined as the ability of a drug/analyte to bind with assay reagents (i.e., capture protein and detection protein). It is a measure of a drug's immunoreactivity to the assay reagents. A reference standard such as from the WHO or another qualified source may be used as reference calibrator.

The potency of a biosimilar product is inevitably the statistical Level 1 comparison and comprises the quantitative measure of the biological activity. Two factors provide a wider range of potency assays—one is the actual variability, which is expected, and the other is the variability due to the testing methodology. As a result, the bioanalytical assays have a wider acceptance criterion (e.g., 50%–150%) than the ligand-binding assay (e.g., 80%–120%). It is always possible to see a higher level of similarity in the ligand-binding assay than in the potency assay. This requires establishing an acceptance criterion of potency based on multiple lots of the originator product. The biosimilar developer must also secure these originator lots with different expiry dates to enable the establishment of a wider range; if samples that were manufactured within a short period are used, the biosimilar developer may face a significant risk of failing the comparable potency test for its product.

It is also worthwhile to consider that the FDA allows the use of only one value per sample, so within-lot variability is authorized to be made part of the establishment of acceptance criteria; however, replicate measures are allowed to ascertain the testing variability.

Potency testing is often done using a parallel line analysis, wherein the dose–response curves from the biosimilar and the originator drug products are compared side by side. The two curves must be as close as possible to being superimposable. If not, then a root cause investigation is performed. The reasons may include that the originator and the biosimilar product do not have the same immunoreactivity toward the assay reagents (e.g., capture antibody, detection antibody). A more detailed analysis will include the evaluation if the epitopes on the biosimilar that react to the assay reagents are similar and then an alternative assay format may be developed. If an adequate cause is not established, this creates a level of residual uncertainty in the mind of the FDA that the efficacy of the two products may not be the same. Some of the corrective steps will include revising manufacturing processes in some instances.

4.13.3 Testing limits

In the side-by-side testing conducted, each test run includes a set of originator calibrators, a set (five levels including lower limit of quantification [LLOQ] and upper limit of quantification [ULOQ]) of originator quality control (QC) samples, a set of biosimilar calibrators, and a set (five levels including LLOQ and ULOQ) of biosimilar QC samples. The calibrators and the QCs for the originator and the biosimilar should first be evaluated separately. Each set of calibrators and their corresponding QCs should meet the predefined acceptance criteria. Once these predefined criteria have been fulfilled, the equivalency between the originator and the biosimilar can then be evaluated. More specifically, these are considered equivalent if the following conditions are met:

- The biosimilar QCs meet predefined acceptance criteria (e.g., ±20% bias [25% bias at LLOQ]) when evaluated against the originator calibration curve.
- The originator QCs meet predefined acceptance criteria (e.g., ±20% bias [25% bias at LLOQ]) when evaluated against the biosimilar calibration curve.
- The percentage difference from the mean between the originator QCs and the biosimilar QCs do not exceed ±20% (25% at LLOQ).

In addition, any trend in bias between the originator and the biosimilar should also be evaluated. The originator and the biosimilar may be considered equivalent if no significant bias or trend is detected. This will indicate that both are equally immunoreactive toward the assay reagents. The equivalency should be established during the initial phases of the method development, prior to evaluating other assay parameters (e.g., selectivity, dilutional linearity, and matrix effect).

If biological similarity cannot be established, two assays may be used: one for the measurement of an originator and one for a biosimilar, with appropriate scientific justification. In this case, all samples should be run in both assays. Robust statistical measures should be developed for meaningful comparison of data from two assays. Data interpretation and acceptance criteria will need to be addressed and documented prior to the sample analysis.

4.13.4 Impact of ADA on PK assessment

It is possible that the presence of ADA can have an effect on the PK evaluation. A further complicating factor is separating the effects of normal assay variability from ADA interference. Several factors should be kept in mind during the PK assay development and during the PK sample analysis.

For the PK method development, it is essential to understand the characteristics of the reagents used. For example, if the capture reagent used is the same as the target, it is possible that neutralizing antibodies could cause interference. Possible ADA interference can be verified by using an ADA positive control (PC) and fortifying it in PK validation samples. The selection of this positive control should be carefully considered so that it reflects, as closely as possible, the potential antibody population in test samples.

During the sample analysis, the PK results can be correlated with the ADA results. A drop in PK with a corresponding positive response in ADA analysis can indicate possible interference. Another possible approach could be to look at the subjects that were positive for neutralizing antibodies. Individual results (e.g., positive PK result for predose samples, failure of incurred sample reproducibility, and nonparallelism of PK samples) should be carefully evaluated and could indicate ADA interference.

4.13.4.1 Immunogenicity assay challenges Immunogenicity testing is a critical component of the safety and the efficacy assessment of biosimilars. Biosimilar guidance suggests that immunogenicity is monitored by tracking the rate of incidence, the time for antibodies to form, the persistence of antibodies, the magnitude of the response, and the type of response.

4.13.5 Assay development

The immunogenicity of biosimilar products is also tested side by side, just like the PK profile, with the originator product, requiring a common point of comparison; however, unlike small molecules, the biological samples used for immunogenicity testing is a mixture of ADAs against the drug. The drug is often used as the capture reagent in the ADA assay. If the biosimilar product is used as a capture reagent, it may not bind and detect ADAs unique to the originator product and vice versa. This lack of cross-reactivity creates a risk of observing false negative results, making a product appear less immunogenic. As a consequence, two assays are validated, one for each of the product very early in the development stage. However, if cross-reactivity is demonstrated with the originator product, then the biosimilar product alone can be used with one assay method, substantially reducing the cost. Single assays are also accepted where the incidence of immunogenicity is low such as filgrastim. Generally, a single assay is more robust since comparing the responses that include the incidence of positive results, isotype distribution, and titer when using two methods can be difficult to validate and conduct. Two assays are more likely to product false negative outcomes. While the ADA studies provide a comparison of immunogenicity, these observations need testing for being clinically meaningful.

4.13.6 Assay controls

A major challenge in developing ADA assay is the availability of PC that establishes sensitivity, specificity, drug tolerance, and assay precision;

these PCs are generated by immunizing animals, preferably nonhuman primates. PCs are used for both assays when required. In those instances where the PTMs are significantly different between the biosimilar candidate and the originator product, separate PCs are recommended. It is noteworthy that a biosimilar product need is the same as the originator product regarding the PTMs; so these are real possibilities in their development. However, the PCs should come from the same species and be processed using identical methods; yet since they come from different animals of the same species, some differences in reactivity, affinity, and avidity are expected. For mAbs where there is a specific immunogenic site, sensitivity of the two controls can be readily made to validate the controls.

When two assays are used, additional matching for factors such as temperature, concentration of capture, and detection reagents is also made. It is important to note that while two assays are being developed, the attempts include temperatures, concentration of capture and detection reagents, and so on. If the format of the assay involves conjugation, then the process should be kept same for both assays.

4.13.7 Specificity and characterization of ADAs

ADAs may induce unwanted side effects, especially in biotechnology-derived pharmaceuticals, such as therapeutic antibodies and growth factors. Hence, ADA has been subjected to increasing scrutiny by the regulatory authorities using immunogenicity safety studies. The ADAs have been observed in preclinical and clinical studies resulting in significant changes in toxicology, PK, and efficacy. These effects arise from the generation of drug-induced (neutralizing) autoantibodies against, e.g., EPO, FVIII (Factor VIII), and insulin; these can be responsible for allergic reactions, or even anaphylactic shock. The adverse immunological reactions may widely vary, depending on how the active ingredients are structured, produced, and applied. For example, the expression of anti-Fc antibodies, anti-idiotypic antibodies, or antibodies against glycosylated antigens may appear. The detection and the characterization assays for ADA must, therefore, be developed, customized, and optimized for each drug.

The ADAs are determined using a formal stepwise approach that includes the following.

- Screening assay (bridging, direct or competitive ELISA, cytokine profile)
- Confirmation assay (determination of specificity)
- Characterization assay (class/isotypes of antibodies, neutralizing yes/no)

The ultimate goal is to correlate the ADA response with clinical observations, to use the comprehensive data to evaluate the differences between the originator and the biosimilar and its impact on safety and efficacy.

The specificity of ADAs is assessed using competitive confirmatory assays utilizing both intact drugs (originator and biosimilar) and a relevant specific domain of the drug. Additionally, potential cross-reactivity to endogenous proteins is considered if the drug contains an endogenous protein sequence.

In those instances where ADAs do not affect the disposition kinetics, additional characterization of ADA is not warranted, but if the disposition profiles are affected, more detailed studies are conducted to demonstrate the similarity of ADAs between the biosimilar and the originator product.

If ADA response is detected, but no PK changes are observed, additional characterization of the positive reaction may not be necessary. If the effects of the ADA interference with the PK assessment are demonstrated differently between the originator and the biosimilar, this would require additional investigation and risk mitigation.

4.13.8 Immunogenicity assays

The biopharmaceutical scientist can choose from several technologies to perform immunogenicity testing. A second antigen-bridging assay has been preferred since such a method, once optimized, can be applied to immunogenicity testing in any host species. Thus, the same IM assay can be used for early animal studies and clinical studies in humans. Each technology platform has its advantages and disadvantages.

ELISA is a well-proven, low-cost, open technology platform for detecting high-affinity ADAs. It has superior drug tolerance, but may miss low-affinity ADAs due to the requirement of high sample dilution and multiple wash steps that may disrupt weakly bound ADA-drug complexes. ELISA can detect ADAs after acid dissociation of drug-complexed antibodies.

A surface plasmon resonance (Biacore) IM assay has been shown to be efficient in the detection of low-affinity ADAs but overall is not as sensitive as ELISA due to the label-free assay configuration and the requirement for sample dilution. It shows higher drug tolerance for low-affinity ADAs, but it cannot be used with acid dissociation of circulating complexes. The method requires investment in costly dedicated instrumentation. Similar problems also exist in the Bio-Layer Interferometry Dip and Read–based IM assays.

Electrochemiluminescence IM assay is very similar to ELISA in performance with the claims of improved sensitivity from the use of an electrochemiluminescent label. However, similar shortcomings with the detection of low-affinity ADAs due to the need for sample dilution and a final wash step still exist in addition to a significantly higher cost of equipment and reagents, when compared to regular ELISA. The method requires investment in costly dedicated instrumentation.

A rapid immunogenicity assay using immunochromatographic test strips is a newly developed IM assay method that requires no sample dilution and wash steps, thus, capable of detecting both high- and low-affinity ADAs. It is very tolerant of acid dissociated samples. ANP's nano intelligent detection system (NIDS)® rapid IM assay can be utilized for not only patient sample testing during clinical trials but, more importantly near-patient monitoring of immunogenic reactions, particularly after the biologic drug/biosimilar is approved (related publication). ANP offers various rapid IM assay products and services using both a handheld reader and a high throughput screening reader.

There are several challenges in detecting ADAs; for example, ADAs in an immune patient may already be bound to the biotherapeutic drug in circulating immune complexes, especially in the presence of the excess drug. Unless dissociated from these complexes, the ADA will not be detectable in any IM assay of any format. The typical approach to this challenge is to perform an acid dissociation pretreatment of the sample to liberate the ADA from the immune complexes, and then after neutralization, immediately run the IM assay. The IM assay is run immediately after neutralization to prevent the immune complexes from reforming.

Endogenous protein interferences can cause erroneous results in immunogenicity tests in whatever format. For mAbs and similar biotherapeutics that function by binding and blocking disease-associated active proteins, the drug's target molecule can create a bridging or a sandwich complex with the drug conjugate reagents in the IM assay. This leads to a false positive result in IM assays in the absence of ADA. Acid dissociation by itself will not resolve this problem. Other approaches that may work involve using a different blocking antibody that will bind interfering target proteins prior to running an immunogenicity assay. Once blocked, the target molecules can no longer form bridging complexes with the drug conjugate reagents. However, these blocking antibodies are dissociated from the target molecules upon acid dissociation, thus, removing their therapeutic effect. If added immediately after the neutralization step in the acid dissociation process, the blocker will not have enough time to bind the target proteins since the IM assay are run immediately.

For drugs where the historical data suggest a low ADA production, the studies are short, allowing a risk-based approach that the FDA allows.

4.14 Interchangeability

A biosimilar product is a biological product that is approved based on a showing that it is highly similar to an FDA-approved biological product, known as a reference product, and has no clinically meaningful differences in terms of safety and effectiveness of the reference product. Only minor differences in clinically inactive components are allowable in biosimilar products.

An interchangeable biological product is biosimilar to an FDA-approved reference product and meets additional standards for interchangeability. An interchangeable biological product may be substituted for the reference product by a pharmacist without the intervention of the healthcare provider who prescribed the reference product.

The FDA requires licensed biosimilar and interchangeable biological products to meet the Agency's rigorous standards of safety and efficacy. That means patients and healthcare professionals will be able to rely on the safety and the effectiveness of the biosimilar or interchangeable product, just as they would the reference product. Subsection (b)(3) of the PHSA 351(k)(3) describes the term *interchangeable* or *interchangeability* in reference to a biological product that is shown to meet the standards described in Subsection (k)(4), meaning that the biological product may be substituted for the reference product without the intervention of the healthcare provider who prescribed the reference product. This is a major commercial event for a biosimilar product. However, to achieve interchangeability, several definitions and concepts should be followed.

A biological product is considered interchangeable with the reference product if

- The biological product is biosimilar to the reference product, and
- It can be expected to produce the same clinical result for any given patient.

In addition, for a biological product that is administered more than once to an individual, the risk in terms of safety or diminished efficacy of alternating or switching between use of the biosimilar and the reference product is not greater than the risk of using the reference product without such alternation or switch. An interchangeable product should be able to be substituted or alternated by a pharmacist, without intervention or even necessary notification of the prescribing doctor, whereas a biosimilar product may yield a comparable outcome as the reference, but may require transitioning or input by a healthcare provider, in order to be switched or alternated with the reference (or not be able to at all,) due to other factors such as excipients. Thus, biosimilarity does not imply interchangeability. Interchangeability is expected to produce the same clinical result in any given patient, which can be interpreted as that the same clinical result can be expected in every single patient. While physicians and hospitals may adopt interchangeability on their own, there remain legal challenges to be resolved in treating a biosimilar product as an interchangeable biosimilar product.

The demonstration of biosimilarity is a stepwise exercise based first on the analytical and functional similarity and then supported with preclinical and clinical data and, if additionally necessary, patient data. The demonstration of interchangeability remains debated in the United States, and the FDA is currently conducting surveys to seek insight into the types of protocols that will allow the statutory evaluation of "no reduced effectiveness" and "no higher side effects" upon switching and alternating. It will take a few years for details of what is considered appropriate to be established, but in the future, it is more likely that these products will be readily substituted, very much the small molecule generic products. Figure 4.14 shows a broader view of interchangeability.

However, taking into consideration the current statutory requirements embedded in the guidance limits what is required to establish interchangeability. Besides the two requirements stated earlier, the statute further states "in a clinical setting," which is construed as testing in patients. These three requirements can be enabled by clinical effectiveness studies (as opposed to clinical efficacy trials) that must be conducted to demonstrate that "switching and alternating" is acceptable.

The concept of *switchability* used for small molecules does not apply to biosimilars. From the FDA's perspectives, interchangeability includes the notion of switching and alternating between a reference licensed product (R) and biosimilar test product (T). The concept of switching is referred to like the switch from not only R to T or T to R (narrow sense of switchability) but also T to T and R to R (broader sense of switchability). As a result, in order to assess switching, biosimilarity for R to T, T to R, T to T, and R to R needs to be assessed based on some biosimilarity criteria under a

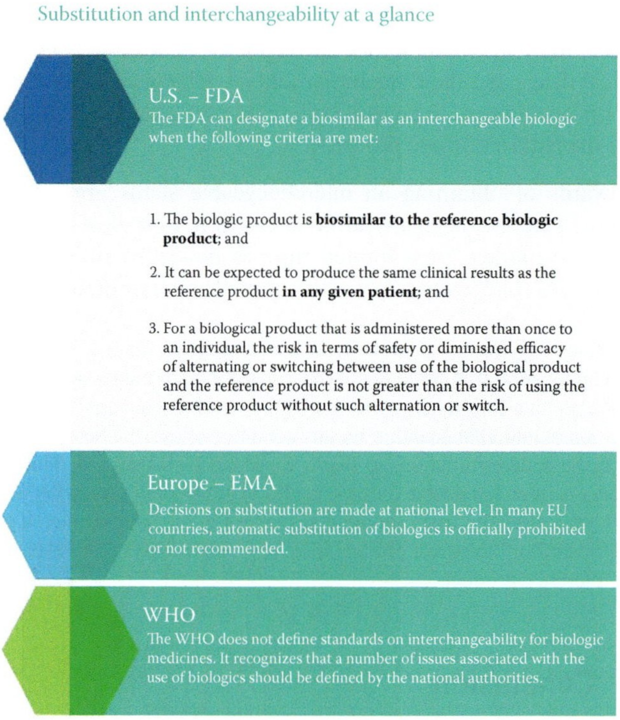
Substitution and interchangeability at a glance
U.S. - FDA
The FDA can designate a biosimilar as an interchangeable biologic when the following criteria are met:
1. The biologic product is biosimilar to the reference biologic product; and
2. It can be expected to produce the same clinical results as the reference product in any given patient; and
3. For a biological product that is administered more than once to an individual, the risk in terms of safety or diminished efficacy of alternating or switching between use of the biological product and the reference product is not greater than the risk of using the reference product without such alternation or switch.
Europe - EMA
Decisions on substitution are made at national level. In many EU countries, automatic substitution of biologics is officially prohibited or not recommended.
WHO
The WHO does not define standards on interchangeability for biologic medicines. It recognizes that a number of issues associated with the use of biologics should be defined by the national authorities.

Figure 4.14 Interchangeability. (Courtesy of Amgen, Thousand Oaks, California, http://www.amgen.com/img/misc/biosimilars_06_large.jpg.)

valid study design. On the other hand, the concept of alternating is referred to as either the switch from T to R and then the switch back to T (i.e., T to R to T) or the switch from R to T and then the switch back to R (i.e., R to T to R). Thus, the difference between the switch from T to R then the switch from R to T and the switch from R to T then the switch from T to R needs to be assessed for addressing the concept of alternating.

The experimental design that can be used to demonstrate interchangeability is ideally a standard at least two-sequence, two-period (2 × 2) crossover design; however, it does not work well with drugs with long half-life. In those instances, a parallel group design is generally preferred. Unfortunately, parallel group design does not provide independent estimates of variance components such as intersubject and intrasubject variabilities and variability due to subject–by-product interaction. This creates a major challenge for assessing biosimilarity and interchangeability (in terms of the concepts of switching and alternating) of biosimilar products under parallel group designs. For establishing switchability, a 4 × 2 crossover design (i.e., TT, RR, TR, RT) is suitable. For demonstrating the similarity during alternating, a two-sequence, three-period dual design (i.e., TRT, RTR) may be useful since it allows a back excursion, the switch from T to R and then back to T (i.e., T to R to T) and from R to T and then back to R (i.e., R to T to R). These can be combined to produce designs such as TT, RR, TRT, and RTR.

Given the highly specific nature of responses anticipated in the use of biological drugs and their biosimilar and interchangeable alternates, the sponsor is encouraged to consult with regulatory agencies with justification for the nature of these protocols.

The rewards of obtaining an interchangeable status are many; even though the outcome is legally difficult to grasp, overall, it means exclusivity in the market for a limited time as described in the following (42 U.S.C. 262(k)(6); https://www.law.cornell.edu/uscode/text/42/262):

> (6) Exclusivity for first interchangeable biological product—Upon review of an application submitted under this subsection relying on the same reference product for which a prior biological product has received a determination of interchangeability for any condition of use, the Secretary shall not make a determination ... that the second or subsequent biological product is interchangeable for any condition of use until the earlier of—
> (A) 1 year after the first commercial marketing of the first interchangeable biosimilar biological product to be approved as interchangeable with that reference product.

4.15 Conclusion

The Biosimilars are additionally required to be evaluated for identity, which is the starting step to establishing whether a product qualifies as a biosimilar candidate (Figure 4.15). The assumption is that if the identities

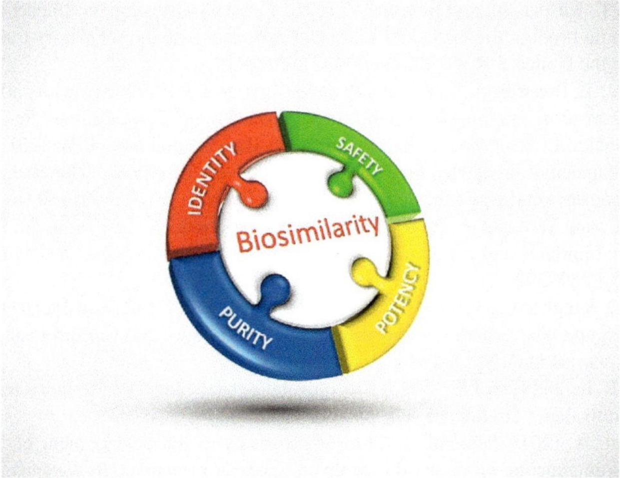

Figure 4.15 Relationship among critical attributes leading to biosimilarity.

match, so would be other attributes of safety, potency, and purity. The fundamental concept of establishing biosimilarity involves a complex, yet tiered approach, that gradually establishes that the biosimilar product will provide a similar outcome as the reference product; the reason why there is an emphasis on substituting studies in patients with other studies such as structural and analytical similarities and clinical pharmacology resides in a statistical concept. When comparing two products, we are essentially performing an NI testing (one-tail); since both products produce highly variable results, establishing NI may require a very large patient population. This is not the case for a new entity, where the comparison is made with a placebo and is thus relatively easy to establish statistical differentiation. Furthermore, since the goal is to award all indications, relying on clinical trials alone will create a scientific logistics issue; however, if it is established that the two products are similar on the basis of the biosimilarity tetrahedron described in this chapter, it becomes scientifically plausible to declare biosimilarity and even interchangeability.

Over the next few years, biosimilar products will become common, yet there will not be a large number of companies competing in this field and one reason for this will be the scientific knowledge required to establish biosimilarity—this is perhaps a higher barrier than even developing a new molecular entity, even in the biological arena.

Bibliography

Abraham, J. (2013 December) Developing oncology biosimilars: An essential approach for the future. *Semin Oncol* 40 Suppl 1: S5–S24.

Ahern, T. J., and Manning, M. C. *Stability of Protein Pharmaceuticals: Part A—Chemical and Physical Pathways of Protein Degradation.* Pharmaceutical Biotechnology Series, Volume 2. New York: Plenum Press; 1992.

Ahmed, I., Kaspar, B., and Sharma, U. (2012 February) Biosimilars: Impact of biologic product life cycle and European experience on the regulatory trajectory in the United States. *Clin Ther* 34 (2): 400–419.

Arakawa, T., Prestrelski, S., Kinney, W., and Carpenter, J. F. (1993) Factors affecting short-term and long-term stabilities of proteins. *Adv Drug Delivery Rev* 10: 1.

Aramadhaka, L. R., Prorock, A., Dragulev, B., Bao, Y., and Fox, J. W. (2013 July) Connectivity maps for biosimilar drug discovery in venoms: The case of Gila monster venom and the anti-diabetes drug Byetta®. *Toxicon* 69: 160–167.

Arato, T., and Yamaguchi, T. (2011 September) Experience of reviewing the follow-on biologics including Somatropin and erythropoietin in Japan. *Biologicals* 39 (5): 289–292.

Beck, A., Sanglier-Cianférani, S., and Van Dorsselaer, A. (2012) Biosimilar, biobetter, and next generation antibody characterization by mass spectrometry. *Anal Chem* 84 (11): 4637–4646.

Berger, R. L., and Hsu, J. C. (1996) Bioequivalence trials: Intersection-union tests and equivalence confidence sets. *Stat Sci* 11: 283–319.

Berghout, A. (2011 September) Clinical programs in the development of similar biotherapeutic products: Rationale and general principles. *Biologicals* 39 (5): 293–296.

Berkowitz, S. A., Engen, J. R., Mazzeo, J. R., and Jones, G. B. (2012) Analytical tools for characterizing biopharmaceuticals and the implications for biosimilars. *Nat Rev Drug Discov* 11 (7): 527–540.

Biologics and biosimilars—An overview. http://www.amgen.com/pdfs/misc/Biologics_and_Biosimilars_Overview.pdf.

Bohlega, S., Al-Shammri, S., Al Sharoqi, I., Dahdaleh, M., Gebeily, S., Inshasi, J., Khalifa, A., Pakdaman, H., Szólics, M., and Yamout, B. (2008 October) Biosimilars: Opinion of an expert panel in the Middle East. *Curr Med Res Opin* 24 (10): 2897–2903.

Borleffs, J. C. et al. (1998) Effect of escalating doses of recombinant human granulocyte colonystimulating factor (filgrastim) on circulating neutrophils in healthy subjects. *Clin Ther* 20: 722–736.

Brewster, M. E., Hora, M. S., Simpkins, J. W., and Bodor, J. (1991) Use of 2-hydroxypropyl-beta-cyclodextrin as a solubilizing and stabilizing excipient for protein drugs. *Pharm Res* 8: 792.

Bristow, A. F., Bird, C., Bolgiano, B., and Thorpe, R. (2012 April) Regulatory requirements for therapeutic proteins: The relationship between the conformation and biological activity of filgrastim. *Pharmeur Bio Sci Notes* 2012: 103–117.

Bui, L. A., and Taylor, C. (2014 February) Developing clinical trials for biosimilars. *Semin Oncol* 41 Suppl 1: S15–S25.

Cai, X. Y., Gouty, D., Baughman, S., Ramakrishnan, M., and Cullen, C. (2011) Recommendations and requirements for the design of bioanalytical testing used in comparability studies for biosimilar development. *Bioanalysis* 3 (5): 535–540.

Cai, X. Y., Thomas, J., Cullen C., and Gouty, D. (2012 September) Challenges of developing and validating immunogenicity assays to support comparability studies for biosimilar drug development. *Bioanalysis* 4 (17): 2169–2177.

Cai, X. Y., Wake, A., and Gouty, D. (2013 March) Analytical and bioanalytical assay challenges to support comparability studies for biosimilar drug development. *Bioanalysis* 5 (5): 517–520.

Calvo, B., and Zuñiga, L. (2012 December 1) The US approach to biosimilars: The long-awaited the FDA approval pathway. *BioDrugs* 26 (6): 357–361.

Camacho, L. H., Frost, C. P., Abella, E., Morrow, P. K., and Whittaker, S. (2014 August) Biosimilars 101: Considerations for U.S. oncologists in clinical practice. *Cancer Med* 3 (4): 889–899.

Casadevall, N., Felix, T., Strober, B. E., and Warnock, D. G. (2014 October) Similar names for similar biologics. *BioDrugs* 28 (5): 439–444.

Chamberlain, P. (2013 March) Assessing immunogenicity of biosimilar therapeutic monoclonal antibodies: Regulatory and bioanalytical considerations. *Bioanalysis* 5 (5): 561–574.
Chen, T. (1992) Formulation concerns of protein drugs. *Drug Dev Ind Pharm* 18: 1311.
Chiu, S. T., Liu, J. P., and Chow, S. C. (2014) Applications of the Bayesian prior information to evaluation of equivalence of similar biological medicinal products. *J Biopharm Stat* 24 (6): 1254–1263.
Chow, S. C. (2013 February 10) Assessing biosimilarity and interchangeability of biosimilar products. *Stat Med* 32 (3): 361–363.
Chow, S. C., Endrenyi, L., and Lachenbruch, P. A. (2013 February 10) Comments on the FDA draft guidance on biosimilar products. *Stat Med* 32 (3): 364–369.
Chow, S. C., Endrenyi, L., Lachenbruch, P. A., and Mentré, F. (2014) Scientific factors and current issues in biosimilar studies. *J Biopharm Stat* 24 (6): 1138–1153.
Chow, S. C., Hsieh, T. C., Chi, E., and Yang, J. (2010 January) A comparison of moment-based and probability-based criteria for assessment of follow-on biologics. *J Biopharm Stat* 20 (1): 31–45.
Chow, S. C., and Liu, J. P. (2010 January) Statistical assessment of biosimilar products. *J Biopharm Stat* 20 (1): 10–30.
Chow, S. C., Lu, Q., Tse, S. K., and Chi, E. (2010 January) Statistical methods for assessment of biosimilarity using biomarker data. *J Biopharm Stat* 20 (1): 90–105.
Chow, S. C., Wang, J., Endrenyi, L., and Lachenbruch, P. A. (2013 February 10) Scientific considerations for assessing biosimilar products. *Stat Med* 32 (3): 370–381.
Chow, S. C., Yang, L. Y., Starr, A., and Chiu, S. T. (2013 February 10) Statistical methods for assessing interchangeability of biosimilars. *Stat Med* 32 (3): 442–448.
Choy, E., and Jacobs, I. A. (2014 February) Biosimilar safety considerations in clinical practice. *Semin Oncol* 41 Suppl 1: S3–S14.
Cleland, J. L., Powell, M. F., and Shire, S. J. (1993) The development of stable protein formulations—A close look at protein aggregation, deamidation and oxidation. *Crit Rev Ther Drug* 11: 60.
Colletti, K. S. (2013 March) Conference report: Bioanalysis-related topics presented at the International Conference and Exhibition on Biowaivers and Biosimilars. *Bioanalysis* 5 (5): 529–531.
Combe, C., Tredree, R. L., and Schellekens, H. (2005 July) Biosimilar epoetins: An analysis based on recently implemented European medicines evaluation agency guidelines on comparability of biopharmaceutical proteins. *Pharmacotherapy* 25 (7): 954–962.
Corbel, M. J., Cortes Castillo Mde, L. (2009 October) Vaccines and biosimilarity: A solution or a problem? *Expert Rev Vaccines* 8 (10): 1439–1449.
Covic, A., and Kuhlmann, M. K. (2007) Biosimilars: Recent developments. *Int Urol Nephrol* 39 (1): 261–266.
Crisino, R. M., and Dulanto, B. (2011 August) Bioanalysis-related highlights from the 2011 AAPS National Biotechnology Conference. *Bioanalysis* 3 (16): 1809–1814.
Dazzi, C. et al. (2000) Relationships between total CD34+ cells reinfused, CD34+ subsets and engraftment kinetics in breast cancer patients. *Haematologica* 85: 396–402.
Declerck, P. J. (2013 February) Biosimilar monoclonal antibodies: A science-based regulatory challenge. *Expert Opin Biol Ther* 13 (2): 153–156.
Defelippis, M. R., Bakaysa, D. L., Bell, M. A., Heady, M. A., Li, S., Pye, S., Youngman, K. M., Radzuik, J., and Frank, B. H. (1998) Preparation and characterization of a cocrystalline suspension of [Lys(B28),Pro(B29)] human insulin analogue. *J Pharm Sci* 87: 170.

DeSilva, B. et al. (2003) Recommendations for the bioanalytical method validation of ligand-binding assays to support pharmacokinetic assessments of macromolecules: Recommendations for the bioanalytical method validation of ligand-binding assays to support pharmacokinetic assessments of macromolecules. *Pharm Res* 20: 1885–1900.

DeVries J. H., Gough, S. C., Kiljanski, J., and Heinemann, L. (2015) Biosimilar insulins: A European perspective. *Diabetes Obes Metab* 17 (5): 445–451.

Djira, G. D. (2010) Relative potency estimation in parallel-line assays—Method comparison and some extensions. *Commun Stat Theory Methods* 39 (7): 1180–1189.

Dorantes Calderón, B., and Montes Escalante, I. M. (2010 March) Biosimilar medicines: Scientific and legal disputes. *Farm Hosp* 34 Suppl 1: 29–44.

Dranitsaris, G., Dorward, K., Hatzimichael, E., and Amir, E. (2013 April) Clinical trial design in biosimilar drug development. *Invest New Drugs* 31 (2): 479–487.

Ebbers, H. C., van Meer, P. J., Moors, E. H., Mantel-Teeuwisse, A. K., Leufkens, H. G., and Schellekens, H. (2013 September) Measures of biosimilarity in monoclonal antibodies in oncology: The case of bevacizumab. *Drug Discov Today* 18 (17–18): 872–879.

EMA (1998) Note for guidance on development of pharmaceutics (CPMP/BWP/328/99). European Medicines Agency, London.

EMA (1999) Development pharmaceutics for biotechnological and biological products: Annex to note for guidance on development pharmaceutics (CPMP/QWP/155/96). European Medicines Agency, London.

EMA (2007) Guidelines on immunogenicity assessment of biotechnology-derived therapeutic proteins: EMA guideline reference EMEA/CHMP/BMWP/14327/2006. European Medicines Agency, London.

EMA (2008) Guidelines on development, production, characterization and specifications for monoclonal antibodies and related products: EMA guideline reference EMEA/CHMP/BWP/157653/2007. European Medicines Agency, London.

EMA. Scientific guidance documents on biosimilar medicines. http://www.ema.europa.eu/ema/index.jsp?curl=pages/regulation/general/general_content_000408.jsp&mid=WC0b01ac058002958c.

Endrenyi, L., Chang, C., Chow, S. C., and Tothfalusi, L. (2013 February 10) On the interchangeability of biologic drug products. *Stat Med* 32 (3): 434–441.

Epstein, M. S., Ehrenpreis, E. D., Kulkarni, P. M., and FDA-Related Matters Committee of the American College of Gastroenterology (2014 December) Biosimilars: The need, the challenge, the future: The FDA perspective. *Am J Gastroenterol* 109 (12): 1856–1859.

Evans, D. R., Romero, J. K., and Westoby, M. (2009) Concentration of proteins and removal of solutes. *Methods Enzymol* 463: 97–120.

Fagain, C. O. (1995). Understanding and increasing protein stability. *Biochim Biophys Acta* 1252: 1.

Fávero-Retto, M. P., Palmieri, L. C., Souza, T. A., Almeida, F. C., and Lima, L. M. (2013 November) Structural meta-analysis of regular human insulin in pharmaceutical formulations. *Eur J Pharm Biopharm* 85 (3 Pt B): 1112–1121.

FDA (1987 February) Guideline for submitting documentation for the stability of human drugs and biologics. FDA, Silver Spring, MD.

FDA (1995 November) Content and format of investigational new drug applications (INDs) for phase 1 studies of drugs, including well-characterized, therapeutic, biotechnology-derived products. FDA, Silver Spring, MD.

FDA (1996 April) Demonstration of comparability of human biological products, including therapeutic biotechnology-derived products. FDA, Silver Spring, MD.

FDA Guidance for Industry (1997 July 24) Changes to an approved application: For specified biotechnology and specified synthetic biological products. 21 CFR 601.12, 314.70; Vol. 62. No. 142.

FDA Guidance for Industry (1997) S6 preclinical safety evaluation of biotechnology-derived pharmaceuticals. FDA, Silver Spring, MD.
FDA Guideline for Industry (1998 June) Stability testing for drug substances and drug products (draft guidances). FDA, Silver Spring, MD.
FDA Guidance for Industry (1998 December) ANDAs: Impurities in drug products (draft guidance). FDA, Silver Spring, MD.
FDA Guidance for Industry (1999 February) For the submission of chemistry, manufacturing and controls and establishment description information for human plasma-derived biological products, animal plasma or serum-derived products. FDA, Silver Spring, MD.
FDA Guidance for Industry (1999 February) INDs for phase 2 and 3 studies of drugs, including specified therapeutic biotechnology-derived products chemistry, manufacturing, and controls content and format (draft guidance). FDA, Silver Spring, MD.
FDA Guidance for Industry (2001) Bioanalytical method validation. FDA, Silver Spring, MD.
FDA Guidance for Industry (2009) Assay development for immunogenicity testing of therapeutic proteins. FDA, Silver Spring, MD.
FDA. FDA briefing document: Oncologic drugs advisory committee meeting. http://www.fda.gov/downloads/AdvisoryCommittees/CommitteesMeetingMaterials/Drugs/OncologicDrugsAdvisoryCommittee/UCM428780.pdf.
FDA—Guidance for Industry: Clinical Pharmacology Data to Support a Demonstration of Biosimilarity to a Reference Product (Draft Guidance). http://www.fda.gov/downloads/Drugs/GuidanceComplianceRegulatoryInformation/Guidances/UCM397017.pdf.
FDA—Guidance for Industry: Comparability Protocols—Protein Drug Products and Biological Products—Chemistry, Manufacturing, and Controls Information. http://www.fda.gov/downloads/Drugs/GuidanceComplianceRegulatoryInformation/Guidances/UCM070262.pdf.
FDA—Guidance for Industry: Formal Meetings between the FDA and Biosimilar Biological Product Sponsors or Applicants (Draft Guidance). http://www.fda.gov/downloads/Drugs/GuidanceComplianceRegulatoryInformation/Guidances/UCM345649.pdf.
FDA—Guidance for Industry: Quality Considerations in Demonstrating Biosimilarity to a Reference Protein Product (Draft Guidance). http://www.fda.gov/downloads/Drugs/GuidanceComplianceRegulatoryInformation/Guidances/UCM291134.pdf.
FDA—Guidance for Industry: Reference Product Exclusivity for Biological Products Filed under Section 351(a) of the PHS Act (Draft Guidance). http://www.fda.gov/downloads/Drugs/GuidanceComplianceRegulatoryInformation/Guidances/UCM407844.pdf.
FDA—Guidance for Industry: Scientific Considerations in Demonstrating Biosimilarity to a Reference Product (Draft Guidance). http://www.fda.gov/downloads/Drugs/GuidanceComplianceRegulatoryInformation/Guidances/UCM291128.pdf.
FDA—Biosimilars: Additional questions, May 2015. http://www.fda.gov/downloads/Drugs/GuidanceComplianceRegulatoryInformation/Guidances/UCM273001.pdf.
FDA—Information on Biosimilars. http://www.fda.gov/drugs/developmentapprovalprocess/howdrugsaredevelopedandapproved/approvalapplications/therapeuticbiologicapplications/biosimilars/default.htm.
FDA—Guidances (Drugs). http://www.fda.gov/Drugs/GuidanceComplianceRegulatoryInformation/Guidances/default.htm.
FDA—Biosimilars: An Update—Focused on Quality Considerations. http://www.fda.gov/downloads/AdvisoryCommittees/CommitteesMeetingMaterials/Drugs/AdvisoryCommitteeforPharmaceuticalScienceandClinicalPharmacology/UCM315764.pdf.

FDA. US-licensed Neupogen labeling approved on September 13, 2013. http://www.accessdata.fda.gov/drugsatfdadocs/label/2013/103353s5157lbl.pdf.

FDA. ZARXIO-Sandoz presentation to the ODAC. http://www.fda.gov/downloads/AdvisoryCommittees/CommitteesMeetingMaterials/Drugs/OncologicDrugsAdvisoryCommittee/UCM428780.pdf.

Feagan, B. G. et al. (2014 July) The challenge of indication extrapolation for infliximab biosimilars. *Biologicals* 42 (4): 177–183.

Francis, G. E., Fisher, D., Delgado, C., Malik, F., Gardiner, A., and Neale, D. (1998) PEGylation of cytokines. *Int J Hematol* 68 (1): 1–18.

Fransson, J., Hallen, D., and Florin-Robertsson, E. (1997) Solvent effects on the solubility and physical stability of human insulin-like growth factor I. *Pharm Res* 14: 606.

Freire, E., Schön, A., Hutchins, B. M., and Brown, R. K. (2013) Chemical denaturation as a tool in the formulation optimization of biologics. *Drug Discov Today* 18 (19–20): 1007–1013.

Fryklund, L., Ritzén, M., Bertilsson, G., and Arnlind, M. H. (2014 May) Is the decision on the use of biosimilar growth hormone based on high quality scientific evidence? *Eur J Clin Pharmacol* 70 (5): 509–517.

Gabrilove, J. L. et al. (1998) Phase I study of granulocyte colony-stimulating factor in patients with transitional cell carcinoma of the urothelium. *J Clin Investig* 82: 1454–1461.

García Alfonso, P. (2010 March) Biosimilar filgrastim: From development to record. *Farm Hosp* 34 Suppl 1: 19–24.

Gascon, P. et al. Development of a new G-CSF product based on biosimilarity assessment. *Ann Oncol* 21: 1419–1429.

Genazzani, A. A., Biggio, G., Caputi, A. P., Del Tacca, M., Drago, F., Fantozzi, R., and Canonico, P. L. (2007) Biosimilar drugs: Concerns and opportunities. *BioDrugs* 21 (6): 351–356.

Goswami, S., Wang, W., Arakawa, T., and Ohtake, S. (2013) Developments and challenges for mAb-based therapeutics *Antibodies* 2: 452–500.

Gsteiger, S., Bretz, F., and Liu, W. (2011 July) Simultaneous confidence bands for nonlinear regression models with application to population pharmacokinetic analyses. *J Biopharm Stat* 21 (4):708–725.

Hadavand, N., Valadkhani, M., and Zarbakhsh, A. (2011 September) Current regulatory and scientific considerations for approving biosimilars in Iran. *Biologicals* 39 (5): 325–327.

Haddadin, R. D. (2011 September) Concept of biosimilar products in Jordan. *Biologicals* 39 (5): 333–335.

Hashii, N., Harazono, A., Kuribayashi, R., Takakura, D., and Kawasaki, N. (2014 April 30) Characterization of N-glycan heterogeneities of erythropoietin products by liquid chromatography/mass spectrometry and multivariate analysis. *Rapid Commun Mass Spectrom* 28 (8): 921–932.

Haverick, M., Mengisen, S., Shameem, M., and Ambrogelly, A. (2014 July–August) Separation of mAbs molecular variants by analytical hydrophobic interaction chromatography HPLC: Overview and applications. *MAbs* 6 (4): 852–858.

Health Canada Guidance. Guidance for sponsors: Information and submission requirements for subsequent entry biologics (SEBs). http://www.hc-sc.gc.ca/dhp-mps/brgtherap/applic-demande/guides/seb-pbu/seb-pbu_2010-eng.php.

Herman, A. C. et al. (1996) Characterization, formulation, and stability of Neupogen (Filgrastim), a recombinant human granulocyte-colony stimulating factor. *Pharm Biotechnol* 9: 303–328.

Herrero Ambrosio, A. (2010 March) Biosimilars: Regulatory status for approval. *Farm Hosp* 34 Suppl 1: 16–18.

Herron, J. N., Jiskoot, W., and Crommelin, D. J. A. *Physical Methods to Characterize Pharmaceutical Proteins*. Pharmaceutical Biotechnology Series, Volume 7. New York: Plenum Press; 1995.

Holloway, C., Mueller-Berghaus, J., Lima, B. S., Lee, S. L., Wyatt, J. S., Nicholas, J. M., Crommelin, D. J. (2012 December) Scientific considerations for complex drugs in light of established and emerging regulatory guidance. *Ann N Y Acad Sci* 1276: 26–36.

Hsieh, T. C., Chow, S. C., Liu, J. P., Hsiao, C. F., and Chi, E. (2010 January) Statistical test for evaluation of biosimilarity in variability of follow-on biologics. *J Biopharm Stat* 20 (1): 75–89.

Hulse, W. L., Gray, J., and Forbes, R. T. (2013 September 10) Evaluating the inter and intra lot variability of protein aggregation behaviour using Taylor dispersion analysis and dynamic light scattering. *Int J Pharm* 453 (2): 351–357.

Hungarian Academy of Sciences (2012) Third international regulatory workshop on A to Z on bioequivalence, bioanalysis, dissolution and biosimilarity. *Acta Pharm Hung* 82 (3): 121–124.

ICH (1994 September 22) Stability testing of new drug substances and products. *Fed Regist* 59 (183): 48754–48759.

ICH (1996 July 10) Final guideline on stability testing of biotechnological/biological products. *Fed Regist* 61 (133): 36466–36469.

ICH (1997 May 16) Guidelines for the photostability testing of new drug substances and products. *Fed Regist* 62 (95): 27115–27122.

ICH (1997) Impurities in new drug products. The ICH Q3B.

ICH (1999) Guidance on specifications: Test procedures and acceptance criteria for biotechnological/biological products. *Fed Regist* 64 (159): 44928–44935.

Inactive Ingredient Guide (1996) Inactive ingredients for currently marketed drug products. FOI Services, Inc. Rockville, MD.

Islam, R. (2014 February) Bioanalytical challenges of biosimilars. *Bioanalysis* 6 (3): 349–356.

Islam, R., Islam, C. Bioanalytical challenges in the development of biosimilars. In: *Bioanalysis of Biotherapeutics*. Gorovits, B. (Ed.). London: Future Science; 2011, 62–75.

Jackisch, C., Scappaticci, F. A., Heinzmann, D., Bisordi, F., Schreitmüller, T., von Minckwitz, G., and Cortés, J. (2014 August) Neoadjuvant breast cancer treatment as a sensitive setting for trastuzumab biosimilar development and extrapolation. *Future Oncol* 28: 1–11.

Jelkmann, W. (2010 October) Biosimilar epoetins and other "follow-on" biologics: Update on the European experiences. *Am J Hematol* 85 (10): 771–780.

Jeske, W. P., Walenga, J. M., Hoppensteadt, D. A., Vandenberg, C., Brubaker, A., Adiguzel, C., Bakhos, M., and Fareed, J. (2008 February) Differentiating low-molecular-weight heparins based on chemical, biological, and pharmacologic properties: Implications for the development of generic versions of low-molecular-weight heparins. *Semin Thromb Hemost* 34 (1): 74–85.

Jones, A. J. S. (1993) Analysis of polypeptides and proteins. *Adv Drug Del Rev* 10: 29.

Kálmán-Szekeres, Z., Olajos, M., and Ganzler, K. (2012 October) Analytical aspects of biosimilarity issues of protein drugs. *J Pharm Biomed Anal* 69: 185–195.

Kang, S. H., and Chow, S. C. (2013 February 10) Statistical assessment of biosimilarity based on relative distance between follow-on biologics. *Stat Med* 32 (3): 382–392.

Kang, S. H., and Kim, Y. (2014) Sample size calculations for the development of biosimilar products. *J Biopharm Stat* 24 (6): 1215–1224.

Karalis, V., and Macheras, P. (2012 August) Current regulatory approaches of bioequivalence testing. *Expert Opin Drug Metab Toxicol* 8 (8): 929–942.

Keizer, R. J., Budde, I. K., Sprengers, P. F., Levi, M., Beijnen, J. H., Huitema, A. D. (2012 February) Model-based evaluation of similarity in pharmacokinetics of two formulations of the blood-derived plasma product c1 esterase inhibitor. *J Clin Pharmacol* 52 (2): 204–213.

Kerpel-Fronius, S. (2012 May) Clinical pharmacology aspects of development and application of biosimilar antibodies. *Magy Onkol* 56 (2): 104–112.

King, G. (2012 November) Quotient bioresearch complete £1.5 million expansion of bioanalytical research facilities. *Bioanalysis* 4 (22): 2666.
Knepp, V. M., Muchnik, A., Oldmark, S., and Kalashnikova, L. (1998) Stability of non-aqueous suspension formulations of plasma derived factor IX and recombinant human alpha interferon at elevated temperatures. *Pharm Res* 15: 1090–1095.
Koyfman, H. (2013 August) Biosimilarity and interchangeability in the Biologics Price Competition and Innovation Act of 2009 and FDA's 2012 draft guidance for industry. *Biotechnol Law Rep* 32 (4): 238–251.
Kuang, B., King, L., and Wang, H. F. (2010) Therapeutic monoclonal antibody concentration monitoring: Free or total? *Bioanalysis* 2 (6): 1125–1140.
Kuczka, K., Harder, S., Picard-Willems, B., Warnke, A., Donath, F., Bianchini, P., Parma, B., and Blume, H. (2008 October) Biomarkers and coagulation tests for assessing the biosimilarity of a generic low-molecular-weight heparin: Results of a study in healthy subjects with enoxaparin. *J Clin Pharmacol* 48 (10): 1189–1196.
Kuhlmann, M., and Covic, A. (2006 October) The protein science of biosimilars. *Nephrol Dial Transplant* 21 Suppl 5: v4–v8.
Kuhlmann, M., and Marre, M. (2010) Lessons learned from biosimilar epoetins and insulins. *Br. J Diabetes Vasc Dis* 10 (2): 90–97.
Kumar, M. et al. (2012) Mass spectrometric distinction of in-source and in-solution pyroglutamate and succinimide in proteins: A case study on rhG-CSF. *J Am Soc Mass Spectrom* doi: 10.1007/s13361-012-0531-7.
Kumar, R., and Singh, J. (2014 July) Biosimilar drugs: Current status. *Int J Appl Basic Med Res* 4 (2): 63–66.
Lapadula, G., and Ferraccioli, G. F. (2012 July–August) Biosimilars in rheumatology: Pharmacological and pharmacoeconomic issues. *Clin Exp Rheumatol* 30 (4 Suppl 73): S102–S106. EPUB (2012 October 18).
Lee, J. F., Litten, J. B., and Grampp, G. (2012 June) Comparability and biosimilarity: Considerations for the healthcare provider. *Curr Med Res Opin* 28 (6): 1053–1058.
Li, Y., Liu, Q., Wood, P., and Johri, A. (2013 February 10) Statistical considerations in biosimilar clinical efficacy trials with asymmetrical margins. *Stat Med* 32 (3): 393–405.
Liao, J. J., and Darken, P. F. (2013 February 10) Comparability of critical quality attributes for establishing biosimilarity. *Stat Med* 32 (3): 462–469.
Lin, J. R., Chow, S. C., Chang, C. H., Lin, Y. C., and Liu, J. P. (2013 February 10) Application of the parallel line assay to assessment of biosimilar products based on binary endpoints. *Stat Med* 32 (3): 449–461.
Lingg, N., Tan, E., Hintersteiner, B., Bardor, M., and Jungbauer, A. (2013 December 6) Highly linear pH gradients for analyzing monoclonal antibody charge heterogeneity in the alkaline range. *J Chromatogr A* 1319: 65–71.
Locatelli, F., and Roger, S. (2006 October) Comparative testing and pharmacovigilance of biosimilars. *Nephrol Dial Transplant* 21 Suppl 5: v13–v6.
Lu, Y., Zhang, Z. Z., and Chow, S. C. (2014) Frequency estimator for assessing of follow-on biologics. *J Biopharm Stat* 24 (6): 1280–1297.
Lubenau, H., Bias, P., Maly, A. K., Siegler, K. E., and Mehltretter, K. (2009) Pharmacokinetic and pharmacodynamic profile of new biosimilar filgrastim XM02 equivalent to marketed filgrastim Neupogen: Single-blind, randomized, crossover trial. *BioDrugs* 23 (1): 43–51.
Maa, Y. F., and Hsu, C. C. (1996). Aggregation of recombinant human growth hormone induced by phenolic compounds. *Int J Pharm* 140: 155.
Manning, M. C., Patel, K., and Borchardt, R. T. (1989) Stability of protein pharmaceuticals. *Pharm Res* 6 (11): 903–916.
Marini, J. C. et al. (2014 November) Systematic verification of bioanalytical similarity between a biosimilar and a reference biotherapeutic: Committee

recommendations for the development and validation of a single ligand-binding assay to support pharmacokinetic assessments. *AAPS J* 16 (6): 1149–1158.
Matthews, B. R. (1999) Regulatory aspects of stability testing in Europe. *Drug Dev Ind Pharm* 25: 831.
McCamish, M., and Woollett, G. (2013 April) The continuum of comparability extends to biosimilarity: How much is enough and what clinical data are necessary? *Clin Pharmacol Ther* 93 (4): 315–317.
Mellstedt, H., Niederwieser, D., and Ludwig, H. (2008 March) The challenge of biosimilars. *Ann Oncol* 19 (3): 411–419.
Minocha, M., and Gobburu, J. (2014 January 1) Drug development and potential regulatory paths for insulin biosimilars. *J Diabetes Sci Technol* 8 (1): 14–19.
Mounho, B., Phillips, A., Holcombe, K., Grampp, G., Lubiniecki, T., Mollerup, I., and Jones, C. (2010) Global regulatory standards for the approval of biosimilars. *Food Drug Law J* 65 (4): 819–837, ii–iii.
Murby, M., Samuelsson, E., Nguyen, T. N., Mignard, L., Power, U., Binz, H., Uhlen, M., and Stahl, S. (1995) Hydrophobicity engineering to increase solubility and stability of a recombinant protein from respiratory synctial virus. *Eur J Biochem* 230 (1): 38–44.
Nagasaki, M., and Ando, Y. (2014) Clinical development and trial design of biosimilar products: A Japanese perspective. *J Biopharm Stat* 24 (6): 1165–1172.
Nellore, R. (2010 January) Regulatory considerations for biosimilars. *Perspect Clin Res* 1 (1): 11–14.
Nema, S., Washkuhn, R. J., and Brendel, R. J. (1997) Excipients and their use in injectable products. *PDA J Pharm Sci Technol* 51: 166.
O'Connor, A., and Rogge, M. (2013 March) Nonclinical development of a biosimilar: The current landscape. *Bioanalysis* 5 (5): 537–544.
Oh, M. J., Hua, S., Kim, B. J., Jeong, H. N., Jeong, S. H., Grimm, R., Yoo, J. S., and An, H. J. (2013 March) Analytical platform for glycomic characterization of recombinant erythropoietin biotherapeutics and biosimilars by MS. *Bioanalysis* 5 (5): 545–559.
Oldfield, P. (2011 July) Differences in bioanalytical method validation for biologically derived macromolecules (biosimilars) compared with small molecules (generics). *Bioanalysis* 3 (14): 1551–1553.
Oldfield, P. (2013 March) A wide angle view of biosimilars from a bioanalytical perspective. *Bioanalysis* 5 (5): 533–535.
Oortwijn, B. D. et al. (2006) Differential glycosylation of polymeric and monoeric IgA: A possible role in glomerular inflammation in IgA nephropathy. *J Am Soc Nephrol* 17 (12): 3529–3539.
Pani, L., Montilla, S., Pimpinella, G., and Bertini Malgarini, R. (2013 October) Biosimilars: The paradox of sharing the same pharmacological action without full chemical identity. *Expert Opin Biol Ther* 13 (10): 1343–1346.
Panopoulus, A. D., and Watowich, S. S. (2008) Granulocyte colony-stimulating factor: Molecular mechanisms of action during steady state and "emergency" hematopoiesis. *Cytokine* 42: 277–288.
Parnham, M. J., Schindler-Horvat, J., and Kozlović, M. (2007 February) Non-clinical safety studies on biosimilar recombinant human erythropoietin. *Basic Clin Pharmacol Toxicol* 100 (2): 73–83.
Pavlovic, M., Girardin, E., Kapetanovic, L., Ho, K., and Trouvin, J. H. (2008) Similar biological medicinal products containing recombinant human growth hormone: European regulation. *Horm Res* 69 (1): 14–21.
Pearlman, R., and Wang, Y. J. *Formulation, Characterization, and Stability of Protein Drugs: Case Histories*. Pharmaceutical Biotechnology Series, Volume 9. New York: Plenum Press; 1996.
PHSA 61 BLA 125553. ODAC Brief EP2006: A proposed biosimilar to Neupogen.

PHSA Section 351(k)(2)(A)(i)(I). As discussed in Section 4.1, the statute provides that the FDA may determine, in the FDA's discretion, that certain studies are unnecessary in a 351(k) application (see Section 351(k)(2) of the PHSA).
PHSA Section 351(k)(2)(A)(i)(IV).
Prync, A. E. et al. (2008 February) Two recombinant human interferon-beta 1a pharmaceutical preparations produce a similar transcriptional response determined using whole genome microarray analysis. *Int J Clin Pharmacol Ther* 46 (2): 64–71.
Pucaj, K., Riddle, K., Taylor, S. R., Ledon, N., and Bolger, G. T. (2014 November) Safety and biosimilarity of ior®EPOCIM compared with Eprex® based on toxicologic, pharmacodynamic, and pharmacokinetic studies in the Sprague–Dawley rat. *J Pharm Sci* 103 (11): 3432–3441.
Pulsipher, M. A. et al. (2014) Lower risk for serious adverse events and no increased risk for cancer after PBSCs BM donation. *Blood* 123: 3655.
Rathore, A. S., and Bhambure, R. (2014 October) Establishing analytical comparability for "biosimilars": Filgrastim as a case study. *Anal Bioanal Chem* 406 (26): 6569–6576.
Roig, M. G., and Kennedy, J. F. (1995) Perspectives for biophysicochemical modifications of enzymes. *J Biomater Sci Polymer Ed* 7: 1.
Rouse, H. (1977) A new look at biosimilarity. *Biorheology* 14 (5–6): 295–298.
Reubsaet, J. L., Beijnen, J. H., Bult, A., van Maanen, R. J., Marchal, J. A., and Underberg, W. J. (1998). Analytical techniques used to study the degradation of proteins and peptides: Chemical instability. *J Pharm Biomed Anal* 17: 955.
Schellekens, H. (2009 May) Assessing the bioequivalence of biosimilars: The Retacrit case. *Drug Discov Today* 14 (9–10): 495–499.
Schiestl, M. (2011 September) A biosimilar industry view on the implementation of the WHO guidelines on evaluating similar biotherapeutic products. *Biologicals* 39 (5): 297–299.
Schiestl, M., Li, J., Abas, A., Vallin, A., Millband, J., Gao, K., Joung, J., Pluschkell, S., Go, T., and Kang, H. N. (2014 March) The role of the quality assessment in the determination of overall biosimilarity: A simulated case study exercise. *Biologicals* 42 (2): 128–132.
Schiestl, M., Stangler, T., Torella, C., Čepeljnik, T., Toll, H., and Grau, R. (2011) Acceptable changes in quality attributes of glycosylated biopharmaceuticals, *Nat Biotechnol* 29: 310–312.
Schneider, C. K. et al. (2012) In support of union biosimilar framework. *Nat Biotechnol* 30 (8): 745–748.
Schneider, C. K. et al. (2012) Setting the stage for biosimilar monoclonal antibodies. *Nat Biotechnol* 30 (12): 1179–1185.
Schön, A., Brown, R. K., Hutchins, B. M., and Freire, E. (2013) Ligand binding analysis and screening by chemical denaturation shift. *Anal Biochem* 443 (1): 52–57.
Schreiber, S., Luger, T., Mittendorf, T., Mrowietz, U., Müller-Ladner, U., Schröder, J., Stallmach, A., and Bokemeyer, B. (2014 November) Evolution of biologicals in inflammation medicine—Biosimilars in gastroenterology, rheumatology and dermatology. *Dtsch Med Wochenschr* 139 (47): 2399–2404.
Shaltout, E. L., Al-Ghobashy, M. A., Fathalla, F. A., and Salem, M. Y. (2014 August) Chromatographic and electrophoretic assessment of Filgrastim biosimilars in pharmaceutical formulations. *J Pharm Biomed Anal* 97: 72–80.
Shankar, G. et al. (2008) Recommendation for the validation of immunoassays used for the detection of host antibodies against biotechnology products. *J Pharm Biomed Anal* 48 (5): 1267–1281.
Shankar, G., Pendley, C., and Stein, K. E. (2007) A risk-based bioanalytical strategy for the assessment of antibody against biological drugs. *Nat Biotechnol* 25 (5): 555–561.

Shin, W., and Kang, S. H. (2014 November 5) Statistical assessment of biosimilarity based on the relative distance between follow-on biologics for binary endpoints. *J Biopharm Stat* 5: 1–13.

Shirafuji, N. et al. (1989) A new bioassay for human granulocyte colony-stimulating factor (hG-CSF) using murine myeloblastic NFS-60 cells as targets and estimation of its levels in sera from normal healthy persons and patients with infectious and hematological disorders. *Exp Hematol* 17: 116–119.

Singleton, C. A. (2014) MS in the analysis of biosimilars. *Bioanalysis* 6 (12): 1627–1637.

Skrlin, A., Radic, I., Vuletic, M., Schwinke, D., Runac, D., Kusalic, T., Paskvan, I., Krsic, M., Bratos, M., and Marinc, S. (2010 September) Comparison of the physicochemical properties of a biosimilar filgrastim with those of reference filgrastim. *Biologicals* 38 (5): 557–566.

Sörgel, F., Lerch, H., and Lauber, T. (2010 December 1) Physicochemical and biologic comparability of a biosimilar granulocyte colony-stimulating factor with its reference product. *BioDrugs* 24 (6): 347–357.

Sörgel, F., Thyroff-Friesinger, U., Vetter, A., Vens-Cappell, B., and Kinzig, M. (2009 June) Biosimilarity of HX575 (human recombinant epoetin alfa) and epoetin beta after multiple subcutaneous administration. *Int J Clin Pharmacol Ther* 47 (6): 391–401.

Sörgel, F., Thyroff-Friesinger, U., Vetter, A., Vens-Cappell, B., and Kinzig, M. (2009) Bioequivalence of HX575 (recombinant human epoetin alfa) and a comparator epoetin alfa after multiple subcutaneous administrations. *Pharmacology* 83 (2): 122–130.

Stroncek, D. F. et al. (1996) Treatment of normal individuals with granulocyte-colony stimulating factor: Donor experiences and the effects on peripheral blood CD34+ cell counts and on the collection of peripheral blood stem cells. *Transfusion* 36: 601–610.

Su, J., Mazzeo, J., Subbarao, N., and Jin, T. (2011 July) Pharmaceutical development of biologics: Fundamentals, challenges and recent advances. *Ther Deliv* 2 (7): 865–871.

Subramanyam, M. (2013 March) Clinical development of biosimilars: An evolving landscape. *Bioanalysis* 5 (5): 575–586.

Suh, S. K., and Park, Y. (2011 September) Regulatory guideline for biosimilar products in Korea. *Biologicals* 39 (5): 336–338.

Sveikata, A., Gumbrevičius, G., Seštakauskas, K., Kregždytė, R., Janulionis, V., and Fokas, V. (2014) Comparison of the pharmacokinetic and pharmacodynamic properties of two recombinant granulocyte colony-stimulating factor formulations after single subcutaneous administration to healthy volunteers. *Medicina (Kaunas)* 50 (3): 144–149.

Szeto, K. J., and Wolanski, M. (2012) Initial steps in the regulation of generic biological drugs: A comparison of U.S. and Canadian regimes. *Food Drug Law J* 67 (2): 131–141, i.

Takahashi, O. et al. (2015) Acetic acid can catalyze succinimide formation from aspartic acid residues by a concerted bond reorganization mechanism: A computational study. *Int J Mol Sci* 16: 1613–1626.

Tamilvanan, S., Raja, N. L., Sa, B., and Basu, S. K. (2010 August) Clinical concerns of immunogenicity produced at cellular levels by biopharmaceuticals following their parenteral administration into human body. *J Drug Target* 18 (7): 489–498.

Tan, Q., Guo, Q., Fang, C., Wang, C., Li, B., Wang, H., Li, J., and Guo, Y. (2012 November–December) Characterization and comparison of commercially available TNF receptor 2-Fc fusion protein products. *MAbs* 4 (6): 761–774.

Tóthfalusi, L., Endrényi, L., and Chow, S. C. (2104 May) Statistical and regulatory considerations in assessments of interchangeability of biological drug products. *Eur J Health Econ* 15 Suppl 1: S5–S11.

Trnka, H., Wu, J. X., Van De Weert, M., Grohganz, H., and Rantanen, J. (2013 December) Fuzzy logic-based expert system for evaluating cake quality of freeze-dried formulations. *J Pharm Sci* 102 (12): 4364–4374.

Tsiftsoglou, A. S., Ruiz, S., and Schneider, C. K. (2013 June) Development and regulation of biosimilars: Current status and future challenges. *BioDrugs* 27 (3): 203–211.

Tsiftsoglou, A. S., Trouvin, J. H., Calvo, G., and Ruiz, S. (2014 November 13) Demonstration of biosimilarity, extrapolation of indications and other challenges related to biosimilars in Europe. *BioDrugs* 28 (6): 479–486.

UNIPORT. http://www.uniprot.org/uniprot/P09919.

U.S. FDA draft guidances: Biosimilars. www.fda.gov/Drugs/DevelopmentApproval Process/HowDrugsareDevelopedandApproved/ApprovalApplications /TherapeuticBiologicApplications/Biosimilars/default.htm.

van Aerts, L. A., De Smet, K., Reichmann, G., Willem van der Laan, J., and Schneider, C. K. (2014 August 5) Biosimilars entering the clinic without animal studies: A paradigm shift in the European Union. *MAbs* 6 (5).

Visser, J., Feuerstein, I., Stangler, T., Schmiederer, T., Fritsch, C., and Schiestl, M. (2013 October) Physicochemical and functional comparability between the proposed biosimilar rituximab GP2013 and originator rituximab. *BioDrugs* 27 (5): 495–507.

Wadhwa, M., and Thorpe, R. (2009 July) The challenges of immunogenicity in developing biosimilar products. *IDrugs* 12 (7): 440–444.

Wadhwa, M., and Thorpe, R. (2013) European perspective on biosimilars. *Bioanalysis* 5 (5): 521–524.

Wang, X., and Chen, L. (2014 August) Challenges in bioanalytical assays for biosimilars. *Bioanalysis* 6 (16): 2111–2113.

Wang, Y. J., and Hanson, M. A. (1988) Parenteral formulations of proteins and peptides: Stability and stabilizers. *J Parent Sci Technol* 42: S4.

Weise, M. et al. (2012) Biosimilars: What clinicians should know. *Blood* 120 (26): 5111–5117.

White, J. T., Golob, M., and Sailstad, J. (2011) Understanding and mitigating impact of immunogenicity on pharmacokinetic assays. *Bioanalysis* 3 (16): 1799–1803.

Wish, J. B. (2014 September 5) The approval process for biosimilar erythropoiesis-stimulating agents. *Clin J Am Soc Nephrol* 9 (9): 1645–1651.

Yamaguchi, T., and Arato, T. (2011 September) Quality, safety and efficacy of follow-on biologics in Japan. *Biologicals* 39 (5): 328–332.

Yang, L. Y., and Lai, C. H. (2014) Estimation and approximation approaches for biosimilar index based on reproducibility probability. *J Biopharm Stat* 24 (6): 1298–1311.

Yang, J., Zhang, N., Chow, S. C., and Chi, E. (2013 February 10) An adapted F-test for homogeneity of variability in follow-on biological products. *Stat Med* 32 (3): 415–423.

Zaia, J. (2010 August) Mass spectrometry and glycomics. *OMICS* 14 (4): 401–418.

Zelenetz, A. D. et al. (2011 September) NCCN biosimilars white paper: Regulatory, scientific, and patient safety perspectives. *J Natl Compr Canc Netw* 9 Suppl 4: S1–S22.

Zhang, A., Tzeng, J. Y., and Chow, S. C. (2103 July 31) Establishment of reference standards in biosimilar studies. *GaBi J* 2 (4): 173–177.

Zhang, A., Tzeng, J. Y., and Chow, S. C. (2013 September 2) Statistical considerations in biosimilar assessment using biosimilarity index. *J Bioequiv Availab* 5 (5): 209–214.

Zhang, N., Yang, J., Chow, S. C., Chi, E. (2014) Nonparametric tests for evaluation of biosimilarity in variability of follow-on biologics. *J Biopharm Stat* 24 (6): 1239–1253.

Zhang, N., Yang, J., Chow, S. C., Endrenyi, L., and Chi, E. (2013 February 10) Impact of variability on the choice of biosimilarity limits in assessing follow-on biologics. *Stat Med* 32 (3): 424–433.

Zink, T. et al. (1994). Structure and dynamics of the human granulocyte colony-stimulating factor determined by NMR spectroscopy: Loop mobility in a four helix bundle protein. *Biochemistry* 33: 8453–8463 and http://www.bmrb.wisc.edu/datalibrary/summary/index.php?bmrbld=18291.

Zuñiga, L., and Calvo, B. (2010 July) Biosimilars: Pharmacovigilance and risk management. *Pharmacoepidemiol Drug Saf* 19 (7): 661–669.

Chapter 5 Biopharmaceutical tools

> Technology is nothing. What's important is that you have faith in people, that they're basically good and smart, and if you give them tools, they'll do wonderful things with them.
>
> **Steve Jobs**

5.1 Background

In the 1980s, when the Hatch–Waxman law came for generic drugs, the biological products were excluded, simply because it was then inconceivable how a similarity could be established, since in most cases, the true structure and composition of many biological products had not been established with certainty; the age of recombinant manufacturing and sophisticated analytics had not yet ushered in, and, as a result, all these drugs were excluded from the generic pathway of approval. Today's analytical instruments can be millions of times more sensitive than what was available just a couple of decades ago.

The biopharmaceutical tools used to characterize stand-alone biologics (that form the subject of 351[a] filing) and the tools used to establish analytical and functional similarities for biosimilars (that form the subject of 351[k] filing) also take a different qualification. The choice of biopharmaceutical tools to establish identity, purity, safety, and potency for biosimilars requires an orthogonal approach since the exact structure that is responsible for the mode of action (MoA) may not always be apparent. It is for this reason that understanding the FDA's stance on biosimilarity requires a review of available biopharmaceutical tools and their appropriate deployment. There has been a recent expansion of analytical tools that now comprise several novel approaches that may be used to provide additional confidence in the similarity of biological products. This chapter is not intended as a primer for analytical methodologies, only their specific use to demonstrate biosimilarity.

5.1.1 The tools

There are numerous analytical methods to evaluate the safety, purity, and potency profiles of a biosimilar, among which are circular dichroism (CD), nuclear magnetic resonance (NMR), immunological tests (ELISA, immunoprecipitation, biosensors, etc.), biological activity from in vitro models (cell culture) and in vivo (animal models), various chromatography techniques (HPLC peptide mapping), electrophoresis methods (sodium dodecyl sulfate [SDS]–PAGE, IEF, capillary zone electrophoresis [CZE]), static and dynamic light diffusion mass spectrometries, x-ray techniques, etc. How the main analytical methods provide information on different orthogonal testing is listed in Table 5.1.

5.1.2 Orthogonal approach

Given that different testing methodologies can yield similar information, the FDA insists on using an orthogonal approach to confirming structural and functional attributes. A good example is that of protein content. The advisory meeting that the FDA held prior to approving the first biosimilar filgrastim product presented the data showing variability in the protein content of the filed product and suggested that the content issue be handled by controlling the manufacturing process; later, more data were added to support that the protein content was within the acceptable range. Generally, an orthogonal approach using both RP-HPLC and ultraviolet (UV) A280 methods to confirm protein content will be desirable.

The basis of using multiple approaches comes from *ICH Q6B: Specifications: Test Procedures and Acceptance Criteria for Biotechnological/Biological Products*. The manufacturer should define the pattern of heterogeneity of the desired product and demonstrate consistency with that of lots used in preclinical and clinical studies.

While the monoclonal antibodies can be thoroughly characterized using the available methods (Figure 5.1), the use of orthogonal strategy proves useful in removing what the FDA calls "residual uncertainty" (Figure 5.2).

5.2 Key methodologies

5.2.1 Mass spectrometry (MS)

MS is used to measure molar mass, molecular structure, and sample purity. As an analytical technique, it has distinct advantages such as increased sensitivity over most other analytical techniques because the analyzer, as a mass-charge filter

- Reduces background interference;
- Has excellent specificity from characteristic fragmentation patterns to identify unknowns;
- Confirms the presence of suspected compounds;
- Gives information about molecular weight;
- Provides information about the isotopic abundance of elements; and
- Gives temporally resolved chemical data.

Table 5.1 Biopharmaceutical Tools Peculiarities and Attributes

Technique	Peculiarity	Attributes
MS		
Hydrogen deuterium exchange MS	Global and local amino acid level structure and peptide backbone	Changes in HOS; dynamic structure
Charge state distribution	Gas-phase global structure	Changes in HOS
Covalent labeling (footprinting)	Global and local amino acid level structure with side chain structure	Changes in HOS; dynamic structure
Ion-mobility spectrometry	Gas-phase global structure	Changes in HOS
Spectroscopy		
UV	Aromatic amino acid environment	Biophysical and HOS; the FDA requires calculation of extinction coefficient
CD	Peptide bond structure and aromatic amino acid environment	Biophysical and HOS; near- and far-UV spectroscopies provide different, secondary and tertiary attributes
Fluorescence spectroscopy	Aromatic amino acid environment; most proteins have the three fluorescing amino acids	Biophysical and HOS; also, ideal test for stressed solution evaluation for fourth-dimensional evaluation; fluorescence microscopy is an emerging field to evaluate
Fourier transform infrared (FTIR) spectroscopy	Peptide bond structure	Biophysical and HOS
NMR	Atomic level resolution via ^{1}H, ^{13}C, ^{15}N NMR	Changes in HOS; dynamic structure evaluation
Chromatography		
IEXC	Surface polar and charge interactions	Biophysical and HOS
Hydrophobic interaction chromatography (HIC)	Surface nonpolar interactions	Biophysical and HOS
Simple interval calculation	Surface interactions with itself	Biophysical and HOS
Affinity	Surface interactions with binding partner, ligand	Biophysical and HOS
Electrophoresis		
Native gel	Global net charge and structure	Biophysical and HOS; aggregation
Native IEF (imaged capillary IEF)	Global net charge	Biophysical and HOS
Native CZE	Global net charge and structure	Biophysical and HOS; aggregation
SDS-gel/capillary	Size, covalent aggregation	Biophysical and HOS; aggregation
Thermodynamics		
DCS	Global and domain structure	Biophysical and HOS
Isothermal titration calorimetry	Protein binding	Biophysical and HOS

(*Continued*)

Table 5.1 (Continued) Biopharmaceutical Tools Peculiarities and Attributes

Technique	Peculiarity	Attributes
Hydrodynamics		
AUC	Global structure via sedimentation, concentration-dependent aggregation, size (hydrodynamic volume), and molecular weight	Biophysical and HOS; changes in HOS
SEC	Global structure, total aggregation, size, hydrodynamic volume	Biophysical and HOS; aggregation
Field flow fractionation (assymmetrical flow FFF, hollow fiber flow FFF)	Global structure, size, aggregation	Biophysical and HOS; aggregation
Viscosity	Aggregation, biophysical	Biophysical and HOS; aggregation
LS	Static light scattering (MW), Dynamic light scattering (D, k_D, η), small-angle x-ray scattering (SAXS)	Biophysical and HOS; aggregates
	Nano-, submicron-, micronsized aggregates	Biophysical and HOS; aggregates
Imaging		
X-ray crystallography	Atomic level resolution (electron density)	Biophysical and HOS
Electron microscopy (cryoelectron microscopy, electron tomography)	Global surface structure, molecular shape	Biophysical and HOS
Solution scattering (SAXS, wide-angle x-ray scattering, small-angle neutron scattering)	Global surface structure, molecular shape	Biophysical and HOS
Chemical Reactions (Covalent, Noncovalent)		
Denaturants	Global structure	Biophysical and HOS
Extrinsic fluorescence	Global surface structure	Biophysical and HOS
Enzymatic digestion	Global structure	Biophysical and HOS
Stress-Induced Spectroscopy		
Intrinsic fluorescence (pH, dielectric constant, temperature, magnetic field, galvanic field, polarity, dielectric constant)	Secondary and tertiary structure; quaternary structure; fourth-dimensional interactions with formulation	Biophysical and HOS

Note: MW, molecular weight.

One of the disadvantages of the method is that it often fails to distinguish between optical and geometrical isomers and the positions of the substituent in *o*-, *m*-, and *p*- positions in an aromatic ring. Also, its scope is limited in identifying hydrocarbons that produce similarly fragmented ions.

In MS, the spectra are used to determine the elemental or the isotopic signature of a sample and the masses of particles and of molecules, and to elucidate the chemical structures of molecules, such as peptides and other chemical compounds. MS works by ionizing chemical compounds

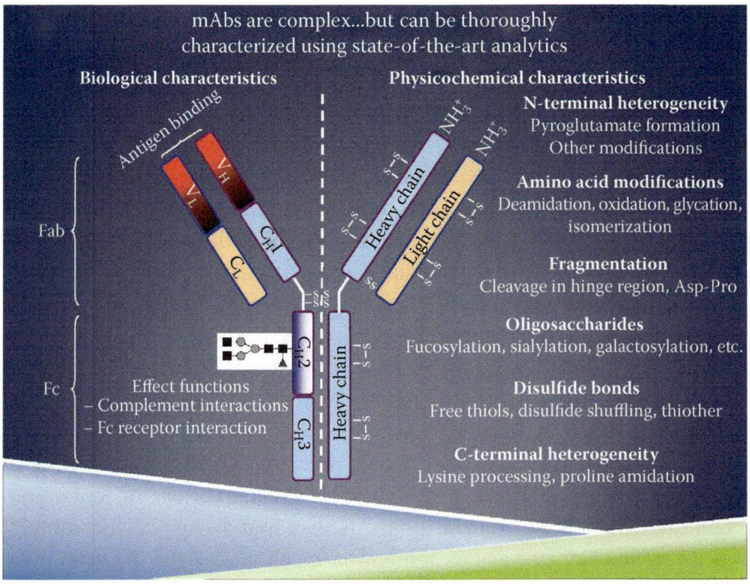

Figure 5.1 Monoclonal antibody characterization techniques. (From FDA—Biosimilars: An update. August 2012. http://www.fda.gov/downloads/AdvisoryCommittees/CommitteesMeetingMaterials/Drugs/AdvisoryCommitteeforPharmaceuticalScienceandClinicalPharmacology/UCM315764.pdf.)

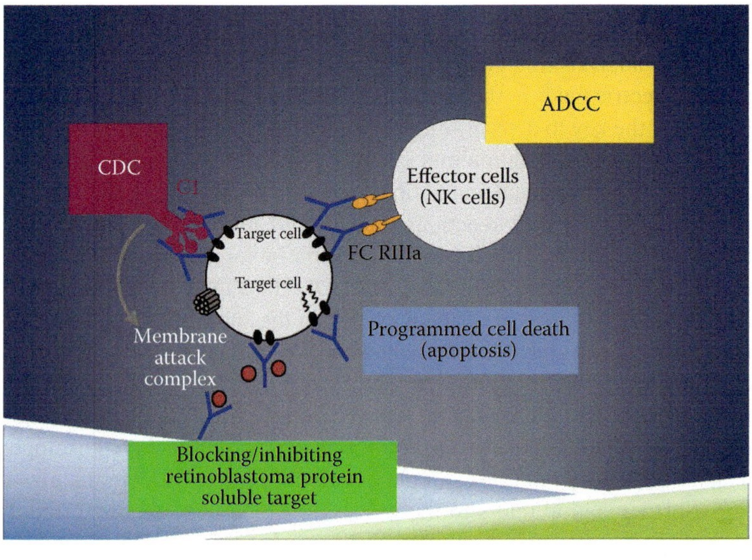

Figure 5.2 Orthogonal assays are addressing multiple functions. (From FDA—Biosimilars: An update. August 2012. http://www.fda.gov/downloads/AdvisoryCommittees/CommitteesMeetingMaterials/Drugs/AdvisoryCommitteeforPharmaceuticalScienceandClinicalPharmacology/UCM315764.pdf.)

to generate charged molecules or molecule fragments and measuring their mass-to-charge ratios (*m/z*). In a typical MS procedure, a sample, which may be solid, liquid, or gas, is ionized, for example, by bombarding it with electrons. This may cause some of the sample's molecules to break into charged fragments. These ions are then separated according to their mass-to-charge ratio, typically by accelerating them and subjecting them to an electric or magnetic field: Ions of the same mass-to-charge ratio will undergo the same amount of deflection. The ions are detected by a mechanism capable of detecting charged particles, such as an electron multiplier. Results are displayed as spectra of the relative abundance of detected ions as a function of the mass-to-charge ratio. The atoms or the molecules in the sample can be identified by correlating the known masses to the identified masses or through a characteristic fragmentation pattern. A mass spectrometer consists of three components: an ion source, a mass analyzer, and a detector. The ionizer converts a portion of the sample into ions. There is a wide variety of ionization techniques, depending on the phase (solid, liquid, gas) of the sample and the efficiency of various ionization mechanisms for the unknown species. An extraction system removes ions from the sample, which are then targeted through the mass analyzer and onto the detector. The differences in masses of the fragments allow the mass analyzer to sort the ions by their mass-to-charge ratio. The detector measures the value of an indicator quantity and thus provides data for calculating the abundances of each ion present. Some detectors also give spatial information, e.g., a multichannel plate.

The ion source is the part of the mass spectrometer that ionizes the material under analysis (the analyte). The ions are then transported by magnetic or electric fields to the mass analyzer. The techniques for ionization have been the key to determining what types of samples can be analyzed by MS. Electron ionization and chemical ionization are used for gases and vapors. In chemical ionization sources, the analyte is ionized by chemical ion–molecule reactions during collisions in the source. Two techniques often used with liquid and solid biological samples include electrospray ionization (ESI) and MALDI. Hard ionization techniques impart high quantities of residual energy in the subject molecule invoking significant degrees of fragmentation (i.e., the systematic rupturing of bonds acts to remove the excess energy, restoring stability to the resulting ion). Resultant ions tend to have *m/z* lower than the molecular mass (other than in the case of proton transfer and not including isotope peaks). The most common example of hard ionization is electron ionization. Soft ionization refers to the processes which impart little residual energy onto the subject molecule and as such result in little fragmentation. Examples include fast atom bombardment, chemical ionization, atmospheric pressure chemical ionization, ESI, and MALDI.

There are many types of mass analyzers, using either static or dynamic fields, or magnetic or electric fields, but all operate according to the above differential equation. Each analyzer type has its strengths and weaknesses. Many mass spectrometers use two or more mass analyzers for MS/MS. There are several important analyzer characteristics. The mass resolving power is the measure of the ability to distinguish two peaks of slightly different *m/z*. The mass accuracy is the ratio of the *m/z* measurement error to the true *m/z*. Mass accuracy is usually measured in ppm or milli mass units. The mass range is the range of *m/z* amenable to analysis by a given analyzer. The linear dynamic range is the range over which an ion signal is linear with the analyte concentration. Speed refers to the time frame of the experiment and is ultimately used to determine the number of spectra per unit time that can be generated.

5.2.2 Spectroscopy

Spectroscopy techniques allow the study of the interaction between matter and electromagnetic radiation. Spectroscopy is used to refer to the measurement of radiation intensity as a function of wavelength and is often used to describe experimental spectroscopic methods. Spectral measurement devices are referred to as spectrometers, spectrophotometers, spectrographs, or spectral analyzers. The central concepts in spectroscopy are a resonance and its corresponding resonant frequency. In quantum mechanical systems, the analogous resonance is a coupling of two quantum mechanical stationary states of one system, such as an atom, via an oscillatory source of energy such as a photon. The coupling of the two states is strongest when the energy of the source matches the energy difference between the two states. The energy E of a photon is related to its frequency η by $E = h/\eta$, where h is Planck's constant, and so a spectrum of the system response versus the photon frequency will peak at the resonant frequency or energy. Particles such as electrons and neutrons have a comparable relationship, the de Broglie relations, between their kinetic energy and their wavelength and frequency and, therefore, can also excite resonant interactions.

The types of spectroscopy are distinguished by the type of radiant energy involved in the interaction. In many applications, the spectrum is determined by measuring changes in the intensity or the frequency of this energy. Electromagnetic radiation was the first source of energy used for spectroscopic studies. Techniques that employ electromagnetic radiation are typically classified by the wavelength region of the spectrum and include microwave, terahertz, infrared, near-infrared, visible and UV, and x-ray and gamma spectroscopy. The types of spectroscopy are also distinguished by the nature of the interaction between the energy and the material. Absorption occurs when energy from the radiative source is absorbed by the material; it is often determined by measuring the fraction of energy transmitted through the material; absorption will decrease the transmitted portion. Emission indicates that radiative energy is released by the material. A material's blackbody spectrum is a spontaneous emission spectrum determined by its temperature; this feature can be measured in the infrared by instruments such as the atmospheric emitted radiance interferometer. Emission can also be induced by other sources of energy such as flames or sparks or electromagnetic radiation in the case of fluorescence.

Elastic scattering and reflection spectroscopies determine how incident radiation is reflected or scattered by a material. Crystallography employs the scattering of high-energy radiation, such as x-rays and electrons, to examine the arrangement of atoms in proteins and solid crystals.

Impedance spectroscopy studies the ability of a medium to impede or slow the transmittance of energy. For optical applications, this is characterized by the index of refraction.

Inelastic scattering phenomena involve an exchange of energy between the radiation and the matter that shifts the wavelength of the scattered radiation. These include Raman and Compton scatterings.

Coherent or resonance spectroscopy is a technique where the radiative energy couples two quantum states of the material in a coherent interaction that is sustained by the radiating field. The coherence can be disrupted by other interactions, such as particle collisions and energy transfer, and so often requires high-intensity radiation to be sustained. NMR spectroscopy is a widely used resonance method, and ultrafast laser methods are also now possible in the infrared and visible spectral regions.

The combination of atoms into molecules leads to the creation of unique types of energetic states and, therefore, unique spectra of the transitions between these states. Molecular spectra can be obtained due to electron spin states (electron paramagnetic resonance), molecular rotations, molecular vibrations, and electronic states. Rotations are collective motions of the atomic nuclei and typically lead to spectra in the microwave and millimeter-wave spectral regions; rotational spectroscopy and microwave spectroscopy are synonymous. Vibrations are relative motions of the atomic nuclei and are studied by both infrared and Raman spectroscopies. Electronic excitations are studied using visible and UV spectroscopies as well as fluorescence spectroscopy.

Nuclei also have distinct energy states that are widely separated and lead to gamma ray spectra. Distinct nuclear spin states can have their energy separated by a magnetic field, and this allows for NMR spectroscopy.

5.2.3 Chromatography

5.2.3.1 Ion-exchange chromatography (IEXC) IEXC is a process that enables the separation of ions and polar molecules based on their affinity to the ion exchanger. It can be used for almost any kind of charged molecule including large proteins, small nucleotides, and amino acids. IEXC retains analyte molecules on the column based on coulombic (ionic) interactions. The stationary phase surface displays ionic functional groups (R-X) that interact with analyte ions of opposite charge. This type of chromatography is further subdivided into cation-exchange chromatography (CIEC) and anion-exchange chromatography (AIEC). The ionic compound consisting of the cationic species M^+ and the anionic species B^- can be retained by the stationary phase. CIEC retains positively charged cations because the stationary phase displays a negatively charged functional group. AIEC retains anions using positively charged functional group. Note that the ion strength of either C^+ or A^- in the mobile phase can be adjusted to shift the equilibrium position and thus the retention time.

5.2.3.2 Reverse-phase chromatography (RPC) RPC, also called hydrophobic chromatography, includes any chromatographic method that uses a hydrophobic stationary phase. The hydrophobic molecules in the polar mobile phase tend to adsorb to the hydrophobic stationary phase, and the hydrophilic molecules in the mobile phase will pass through the column and they are eluted first. Hydrophobic molecules can be eluted from the column by decreasing the polarity of the mobile phase using an organic (nonpolar) solvent, which reduces hydrophobic interactions. The more hydrophobic the molecule, the more strongly it will bind to the stationary phase and the higher the concentration of organic solvent that will be required to elute the molecule.

5.2.3.3 High-performance IEXC (HP-IEXC) Analytical HPLC offers a high level of resolution and precision making the technology available for identity, purity, and quantity determinations. HP-IEXC is based on highly specific analytical columns comprising monodisperse particles with a diameter of 5–10 μm separating proteins according to their electrical charge. The resolution may be comparable to that of HP-RPC, and the technology will apply to almost all types of globular proteins. The HP-IEXC is used for the detection of target protein–related compounds (e.g., des-amido forms, oxidized forms, scrambled forms, cleaved forms), which may be present in amounts from 1 ppt and upward. The resulting UV diagram provides an impurity profile within the relatively narrow window offered by the technology, but it should be kept in mind that not all impurities are detected by this or similar methods. Impurities present in 0.1% or higher should be fully characterized no later than phase 3 of the manufacture. HP-IEXC offers two separation modes: CIEC and AIEC. In CIEC, positively charged biomolecules are typically retained due to interaction with negatively charged groups (e.g., sulfonic acid) on the surface of the chromatographic resin. The buffer pH must favor a net charge of the biomolecule lower than pI in order to maintain separation. CIEC primarily retains biomolecules by the interaction with histidine, lysine, and arginine (pK_as of about 6.5, 10, and 12, respectively). In AIEC, negatively charged biomolecules are typically kept due to interaction with positively charged groups (e.g., quaternary amine) on the surface of the chromatographic resin. The buffer pH must favor a net charge of the biomolecule higher than pI in order to maintain separation. AIEC primarily retains biomolecules by the interaction with aspartic or glutamic acid side chains (pK_a about 4.4). The separation is affected by the temperature (due to structural changes in the protein molecule), the presence of displacer ions such as Na and Cl, the presence of denaturing agents, the presence of organic solvents, and the hydrophobic interactions with the resin. HP-IEXC is used for in-process control analysis of target protein identity (retention time), quantity (peak area), and purity (215 or 280 nm profile). The method is also used for drug substance/product impurity profiles and determination of quantity.

5.2.3.4 HP-RPC The HP-RPC is based on highly specific analytical columns comprising monodisperse particles with a diameter of 5–10 μm separating proteins according to their hydrophobicity. The high-resolution methodology is restricted to the analysis of hydrophilic or semihydrophobic proteins of a molecular weight of 3000–100,000. The retention of molecules of interest can be controlled by manipulating the properties of the mobile phase, and the separation of molecules with only small differences in hydrophobicity can be performed. The HP-RPC is used for the detection of target protein–related compounds (e.g., des-amido forms, oxidized forms, scrambled forms, cleaved forms), which may be present in amounts from 1 ppt and upward. The resulting UV diagram is said to provide an impurity profile within the relatively narrow window offered by the technology, but it should be kept in mind that not all impurities are detected by this or similar methods. Impurities present in 0.1% or higher should be fully characterized no later than phase 3 of the manufacture. HP-RPC is used for in-process control analysis of target protein identity (retention time), quantity (peak area), and purity (215 or 280 nm profile). The method is also used for drug substance/product impurity profiles and determination of quantity.

5.2.3.5 High-performance size exclusion chromatography (HP-SEC) HP-SEC is based on highly specific analytical columns comprising uniform particles of a given diameter depending on the molecular weight of the target protein. The principal feature of SEC is its gentle noninteraction with the sample, enabling high retention of biological activity while separating multimers that are not easily distinguished by other chromatographic methods.

The resolution is less than that of HP-IEC and HP-RPC techniques. The technology applies to almost all types of globular proteins. HP-SEC can be directly coupled to ESI and MS by means of ammonium formate buffer (typically 50 mM) making a direct determination of molecular weights possible.

HP-SEC is used for detection of di- and polymeric target protein content in the drug substance/product. It is a purity analysis.

5.2.4 Electrophoresis

5.2.4.1 SDS-PAGE PAGE describes a technique widely used to separate biological macromolecules, usually proteins or nucleic acids, according to their electrophoretic mobility. Mobility is a function of the length, the conformation, and the charge of the molecule. As with all forms of gel electrophoresis, molecules may be run in their native state, preserving the HOS, or a chemical denaturant may be added to remove this structure and turn the molecule into an unstructured linear chain whose mobility depends only on its length and mass-to-charge ratio. For nucleic acids, urea is the most commonly used denaturant. For proteins, SDS is an anionic detergent applied to the protein sample to linearize proteins and to impart a negative charge to linearize proteins. In most proteins, the binding of SDS to the polypeptide chain imparts an even distribution of charge per unit mass, thereby resulting in a fractionation by approximate size during electrophoresis. Proteins that have a greater hydrophobic content, for instance, many membrane proteins and those that interact with surfactants in their native environment, are intrinsically harder to accurately treat using this method, due to the greater variability in the ratio of bound SDS.

5.2.4.2 2D-SDS PAGE Two-dimensional gel electrophoresis, abbreviated as 2DE or 2D electrophoresis, is a form of gel electrophoresis commonly used to analyze proteins. Mixtures of proteins are separated by two properties in two dimensions on 2D gels. 2DE was first independently introduced by O'Farrell and Klose in 1975. 2DE begins with one-dimensional (1D) electrophoresis but then separates the molecules by a second property in a direction 90° from the first. Because it is unlikely that two molecules will be similar in two distinct properties, molecules are more effectively separated in 2DE than in 1D electrophoresis. The two dimensions that proteins are separated by using this technique can be the pI, a protein complex mass in the native state and protein mass.

5.2.4.3 Native electrofocusing Native electrophoresis is one of the electrophoretic methods comprising SDS-PAGE, native electrophoresis, IEF, 2DE, and CE. One-dimensional SDS-PAGE offers separation of proteins according to their molecular weight. Samples run under denaturing, but nonreducing conditions will provide information of presence of other molecular species and of disulfide intermolecular di- and polymers. Samples run under denaturing and reducing conditions will provide information on monomeric compounds. Notice that in the latter procedure, it is common practice to boil the sample in the denaturing and reducing buffers before application. The boiling procedure must not be used if information of aggregates is required (denaturing but nonreducing conditions). Native electrophoresis separates proteins according to charge, molecular weight, shape, and other factors (samples are typically applied under conditions maintaining the tertiary structure).

IEF separates proteins according to the pI (samples may be implemented under native or denaturing conditions). The method offers very high resolution and it is often used to provide information of presence of closely related derivatives (e.g., des-amido forms) or presence of glycosylated derivatives of the target protein. 2DE separates proteins according to the protein's pI (first dimension) and its molecular weight (second dimension). The method is a combination of IEF and SDS-PAGE. The resulting coordinate (pI, molecular weight) provides a unique identification of the protein. Differences in PTMs (e.g., phosphorylation) will often result in separate spots (slightly different pI and molecular weight). CE offers similar separation technologies. The CE methods can be used as a purity analysis. In native electrophoresis, proteins are separated according to charge, shape, and molecular weight in the absence of denaturants, ampholytes, or other reagents, which can influence the molecular properties or the electric field. The sample is typically transferred to or solubilized in 5% (w/v) sucrose or dilute gel buffer (1–5 mM). The gel pH and the pI of the protein(s) to be analyzed must match, as the net charge of the protein(s) may change from positive to negative or negative to positive affecting the protein's ability to enter the gel (i.e., if gel pH < protein pH, the protein will have a net positive charge; if gel pH > protein pH, the protein will have a net negative charge). Note that severe solubility problems can be experienced for certain proteins in the absence of denaturing and solubilizing agents such as urea or SDS. IEF standards can be used for native electrophoresis as well. Coomassie blue and silver staining are the two most common staining methods used for band detection on slab gels. Coomassie staining has a sensitivity of 0.05 to 0.5 pg protein per band. Silver staining is about 10–100 times more sensitive at enabling detection of 1–5 ng of protein per band. Native electrophoresis is used as a target protein identity method and to evaluate product-related impurities (e.g., des-amido forms, oxidized forms) during process development. One should, in general, be careful to use electrophoretic methods as purity analyses due to difficulties in quantifying the method.

5.2.4.4 Western blot (WB) WB (sometimes called protein immunoblot) is used to detect specific proteins; it uses gel electrophoresis to separate native proteins by 3D structure or denatured proteins by the length of the polypeptide. The proteins are then transferred to a membrane (typically nitrocellulose or polyvinylidene fluoride), where they are stained with antibodies specific for the target protein. The gel electrophoresis step is included in WB analysis to resolve the issue of the cross-reactivity of antibodies. There are now many reagent companies that specialize in providing antibodies (both monoclonal and polyclonal antibodies) against tens of thousands of different proteins. Commercial antibodies can be expensive, although the unbound antibody can be reused between experiments. This method is used in the fields of molecular biology, immunogenetics, and other molecular biology disciplines.

A number of search engines, such as CiteAb, are available that can help researchers find suitable antibodies for use in western blotting. Other related techniques include dot blot analysis, immunohistochemistry, and immunocytochemistry where antibodies are used to detect proteins in tissues and cells by immunostaining and ELISA.

5.3 Choosing a proper tool

The choice of biopharmaceutical tools is related to the complexity of the protein; the goal remains the same, to establish similarity of primary and secondary structures, bioactivity, safety, and purity.

5.3.1 Identity

As mentioned earlier, identity is not an attribute for new molecules as their identity is developed or described. For biosimilars, the first step is to establish that the biosimilar and the originator molecules have the same identity. In reality, it will be appropriate not to call it a molecule but an entity, since this may include several variants, which when combined form the total identity of the biosimilar drug. Almost always, if this stage of development leaves any residual uncertainty, the sponsor will be required to file a 351(a) or the full BLA.

The identity attributes are such characterizations as the primary, secondary, tertiary, and quaternary structures of the molecule; these can be tested with MS, ELISA, capillary IEF, differential scanning calorimetry (DSC), etc. Also included in the identity are all PTMs, such as in the case of monoclonal antibodies, and finally, an identity test where the molecule shows binding to a molecule-specific antibody, such as in an SDS-PAGE, ideally, in a 2D staging.

All biological products can be divided into two distinct categories: one that does not involve PTM and the other that does undergo PTM. The PTMs always lead to a mixture of products, variants, that combine to form the product. Whereas the exact significance of the distribution of these variants is not known, the agencies are reluctant to allow a lot of variance in these patterns, even if the variants may not be related to the MoA or the side effects.

5.3.1.1 Primary structure This includes all attributes related to the amino acid sequence and any or all PTMs including glycans. The common methods used include whole protein man spectroscopy (MS), hydrophobic interaction chromatography (HIC) LC–MS, peptide map, disulfide structure, glycan map, pI, extinction coefficient, and immune-based identity. These methods should be sensitive and resolving. Whereas the methods need not be fully validated, they must be sufficiently reliable. Some methods such as NMR are difficult to validate, particularly, if these testings are outsourced.

An example of the difference may be in the glycosylation pattern. Knowing that differences in fucosylation and high mannose can impact ADCC function; these differences are significant and must be resolved before the biosimilar product development moves forward. The causes of these variations can be traced back to the choice of the host cell to the bioprocessing conditions. Since the biosimilar product developer is likely to claim extrapolation of indications, which means asserting similarity for all MOAs, the matching of glycosylation pattern, even if it is not totally relevant, will always be required to remove any residual uncertainty of biosimilarity. The reference product developers know this well and have provided broad protection to their process that results in a particular glycan pattern. This is one good example to demonstrate the need for the biosimilar product developer to engage early in the IP evaluation of the proposed biosimilar product.

For the nonglycosylated proteins, the structural challenges may be less onerous, yet there remain process-related impurity profiles that will require optimization of upstream processing to match these profiles early in the development stage.

5.3.1.2 Sequencing Protein sequencing is a technique to determine the amino acid sequence of a protein, as well as which conformation the protein adopts and the extent to which it is complexed with any nonpeptide molecules. The two major direct methods of protein sequencing are MS and the Edman degradation reaction (N-terminal as well). It is also possible to generate an amino acid sequence from the DNA or mRNA sequence encoding the protein if this is known. However, there are many other reactions that can be used to gain more limited information about protein sequences, and can be used as preliminaries to the aforementioned methods of sequencing or to overcome specific inadequacies within them. The mass of the intact met-GCSF protein is determined by MS (ESI MS and MALDI-MS).

5.3.1.3 Extinction coefficient The extinction coefficient method is based on the absorbance of tyrosine, tryptophan, and phenylalanine residues at 275–280 nm (UV region). Phenylalanine is only weakly absorbing and is usually neglected for most purposes. The protein structure is not affected by the method making on-line measurement a possibility. Pigments, organic cofactors, and phenolic compounds interfere with the assay. The UV absorbance method is used for determining the total protein in semipurified and purified samples. The assay may be used as an on-line in-process control method, for determining the total protein in the intermediary samples and in the drug substance/product.

The extinction coefficient can be determined by two methods: amino acid analysis and UV light absorption at 280 nm. This is in line with ICH Q6B, which recommends determining the coefficient (sometimes referred to as molar absorptivity) by a combination of the two. This method is important because, in complex solutions, proteins are not the only molecules that absorb UV light. Other compounds can skew the results, but their interference is minimized when the absorbance is measured at the UV level. Note that presence of nucleic acids in the sample will interfere with the absorbance; the extinction coefficient of a protein is pH dependent.

In the past, the extinction coefficient was determined via a number of experimental procedures that tended to be very laborious and error prone. Today, nearly all protein extinction coefficients are assessed using empirical equations that utilize the average molar extinction coefficients determined from a collection of published literature data for the three key chromophores that contribute to the UV absorbance at 280 nm (tyrosine, tryptophan, and disulfide bond), in conjunction with known amino acid sequence of the product drug of interest:

$$\text{Protein} \times \text{molar extinction coefficient at}$$
$$280\ \text{nm} = \varepsilon_{\text{tyr}}(n_{\text{tyr}}) + \varepsilon_{\text{try}}(n_{\text{try}}) + \varepsilon_{\text{disulf}}(n_{\text{disulf}}),$$

wherein ε is the extinction coefficient and n is the number of moles.

The accuracy of the extinction coefficient generated from this empirical formula has been assessed at about 5%, but could be as great as 10% particularly if the protein has an unusual amino acid composition. The FDA recommends determining the extinction coefficient using an orthogonal measurement such as using analytical centrifuge and SEC with LS, UV, and refractometric detection.

Once the extinction coefficient is determined, it can be combined with other attributes of the protein, such as amino acid composition, to improve the robustness of the measurement of the concentration of protein in the samples.

5.3.1.4 Amino acid analysis (AAA) AAA is done to determine the amino acid composition of a protein without using an external standard. It can be applied in many ways to reveal different aspects of the protein. In combination with UV-absorbance measurements; it can be used directly to determine the extinction coefficient of a protein. By omitting hydrolysis, it can be used to quantify free amino acids, for example, in cell culture media. It can quantify unusual amino acids such as norleucine (encountered in *E. coli* fermentations) or hydroxyproline and lysine. The concentration based on mass can be combined with MALDI-TOF to reveal the intact mass of the protein.

5.3.1.5 Peptide mapping Peptide mapping is commonly undertaken to analyze the protein's primary structure after cleavage of the protein into proteolytic peptides. The power of peptide mapping lies in the large number of site-specific molecular features that can be detected. When using one digestion enzyme (for example, trypsin), peptide mapping is typically carried out for protein identification. The analysis is performed using MALDI-MS/MS or LC-ESI-MS/MS, for example, during protein identification after electrophoreses, such as 1D or 2D PAGE. When using multiple enzymes, peptide mapping is applied for the confirmation of a complete amino acid sequence, for example, when confirming the amino acid sequence of a biosimilar and comparing it with the originator molecule. Depending on the experimental setup, peptide mapping can also be used to determine the N- and C-termini of a protein. This is sometimes crucial information for our clients, for example, in the case of monoclonal antibodies, where the truncation level of the C-terminal lysine can be monitored. Proteins and peptides are ionized and fragmented in the mass spectrometer. The resulting MS/MS spectra are used to sequence the individual amino acids in order of their appearance in a protein or peptide. In combination with additional sample preparation, peptide mapping can also be used to determine the degree of deamidation or oxidation for each affected amino acid, glycosylation sites and structure, N-glycosylation sites, and disulfide linkages.

5.3.1.6 Terminal sequence The N- and C-terminal sequencing can reveal a great deal of information about proteins and antibodies at any stage of the drug development process. It is also performed to demonstrate consistency and comparability between lots. It can determine the N-terminal blockage or signal peptide cleavage. The level of C-terminal lysine truncation of monoclonal antibodies is a critical quality attribute and, therefore, needs to be closely monitored. When done by MALDI-in source decay (ISD), N- and C-terminal sequencings can be specifically used to monitor terminal amino acids for modifications such as glycosylation, disulfide bridging, and oxidation. With the digestion strategy, we can use peptide mapping with LC-ESI-MS/MS to identify and quantify the N- and C-terminal sequence variants.

5.3.1.7 Disulfide link The disulfide linkages are an important structural feature of many proteins. Intrachain bonds form or stabilize the tertiary structure of a protein (for example, the zinc-binding domain of zinc-finger proteins) and interchain disulfide bonds covalently link protein subunits together, (for example, the insulin A and B chains). The processes for identifying disulfide linkages include investigating the differential appearance of the linked peptides before and after reduction of the disulfide bond and analyzing the fragment spectra of the linked peptides using MS. Peptide mapping may be helpful to confirm the primary structure and aid in determining the most appropriate enzymatic digestion strategy for the disulfide bridge analysis. N- and C-terminal sequencing using MALDI-ISD can be used to determine the presence of free sulfhydryl groups or disulfide linkages within these regions. Finally, electrophoresis, such as reducing and nonreducing SDS-PAGE to identify disulfide-linked subunits of a protein, may also be undertaken.

5.3.1.8 Glycosylation MAbs, having high selectivity and specificity, constitute a large and growing portion of the biosimilars. The majority of marketed mAbs belong to the IgG class. IgGs, which consist of two heavy chains and two light chains linked by a total of 16 inter- or intramolecular disulfide bonds. The two heavy chains are linked by disulfide bonds, and each heavy chain is disulfide bonded to a light chain. IgGs include Fab and Fc regions: The Fab is responsible for binding to the antigen, while the Fc binds to Fcγ receptors, which regulate immune responses.

Glycosylation is a common PTM for IgG antibodies produced by mammalian cells such as CHO cells, which are frequently used for production. IgG1 molecules contain a single N-linked glycan at Asn297 in each of the two heavy chains. During the synthesis of N-glycans, multiple sugar moieties can be added to form different glycoforms, e.g., G0, G1, G2 afucosylated complex. Glycosylation plays an important role in CDC and ADCC functions through modulating the binding to the Fcγ receptor. Particular glycoforms may be necessary to achieve therapeutic efficacy. These glycoforms may be targeted by glycosylation engineering but may also be affected by cell culture conditions.

Glycan testing is a complex and comprehensive analytical exercise. All glycan patterns can be judged from 2D PAGE analysis and tested for monosaccharides and sialic acid content. The N-glycans and O-glycans require determination of the site of glycosylation and profiling by MALDI and HPLC that allows determination of the content of each glycan. The structural heterogeneity of a glycoprotein can be ascertained using IEF or 2D PAGE. This is because sialic acids will lead to a shift in the pI of the glycoprotein, which can be determined. The cores of N- and O-linked glycans are largely composed of neutral monosaccharide building blocks, joined together by a specific stereochemistry. The stoichiometry and the identity of these building blocks are quantitatively analyzed by using high-performance anion-exchange chromatography with pulsed amperometric detection (HPAEC-PAD). This allows analysis at both N- and O-linked glycans in a single experiment. Usually, N-linked glycans are attached to the protein backbone by an N-acetylglucosamine and O-linked glycans by an O-N-acetylgalactosamine. Other typical neutral monosaccharides involved in N-linked glycosylation and O-linked glycosylation are fucose, galactose, and mannose. More specific testings may include analysis of monosaccharides released by acidic hydrolysis with HPAEC-PAD, investigation of intact N- or O-linked glycans by HPAEC-PAD, LC-ESI-MS or MALDI-MS, or visualization of the structural heterogeneity of a glycoprotein using 2D PAGE or intact mass.

Sialic acids are negatively charged, terminal monosaccharides and are important structural constituents of many glycans. The number of sialic acid molecules present impacts the activity and the serum stability of many glycoproteins. As different types of sialic acid can be incorporated into the glycan structure, it is important to be able to determine the presence of correct versus undesired sialic acid structures. Once sialic acids are released by acidic hydrolysis, it can be analyzed by HPAEC-PAD; also, N- and O-linked glycans carrying sialic acids can be tested by using HPAEC-PAD, LC-ESI-MS, or MALDI-MS.

Whereas most of recombinant product would undergo similar testing protocols, there are specifically recommended tests that may be required for the monoclonal antibodies. Some examples of these tests include the following:

- Heavy chain and light chain molecular weight determination by MS
- Peptide mapping by MS of heavy and light chains
- N- and C-terminal sequencing of heavy and light chains by MALDI-ISD
- Complementarity-determining region sequencing of variable complementary determining regions
- PTM analysis; deamidation, oxidation, pyroglutamate, N-glycosylation
- For most monoclonal antibodies, the degree of Fc- and ADCC-binding profiles will be required for similarity determination even if these do not affect the functional response

It is well known that the terminal functional groups in protein structure may not have a significant impact on the efficacy of the molecule, but it leaves one uncertain whether they would have any potential immunogenic response; the same holds true for disulfide bonding and other intramolecular interactions. In those instances where such changes are determined earlier such as through MS and CD, the sponsor may choose the 351(a) route instead to avoid more extensive analytical comparison.

5.3.2 HOS

The integrity of the secondary, tertiary, and quaternary structures is important to establish similarity. Common methods used include FTIR, near-UV spectroscopy, CD, and DSC. These methods should be sensitive and have high resolution resolving. It should be realized that the reference product extinction coefficient is not always available in public and must be determined. Secondary and tertiary structures are best evaluated using far- and near-UV CD, and 1D and 2D NMR. Far- and near-UV CD spectroscopy provides information about secondary (alpha-helix, beta-sheet, and random coil structures) and tertiary structure, respectively. In addition to similar CD spectra, comparison of transition point (specific ellipticity = 0) and ratio of specific ellipticity ($\theta_{R208}/\theta_{R222}$) data derived from the far-UV CD spectra can be used to demonstrate a high level of similarity. ^{1}H NMR spectroscopy also provides information about the 3D structure of the protein. No significant difference in the NMR spectra of the test product compared to the reference product is required as judged by the number, position, and intensity of peaks. To further support HOS similarity, natural isotope abundance 2D NMR (^{1}H–^{15}N heteronuclear single quantum coherence) spectra can be used. ^{1}H–^{15}N NMR provides better resolution than ^{1}H NMR, and that is considered a structural fingerprint of the protein.

5.3.3 Effectiveness

5.3.3.1 Bioactivity The biological activity describes the ability or the capacity of the drug substance to achieve a defined biological effect. Examples of procedures used to measure the biological activity include animal-based biological assays, cell culture–based biological assays, biochemical assays, and ligand- and receptor-binding assays. A biologic assay may be replaced by physicochemical tests provided sufficient information and correlation between the bioassay and said tests can be given and there exists a well-established manufacturing history (ICH *Harmonized Tripartite Guideline Specifications: Test Procedures and Acceptance Criteria for Biotechnological Products [Q6B]* on March 10, 1999). In some cases, the specific biological activity may provide additional useful information.

5.3.3.2 Protein content The quantity of the target protein is determined as the total peptide/protein content in a given sample excluding any inactive derivatives such as des-amido forms, oxidized forms, polymeric forms. High-performance chromatographic methods are used to quantitate both the target protein as well as its derivatives using UV detection and determination of peak areas. If the extinction coefficient is not known (e.g., analogues), amino acid or Kjeldahl analysis is used as a primary reference method. Bioassays are often replaced with quantity determination partly because of the usual high costs associated with biological assays and partly because of the much higher accuracy of quantitative assays. The commonly used quantity methods are amino acid analysis, Kjeldahl analysis, UV spectrometry, and high-performance chromatographic procedures.

5.3.4 Purity

Protein purity has been historically linked to the specific biological activity in terms of units of biological activity per mass unit of the product. The purest product was that of the highest specific biological activity. In contrast to drugs based on small molecules, which could be controlled on the drug product level, protein-based pharmaceuticals were closely linked to the process due to the complexity of the active pharmaceutical ingredient and the lack of proper characterization of the final product. With the introduction of recombinant technology and modern analytical methods, a much better drug substance/product characterization became possible resulting in the well-characterized protein concept and the widespread use of comparability studies. The importance of a stronger focus on the presence of adventitious agents and specific impurities was also recognized, as the presence of even minor amounts of toxic, immunogenic, or adventitious compounds proved to have severe side effects. Unless otherwise specified, the level of acceptable impurities depends on the nature of the drug product and the dose.

5.3.4.1 Endotoxins Endotoxins come from Gram-negative bacteria (e.g., *E. coli*) if they are used as the expressions system. The presence of endotoxins indicates bacterial contamination in raw materials, columns, water, and buffers. Endotoxins strongly bind to anion-exchange media even at high ionic strength and thus hydrophobic interaction chromatography and CIEC are used for their removal provided the target protein binds to the matrix. Binding of the target protein to CEX also allows effective endotoxin clearance. SEC can remove endotoxins provided the differences in molecular weight between the endotoxins and the protein are sufficient. However, SEC may be an unpredictable method since endotoxins range in size from subunits of 10–20 kDa in the presence of detergents to vesicles of 0.1 pm in diameter in the presence of divalent cations. In the absence of significant levels of divalent cations and surface-active agents, they dissociate into micelles of 300–1000 kDa.

Traditional inactivation methods (CIP) against endotoxins include acid hydrolysis, base hydrolysis, oxidation, alkylation, and heat and ionizing radiation. The use of a concentration-dependent matrix of sodium hydroxide is recommended for the removal endotoxins from chromatographic columns; endotoxins are destroyed by exposure to NaOH or peracetic acid but are not affected by ethanol.

5.3.4.1.1 Nucleic acids Nucleic acid contamination comes from host cell DNA/RNA or retroviral RNA. Molecules with more than 150–200 base pairs will behave as flexible coils in SEC, while molecules up to 18 base pairs behave as globular proteins. In between, the rigid rod structure should be expected. Their presence results in increased viscosity of the solution. Circular DNA is often supercoiled and will elute as a molecule of smaller size. Preventive action nucleic acid–free biopharmaceutical products are obtained by using nucleases (e.g., Benzonase) and/or by minimizing the release of nucleic acids from the host cell organism. AEIC has been shown to be effective in binding the highly charged nucleic acids at ionic strength at which most proteins elute. Due to the net negative charge and hydrophilic-binding character of the target protein to a CEX, hydrophobic interaction or affinity matrix may reduce the nucleic acid content. DNA binds to hydroxyapatite at low to moderate phosphate concentrations. Precipitation of nucleic acids with polyethyleneimine or magnesium chloride has been reported. The use of 1 M NaOH is recommended (make sure that equipment, filters, and chromatographic media are not affected by NaOH) for CIP. Nucleic acids are detected by monitoring absorption of light at 260 nm. The residual content of drug substance and/or drug product is usually measured by polymerase chain reaction (PCR) or amplification techniques. The maximum allowable content of nucleic acid per dose has been under continuous evaluation of the initially proposed content of 10 pg per dose suggested by CBER. WHO has stated that 100 pg per dose is acceptable. CBER now states that "lot-to-lot testing for DNA content in biological products produced in cell lines should be performed, and lot release limits established that reflect a level of purity that can be achieved reasonably and consistent."

5.3.4.2 HCPs HCPs come from the host organism and constitute a major purification problem due to variability structure and surface properties. The amount released into the culture medium depends on the expression system used, the culture conditions, and whether the cells are disrupted or not in order to intracellularly extract expressed target protein. Notice that foreign cellular proteins can be introduced by means of recombinantly derived raw materials (e.g., enzymes) used in the downstream process. The range of preventive actions includes use of expression systems with direct expression of the target protein to the culture medium, gentle handling of intact cells, and purification procedures such as chromatography, filtration, precipitation, and crystallization. If milk from transgenic animals is used as the product source, the presence of the animal equivalent of the target protein should be of concern (as it might copurify with the target protein). Protein impurities should be considered on a case-by-case basis and be relegated to process validation rather than final product testing. Due to molecular diversity, no specific purification method can be recommended, as the separation depends on the difference in affinity (selectivity) between the HCP and the target protein for chosen chromatographic media and operating conditions. The use of a combination of different chromatographic principles is recommended. Most proteins will be removed (CIP) by means of 0.1–1 M NaOH (make sure that equipment, filters, and chromatographic media are not affected by NaOH). Several analytical methods have been used to monitor HCP including SDS-PAGE, 2DE, WB, and immunoassays. SDS-PAGE separates molecules according to the molecular weight of the protein. The method, which is semiquantitative, has a sensitivity of 100 pg/band (silver staining). 2-DE (IEF in combination with SDS-PAGE) provides the most powerful separation of protein mixtures. The method, which is semiquantitative, provides the widest window of the methods used with a sensitivity of 100 pg/spot. The WB method provides information about immunological identity. The sensitivity is 0.1–1 ng/band and the method is qualitative. Immunoassays are widely used for HCP analysis in drug substances and drug products. The method depends on the nature and the quality of antibodies used, and not all proteins (regardless of quantity) are detected. The method also provides the highest sensitivity (<0.1 ng/mL). Two types of assays have been used to detect HCPs: generic and specific assays. In generic assays, the HCPs typical for a given expression system are detected. If the assays are based on competently produced antibodies raised against cell lysates, the quality may be adequate or better than those produced by individual companies. Generic assays are typically used during process development, as process specific assays by definition are not available before the process has been locked. However, it is also recommended to use generic HCP assays for lot release for several reasons. Firstly, the protein patterns are highly conserved among strains and secondly, a generic HCP assay will be a strong tool for detection of variations in the process, which could lead to a different impurity profile. Process-specific assays are directed against HCPs copurifying with the target protein. The assays are typically developed for purifying the cell lysate without target protein using the exact process to be used for the licensed product. By definition, the process-specific assay cannot be developed before the process is locked. The assay, which typically takes one to two years to develop, may thus be a time-delaying factor. The process-specific assays provide a much narrower window than generic assays do and their value as lot-release test has recently been challenged because these assays will most probably fail to detect atypical HCP contaminants. There are some significant differences between WB technology and immunoassays. In WB, the denaturation and solubilization steps can destroy some native epitopes while the immunoassay technology relies on reaction with the native protein. The immunoassay technology provides an objective result while the WB depends on a subjective interpretation. Finally, the sensitivity of immunoassays is generally higher than that of WB assays. None of the methods mentioned are quantitative. They are at best semi-quantitative. Even the commonly used HCP immunoassay lack the linear accuracy applied to single analyte immunoassays, due to variance in relative affinities between antibodies and HCP antigens and HCP concentrations. Instead, assay results are correlated with clinical conditions and to process control. The amount of HCP to be accepted depends on the antigenicity of the copurifying proteins. Recognizing the complexity of the task and the inability of quantitative measurements it is not possible to state a generally acceptable level.

5.3.4.3 Viruses Virus contamination comes from the host cell, the culture medium, and the infections during manufacture. The host cell may contain a genomic virus or virus vectors used to transform the cell line. The type of viral genome and/or vector depends on the cell line history. Continuous cell lines are extensively characterized, but chronic or latent viruses may be present. The retroviruses associated with continuous cell lines are noninfectious but oncogenic. The Epstein–Barr virus or the Sendai virus is often used for cell transformations. Contaminants such as bovine viral diarrhea virus, infectious bovine rhinotracheitis, reovirus, PI-3, bovine leukemia virus, and bovine polyomavirus should be expected from serum-supplemented media. Virus control is executed on several levels. The cell line history reveals all information on the origin and identity of the cell line and the host genome vectors used to establish the cell line. The master cell bank is extensively characterized using viral identity tests, in vitro tests, and in vivo tests to assure freedom of adventitious viruses. The end-of-production test of the cell culture is carried out to assure that the cells are free of viruses. Viruses are brought into the process from the environment because of either contaminated equipment, infected raw materials, water, or because of nonsterile handling procedures. Working in closed systems and avoiding of raw materials of animal origin will help reduce the risk of infection. Strict control of equipment cleaning and sanitization procedures during processing will also help in reducing contamination risk. Removal of viruses may be inactivated by heat, radiation, chemical compound, or low pH, or removed by chromatography or filtration techniques. Due to molecular diversity, no specific chromatographic purification method can be recommended, and virus reduction factors must be determined for selected unit operations. Nanofiltration is a very efficient virus removal step often resulting in logarithmic reduction factors of 5–8. A commonly used reagent for cleaning chromatographic media is 0.1–1 M NaOH. Viruses can be successfully destroyed with peracetic acid (make sure that equipment, filters, and chromatographic media are not affected by NaOH or peracetic acid). A variety of purity analyses are available: monolayer cultures, test for pathogen viruses not able to grow in cell cultures in both animals and eggs, test for retroviruses, endogenous viruses, or viral nucleic acid, and test for selected viruses using mouse, rat, and hamster antibody production tests. It is necessary to document the utilization of adequate virus removal and inactivation strategies to ensure the exclusion of contaminating viruses. Different MoAs should ensure overlapping and complementary levels of protection. The purification process is validated with respect to virus removal and inactivation. The final product is rarely tested if continuous mammalian cell lines have been used as an expression system.

5.3.4.4 Prions Prions come from transmissible spongiform encephalopathies including scrapie in sheep and goats, chronic wasting disease in mule deer and elk, bovine spongiform encephalopathy (BSE) in cattle, Kuru, and Creutzfeldt-Jakob disease in humans. The disease-causing agents (prions) generally replicate in infected individuals without evidence of infection detectable by available diagnostic tests applicable in vivo. The primary source of contamination of a recombinant product is the use of animal-derived raw materials, which could harbor bovine prions (BSE agent). Currently, there are no assays that are sensitive or specific enough to test raw materials or sources and the only reliable prevention is to include barriers, such as avoidance of animal or human raw materials (e.g., trypsin, serum, transferrin, bovine/human serum albumin, protein supplements, peptones). However, this is not always possible (e.g., in the propagation of cells for the establishment of cell banks), and inactivation and removal procedures during downstream processing become of interest. Milk is unlikely to present any risk of prion contamination. Filtration has to be proven efficient in the removal of prion particles. Thus, size exclusion partitioning of abnormal prion particles using normal flow filtration or tangential flow filtration resulted in significant reduction of the infectious agent. The most effective inactivation methods include chloride dioxide, glutaraldehyde, 4 M guanidium thiocyanate, sodium dichloroisocyanurate, sodium metaperiodate, 6 M urea, and autoclaving at 121°C for 15 minutes, several of which will not be suited if the target protein is present. Biological assays such as in vivo infection of susceptible animals are time consuming (months to years). They will not be of practical use in the test of biopharmaceutical products. The best semiquantitative biochemical assays include WB, capillary immunoelectrophoresis, conformation-dependent immunoassay, and dissociation-enhanced, time-resolved fluoroimmunoassay. The infectious dose is not known. Acceptable criteria must be decided upon on a case-by-case basis.

5.3.4.5 Proteolytic enzymes Proteolytic enzymes are released to the medium because of cell death, mechanical stress, or induced cell lysis. Their presence should be expected during fermentation and initial downstream unit operations. Measures are taken to work fast at low temperatures and to avoid working near the pH optimum of the enzyme. The most rewarding strategy is to prevent proteolysis already during fermentation either by use of mutant strains or by optimizing the conditions toward minimum enzymatic activity. Most enzymes of the vacuoles and lysosomes will be minimally active at slightly alkaline pH (7–9), a pH interval strongly recommended for extraction of proteins expressed in bacteria. Proteins are probably more resistant toward proteolytic attacks in their native state and stabilizing factors (e.g., cofactor, correct parameter interval, cosolvent) should always be considered optimized. The use of protein inhibitors is not recommended for safety reasons. Proteolytic enzymes are typically removed during the capture and intermediary purification steps and they are rarely copurified with the target protein throughout the downstream process. Despite the variety of enzymes present in the cell cytosol, proteolytic enzymes rarely constitute a problem in final products. Selective removal (e.g., affinity chromatography) of specific enzymes should be considered. Most proteins will be removed by means of 0.1–1 M NaOH (make sure that equipment, filters, and chromatographic media are not affected by NaOH). Suited analytical methods for early control are SDS-PAGE and western blotting. Purified preparations may be analyzed by means of HP-IEC, HP-RPC, MS, and peptide mapping. Ascertain that the degradation observed is not a function of the analytical assay. Enzyme inhibitors can be used for prevention of enzymatic activity in analytical assays.

5.3.4.6 Lipids Lipids (lipoproteins, triglycerides, phospholipids, cholesterol) are brought to the medium by cell lysis. If transgenic animals are used, the protein is expressed in the milk containing up to 4% fat. Lipids can be removed from the feedstock by centrifugation, by specific adsorption to hydrophobic compounds such as Hyflow by precipitation with dextran sulfate, by binding to anion exchangers, or by affinity chromatography allowing for specific binding of the target protein. Lipids will bind to hydrophobic media and surfaces. Lipids are retarded (two to three column volumes) by adsorption to Sephadex. Milk fat is usually removed by centrifugation. Lipids are removed by means of NaOH or organic solvents (make sure that equipment, filters, and chromatographic media are not affected by NaOH or organic solvents).

5.3.4.7 Microbial agents Microbial agents and fungi come from infection of the bioreactor during cell culture. Other sources are contaminated water, buffers, raw materials, chromatographic columns, and equipment. Fermentation and cell culture bioreactors are prone to microbial infections. As the use of antibiotics in large-scale operations should be avoided, strict demands on the design of bioreactors and handling procedures are the key measures to avoid microbial infections. Test for microorganisms at the end of production assures that no infections have taken place during culture. The nature of samples and buffers used during downstream processing make these excellent growth substrates for microorganisms. For that reason, water quality control, sterile filtration of buffers prior to use, sterile filtration of intermediary products, and effective cleaning and sanitization procedures are key elements of the downstream operations. Filtration through 0.22 μm filters. Bacterial spores are typically removed by means of 0.1 μm filters. Cleaning with 60%–70% v/v ethanol is a commonly used disinfectant against microbial agents; often 20% v/v ethanol is used as a storage solution for chromatographic resins, but the solution has no sporicidal effect, while 0.1–1.0 M NaOH is widely used to kill microorganisms. Peracetic acid has both bacterial and sporicidal effects. Viable cells can be identified by spread out of the cell suspension or sample solution on agar plates.

5.3.4.8 Mycoplasma Mycoplasmas have long been recognized as a contaminant of continuous cell cultures caused by an infection of the cell line or the bioreactor. Working in closed systems under good manufacturing practices (GMPs) will reduce the risk of infection. The end-of-production test includes screening for mycoplasma. Mycoplasmas are extremely sensitive to osmotic shock and pH extremes and should not constitute a problem in downstream processing provided sanitization and cleaning in place procedures are carried out according to GMPs. Mycoplasmas are resistant to most antibiotics. Frequent testing (at every passage) is recommended. The cell culture is discarded upon infection. Cleaning with 0.1–1 M NaOH will inactivate the mycoplasma. Mycoplasmas are difficult to detect; the only reliable way of demonstrating infection is by agar plating, fluorescent dyeing of DNA, or by PCR. Recently, a selective biochemical test that exploits the activity of certain mycoplasma enzymes has been made commercially available.

5.3.4.9 Des-amido forms Des-amido forms are target protein derivatives in which one or several of the glutaminyl or asparaginyl amino acid residues are converted to the corresponding acids (glutamyl and aspargyl). The deamidation reaction is slow at pH 3–5, at low temperatures, and at low conductivity. Deamidated forms are removed by HP-IEC and HP-RPC. Des-amido forms are detected by analytical HP-IEC,

HP-RPC, native PAGE, IEF, MS, or CE. The content accepted depends on the nature of the drug product and the dose.

5.3.4.10 Oxidized forms Oxidized forms are target protein derivatives in which one or several Met, Cys, His, Trp, and Tyr residues have been oxidized. The oxidation of cysteinyl residues results in the formation of a disulfide bond (cystinyl residue). The oxidation reaction is slow at low pH and low temperature. The formation of disulfide bonds will take place above 0 mV. Oxidized forms are removed by HP-IEC and HP-RPC. Disulfide aggregates can be removed by SEC. Oxidized forms are detected by analytical HP-IEC, HP-RPC, native PAGE, IEF, MS, or CE. The content accepted depends on the nature of the drug product and the dose.

5.3.4.11 Carbamylated forms Carbamylated forms are target protein derivatives in which one or several primary amino, sulfhydryl, carboxyl, phenolic hydroxyl, imidazole, and phosphate groups react with cyanate to form a derivative. The blocking may change the pI of the protein. Cyanate is spontaneously formed in urea solutions, which is the primary source. The formation is slow at low temperatures, but it is nevertheless strongly recommended to purify the urea solution by means of mixed ion exchangers before use. Carbamylated forms are removed by HP-IEC and HP-RPC and detected by analytical HP-IEC, HP-RPC, native PAGE, IEF, MS, or CE. The content accepted depends on the nature of the drug product and the dose.

5.3.4.12 Aggregates Aggregates are target protein derivatives in which two or more molecules is linked together either by covalent interdisulfide bonds or by hydrophobic interaction. Target protein aggregates are formed as a result of hydrophobic intermolecular reactions or because of intermolecular disulfide bond formation under oxidizing conditions. Aggregates are very often antigenic resulting in the formation of target protein antibodies. Proteins exposed to even mildly denaturing conditions may partially unfold resulting in exposure of hydrophobic residues to the aqueous solvent favoring aggregation. The aggregation process is assumed to be controlled by the initial dimerization step in a second-order reaction. Consequently, high protein concentrations will increase the aggregation rate. Intermolecular disulfide bond formation between cysteinyl residues takes place at alkaline pH under oxidizing conditions. Proteins with reactive-free thiol groups should be purified under reducing conditions (typically 1–10 mM reducing agent) in the presence of ethylenediaminetetraacetic acid. Even proteins with disulfide bonds may participate in intermolecular disulfide bond reactions due to disulfide bond shuffling at neutral and alkaline pH. The aggregation reaction based on intermolecular disulfide bond formation is prevented at $pH < 6$ and under reducing conditions. The hydrophobic aggregation reaction strongly depends on the hydrophobicity of the molecule. Preventive actions are taken to keep the protein in its native conformation during processing in order to avoid unfolding and exposure of hydrophobic sites. Hydrophobic proteins (e.g., certain membrane proteins) may be kept soluble by the addition of specific cosolvents (e.g., detergents). Aggregates may be removed by filtration or SEC. Disulfide-based aggregates can be detected by nonreducing (no boiling of the sample) 1D-SDS, HP-SEC, MS, or CE. Hydrophobic aggregates may be detected by HP-SEC. The content accepted depends on the nature of the drug product and the dose.

5.3.4.13 Scrambled forms Scrambled forms are target protein molecules with a disulfide bond pattern different from that of the native molecule. Scrambled forms are typically formed during in vitro folding of proteins, but disulfide bond shuffling at neutral pH or above also occurs. This requires studies on control of protein stability during downstream processing. The formation of scrambled forms is closely linked to the folding procedure. The best preventive action is to optimize said procedure. As the folding reaction is protein specific, no general rules can be given. Scrambled forms are removed by HP-IEC and HP-RPC. Scrambled forms are detected by analytical HP-IEC, HP-RPC, CE, or peptide mapping. The content accepted depends on the nature of the drug product and the dose.

5.3.4.14 Cleaved forms Cleaved forms are typically used for target protein derivatives with almost identical molecular weight (plus or minus a few hundred daltons), where a peptide bond is cleaved resulting in loss of an N- or C-terminal site or where an internal peptide bond is cleaved; simultaneously, the resulting fragments are kept together by means of disulfide bonds. Gentle handling of cells, low temperatures, and working in pH intervals where enzymatic activity is low reduce proteolysis. The use of enzyme inhibitors is not recommended for safety reasons. Removal of proteolytic enzymes during capture prevents the formation of cleaved forms as well. Cleaved forms are removed by HP-IEC and HP-RPC. Detection cleaved forms are detected by analytical HP-IEC, HP-RPC, native PAGE, IEF, MS, peptide mapping, or CE.

5.4 Novel methods

Stress testing proteins under various conditions and examining a change in their behavior is one of the several new methods that are being developed. A proprietary and patented (pending) testing method developed by Therapeutic Proteins International, LLC (Chicago) makes the following claims:

1. A method of comparing structural similarity of a first biomolecule to a second biomolecule, the method comprising
    - altering a concentration of one or more components in a solution comprising a first biomolecule;

- measuring at least one of a fluorescence emission wavelength and/or an intensity of fluorescence emission of the first biomolecule in the solution; and
- comparing the fluorescence emission wavelength and/or the intensity of fluorescence of the first biomolecule in the solution to a fluorescence emission wavelength and/or an intensity of fluorescence emission in a second solution comprising a second biomolecule having the same concentration of the one or more components.

Figures 5.3 and 5.4 show the results of using three different concentrations of a nonionic surfactant to alter the dielectric stress. There is a significant shift in the maximum fluorescence as well as the intensity of fluorescence. Since both test and reference proteins demonstrate equivalent shifts, this provides an additional proof of similarity.

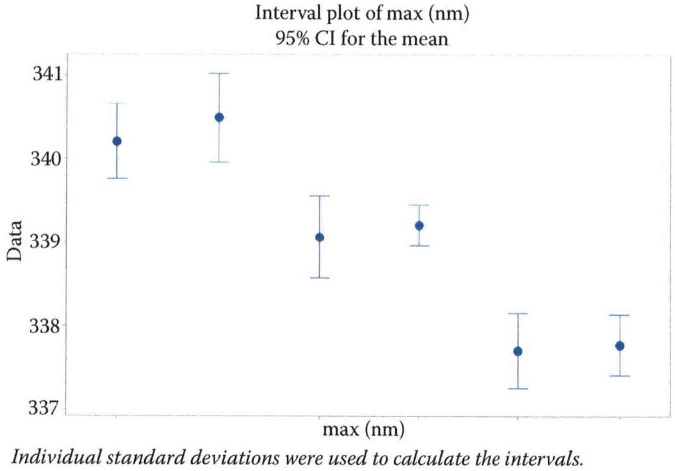

Figure 5.3 Interval plot—four-dimensional (4D) test for shift in λ_{max}.

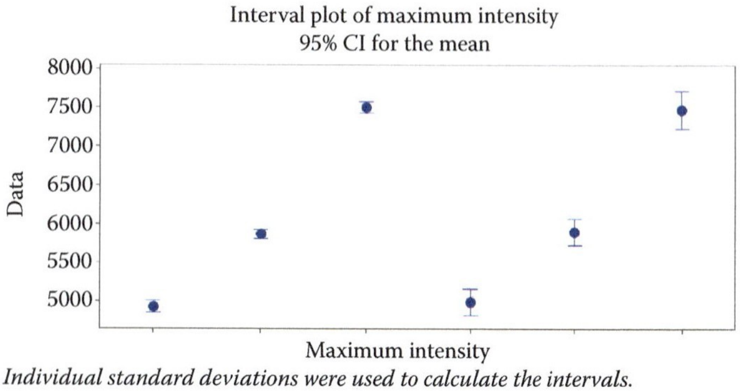

Figure 5.4 Interval plot for maximum intensity changes in the 4D test.

Bibliography

Apte, A. and Meitei, N. S. (2009) Bioinformatics in glycomics: Glycan characterization with mass spectrometric data using simglycan. *Methods Mol Biol* 600: 269–281.

Blow, N. (2009) Glycobiology: A spoonful of sugar. *Nature* 457 (7229): 617–620.

Boyd, R. K. (1994) Linked-scan techniques for MS/MS using tandem-in-space instruments. *Mass Spectrom Rev* 13 (5–6): 359–410.

Bruins, A. P. (1991) Mass spectrometry with ion sources operating at atmospheric pressure. *Mass Spectrom Rev* 10 (1): 53–77.

Comisarow, M. B. and Marshall, A. G. (1974) Fourier transform ion cyclotron resonance spectroscopy. *Chem Phys Lett* 25 (2): 282–283.

Cottrell, J. S. and Greathead, R. J. (1986) Extending the mass range of a sector mass spectrometer. *Mass Spectrom Rev* 5 (3): 215–247.

Covey, T. R., Lee, E. D., and Henion, J. D. (1986) Mass spectrometry for the determination of drugs in biological samples. *Anal Chem* 58 (12): 2453–2460.

Covey, T. R., Crowther, J. B., Dewey, E. A., and Henion, J. D. (1985) Mass spectrometry determination of drugs and their metabolites in biological fluids. *Anal Chem* 57 (2): 474–481.

Dass, C., *Principles and Practice of Biological Mass Spectrometry*. New York: John Wiley & Sons. ISBN 0-471-33053-1; 2001.

Dass, C., *Fundamentals of Contemporary Mass Spectrometry*. New York: John Wiley & Sons. p. 5. ISBN 978-0-470-11848-1; 2007.

Downard, K., *Mass Spectrometry—A Foundation Course*. Cambridge, UK: Royal Society of Chemistry. ISBN 0-85404-609-7; 2004.

Downard, K. M. (2007) Francis William Aston—The man behind the mass spectrograph. *Eur J Mass Spectrom* 13 (3): 177–190.

Dubois, F., Knochenmuss, R., Zenobi, R., Brunelle, A., Deprun, C., and Le Beyec, Y. (1999) A comparison between ion-to-photon and microchannel plate detectors. *Rapid Commun Mass Spectrom* 13 (9): 786–791.

de Hoffman, E. and Stroobant, V., *Mass Spectrometry: Principles and Applications* (Second ed.). New York: John Wiley & Sons. ISBN 0-471-48566-7; 2001.

Eiceman, G. A., Gas chromatography. In R. A. Meyers (Ed.), *Encyclopedia of Analytical Chemistry: Applications, Theory, and Instrumentation*. Chichester, England: Wiley. p. 10627. ISBN 0-471-97670-9; 2000.

FDA—Biosimilars: An update. August 2012. http://www.fda.gov/downloads/AdvisoryCommittees/CommitteesMeetingMaterials/Drugs/AdvisoryCommitteeforPharmaceuticalScienceandClinicalPharmacology/UCM315764.pdf.

Fenn, J. B., Mann, M., Meng, C. K., Wong, S. F., and Whitehouse, C. M. (1989) Electrospray ionization for mass spectrometry of large biomolecules. *Science* 246 (4926): 64–71.

Franchetti, V., Solka, B. H., Baitinger, W. E., Amy, J. W., and Cooks, R. G. (1977) Soft landing of ions as a means of surface modification. *Mass Spectrom Ion Phys* 23 (1): 29–35.

Gothard, J. W. W., Busst, C. M., Branthwaite, M. A., Davies, N. J. H., and Denison, D. M. (1980) Applications of respiratory mass spectrometry to intensive care. *Anaesthesia* 35 (9): 890–895.

Gross, J. H., *Mass Spectrometry: A Textbook*. Berlin, Germany: Springer-Verlag. ISBN 3-540-40739-1; 2006.

Harper, D. (2001 November) Spectrum. *Online Etymology Dictionary*. http://www.etymonline.com/.

Harvey, D., Dwek, R. A., and Rudd, P. M., Determining the structure of glycan moieties by mass spectrometry. *Current Protocols in Protein Science*. Chapter 12: 12.7–12.7.15. New York: John Wiley & Sons; 2000.

Hoffman, J. Chaney, R., and Hammack, H. (2008) Phoenix Mars mission—The thermal evolved gas analyzer. *J Am Soc Mass Spectrom* 19 (10): 1377–1383.

Hsieh, Y. and Korfmacher, W. A. (2006) Systems for drug metabolism and pharmacokinetic screening. *Curr Drug Metab* 7 (5): 479–489.
Hu, Q., Noll, R. J., Li, H., Makarov, A., Hardman, M., and Graham Cooks, R. (2005) The orbitrap: A new mass spectrometer. *J Mass Spectrom* 40 (4): 430–443.
Kandiah, M. and Urban, P. L. (2013) Advances in ultrasensitive mass spectrometry of organic molecules. *Chem Soc Rev* 42 (12): 5299–5322.
Karas, M., Bachman, D., Bahr, U., and Hillenkamp, F. (1987) Matrix-assisted ultraviolet laser desorption of non-volatile compounds. *Int J Mass Spectrom Ion Proc* 78: 53–68.
Lammert, S. A., Rockwood, A. A., Wang, M., and Lee, M. L. (2006) Miniature toroidal radio frequency ion trap mass analyzer. *J Am Soc Mass Spectrom* 17 (7): 916–922.
Loo, J. A., Udseth, H. R., and Smith, R. D. (1989 June) Peptide and protein analysis by electrospray ionization-mass spectrometry and capillary electrophoresis-mass spectrometry. *Anal Biochem* 179 (2): 404–412.
Maher, S., Jjunju, F. P. M., and Taylor, S. (2015) 100 years of mass spectrometry: Perspectives and future trends. *Rev Mod Phys* 87 (1): 113–135.
March, R. E. (2000) Quadrupole ion trap mass spectrometry: A view at the turn of the century. *Int J Mass Spectrom* 200 (1–3): 285–312.
Marshall, A. G., Hendrickson, C. L., and Jackson, G. S. (1998) Fourier transform ion cyclotron resonance mass spectrometry: A primer. *Mass Spectrom Rev* 17 (1): 1–34.
Matz, L. M., Asbury, G. R., and Hill, H. H. (2002) Two-dimensional separations with electrospray ionization ambient pressure high-resolution ion mobility spectrometry/quadrupole mass spectrometry. *Rapid Commun Mass Spectrom* 16 (7): 670–675.
Maxwell, E. J. and Chen, D. D. (2008 October) Twenty years of interface development for capillary electrophoresis-electrospray ionization-mass spectrometry. *Anal Chim Acta* 627 (1): 25–33.
Mistrik, R., A new concept for the interpretation of mass spectra based on a combination of a fragmentation mechanism database and a computer expert system. In Ashcroft, A. E., Brenton, G., and Monaghan, J. J. (Eds.), *Advances in Mass Spectrometry*. Amsterdam, Netherlands: Elsevier. Vol. 16, p. 821; 2004.
Muzikar, P. et al. (2003) Accelerator mass spectrometry in geologic research. *Geol Soc Am Bull* 115: 643–654.
Park, M. A., Callahan, J. H., and Vertes, A. (1994) An inductive detector for time-of-flight mass spectrometry. *Rapid Commun Mass Spectrom* 8 (4): 317–322.
Parkins, W. E. (2005) The uranium bomb, the calutron, and the space-charge problem. *Phys Today* 58 (5): 45–51.
Paul, W. and Steinwedel, H. (1953) Ein neues massenspektrometer ohne magnetfeld. *Z Naturforschung A* 8 (7): 448–450.
Petrie, S. and Bohme, D. K. (2007) Ions in space. *Mass Spectrom Rev* 26 (2): 258–280.
Price, P. (1991) Standard definitions of terms relating to mass spectrometry: A report from the Committee on Measurements and Standards of the American Society for Mass Spectrometry. *J Am Soc Mass Spectrom* 2 (4): 336–348.
Riker, J. B. and Haberman, B. (1976) Expired gas monitoring by mass spectrometry in a respiratory intensive care unit. *Crit Care Med* 4 (5): 223–229.
Schwartz, J. C., Senko, M. W., and Syka, J. E. P. (2002) A two-dimensional quadrupole ion trap mass spectrometer. *J Am Soc Mass Spectrom* 13 (6): 659–669.
Sheldon, M. T., Mistrik, R., and Croley, T. R. (2009) Determination of ion structures in structurally related compounds using precursor ion fingerprinting. *J Am Soc Mass Spectrom* 20 (3): 370–376.
Siri, W. (1947) Mass spectroscope for analysis in the low-mass range. *Rev Sci Instrum* 18 (8): 540–545.
Siuzdak, G. *Mass Spectrometry for Biotechnology*. Boston: Academic Press. ISBN 0-12-647471-0; 1996.

Sobott, F., *Biological Mass Spectrometry*. Boca Raton, FL: CRC Press. ISBN 1439895279; 2014.
Sowell, R. A., Koeniger, S. L., Valentine, S. J., Moon, M. H., and Clemmer, D. E. (2004) Nanoflow LC/IMS-MS and LC/IMS-CID/MS of protein mixtures. *J Am Soc Mass Spectrom* 15 (9): 1341–1353.
Sparkman, O. D., *Mass Spectrometry Desk Reference*. Pittsburgh, PA: Global View Pub. ISBN 0-9660813-9-0; 2006.
Squires, G. (1998) Francis Aston and the mass spectrograph. *Dalton Trans* (23): 3893–3900.
Tanaka, K., Waki, H., Ido, Y., Akita, S., Yoshida, Y., and Yoshida, T. (1988) Protein and polymer analyses up to m/z 100 000 by laser ionization time-of flight mass spectrometry. *Rapid Commun Mass Spectrom* 2 (20): 151–153.
Thomson, J. J., *Rays of Positive Electricity and Their Application to Chemical Analysis*. London: Longman's Green and Company; 1913.
Tuniz, C., *Accelerator Mass Spectrometry: Ultrasensitive Analysis for Global Science*. Boca Raton, FL: CRC Press. ISBN 0-8493-4538-3; 1998.
Tureček, F. and McLafferty, F. W., *Interpretation of Mass Spectra*. Sausalito, CA: University Science Books. ISBN 0-935702-25-3; 1993.
Verbeck, G., Hoffmann, W., and Walton, B. (2012) Soft-landing preparative mass spectrometry. *Analyst* 137 (19): 4393–4407.
Verbeck, G. F., Ruotolo, B. T., Sawyer, H. A., Gillig, K. J., and Russell, D. H. G. (2002) A fundamental introduction to ion mobility mass spectrometry applied to the analysis of biomolecules. *J Biomol Tech* 13 (2): 56–61. PMC 2279851. PMID 19498967.
Watson, J. T. and Sparkman, O. D., *Introduction to Mass Spectrometry: Instrumentation, Applications, and Strategies for Data Interpretation* (Fourth ed.). Chichester, England: John Wiley & Sons. ISBN 978-0-470-51634-8; 2007.
Wollnik, H. (1993) Time-of-flight mass analyzers. *Mass Spectrom Rev* 12 (2): 89–114.

Chapter 6 Critical quality attributes

The attributes of God tell us what He is and who He is.

William Ames

6.1 Background

The demonstration of biosimilarity begins with selecting critical quality attributes (CQAs), which are likely to have a direct impact on the four pillars of the biosimilarity tetrahedron (Chapter 4): identity, purity, potency, and safety. Whereas the importance of immunogenicity, safety, and efficacy (effectiveness) is compared head to head in biosimilarity assessments, it is not possible to provide an equal level of comparison for every quality attribute; it is for this reason that the regulatory agencies require biosimilar developers first to produce a matrix of CQAs. These attributes are selected from a risk-based exercise that identifies these in accordance with guidances such as ICH Guidelines Q8–Q11 that deal in the subjects of variation guidance, concepts, design space, process, design specifications, CQAs, control strategy, and ability to develop. Figure 6.1 provides a schematic representation of how each of the guidance is interrelated with their supporting elements for the quality risk assessment.

The quality target product profile (QTPP) is defined as a "prospective and dynamic summary of the quality characteristics of the molecule that ideally will be achieved to ensure that the desired quality, and thus the safety and efficacy, of a drug product, are realized." Once QTPP is established for the target molecule, it is used for comparative analysis to assist in the development process and final process design. The biosimilar product is designed, developed, and manufactured according to QTPP with specification consistent with the desired in vivo performance of the product, linking process, a product with patient benefit.

The aim of pharmaceutical development is to design a quality product and its manufacturing process to consistently deliver the intended performance of the product. The information and the knowledge gained from pharmaceutical development studies and manufacturing experience provide scientific understanding to support the establishment of the design space, specifications, and manufacturing controls. Figure 6.2 describes the interrelationship among the various distinct steps involved in implementing quality-by-design (QbD) paradigm for biosimilar products.

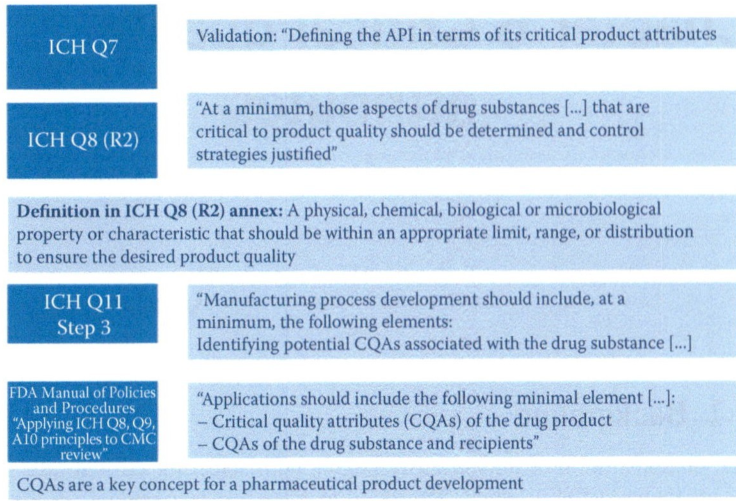

Figure 6.1 Quality expectations of ICH and the FDA guidance.

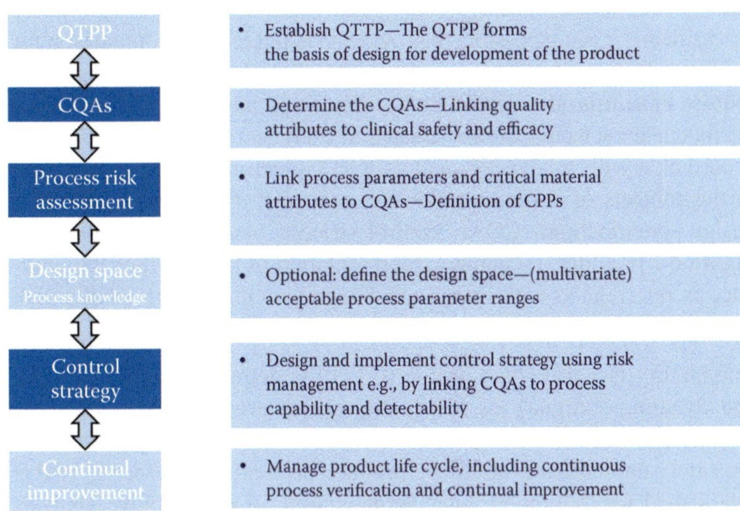

Figure 6.2 QbD connectivity (ICH Q8 RS2).

In the mind of the FDA, when there is no residual uncertainty left and that there is no clinically meaningful difference between a biosimilar candidate and the originator product, the biosimilar product is declared as having a high level of biosimilarity—the product is declared biosimilar. How this target is reached through a risk-based approach in accordance with the QbD paradigm, which promotes pharmaceutical development based on risk management and sound science.

The CQA identification takes three different approaches. For a standalone new product, the CQAs are established through confirmed studies,

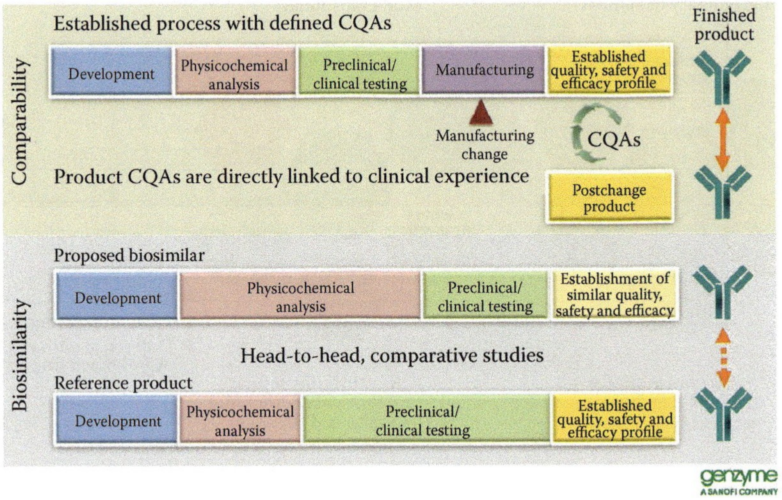

Figure 6.3 Comparison of CQAs identification in comparability protocol and biosimilars development. (From FDA—Biosimilar: An update, 2012. http://www.fda.gov/downloads/AdvisoryCommittees/CommitteesMeetingMaterials/Drugs/AdvisoryCommitteeforPharmaceuticalScienceandClinicalPharmacology/UCM315764.pdf.)

the CQAs for comparability protocols are established through historical data from previous batches and the CQAs for biosimilars are based on a thorough reverse engineering of the originator product, a literature review, and a scientific assessment of the linking of attributes to patient safety.

The QbD for biosimilars takes a route different from that used for new products since biosimilar development is based on the characteristics of the originator product and relies on existing prior experience with the same drug substance and product. There is also a difference between the comparability protocol risk assessment and the biosimilar risk assessment (Figure 6.3).

6.2 Workflow

The QbD workflow starts with the definition of the targeted clinical performance in the QTPP document, the basis of the manufacturing process to deliver a product that meets these quality specifications. Linking process understanding to product understanding and ultimately to the desired QTPP is, therefore, a cornerstone of QbD approaches. Structural characterization is the core to assess the CQAs of biosimilar products. First, it applies to the characterization of the reference product to establish QTPP then connecting the QTPP to CQAs, which is achieved for biosimilars from a scientific understanding of the MOA as well as safety

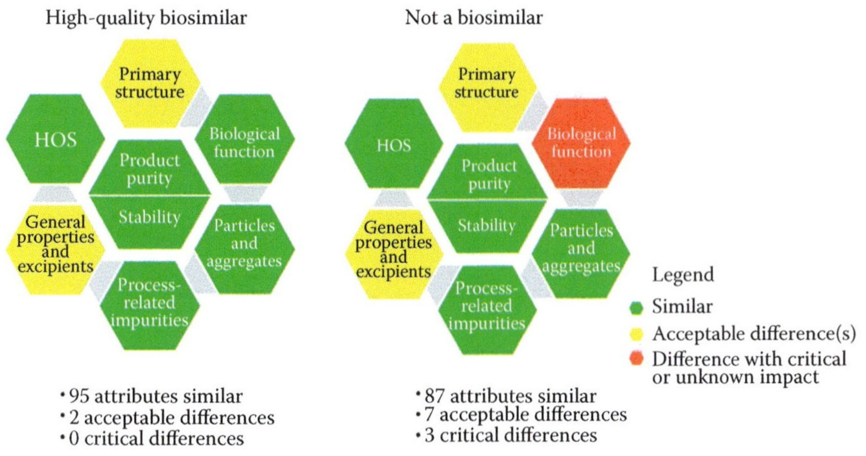

Figure 6.4 The role of critical difference in establishing biosimilarity. (From Amgen Inc., Critical quality attributes, http://www.amgenbiosimilars.com/the-science/critical-quality-attributes/. With permission.)

and immunogenicity profiles. Note that for stand-alone development, a stand-alone molecule undergoes repeated clinical and nonclinical testing to determine CQAs. Once the CQAs are established, the risk analysis begins—how to assure that during commercial manufacturing, the CQAs shall remain within limits. Since it is not expected that all attributes will be the same, how similar is similar is depicted in Figure 6.4, where variation in CQAs leads to nonsimilarity.

The risk assessments are identified as logical linkages between product development stages and as tools to integrate prior existing product knowledge. The risk assessment process as defined by the ICH for Quality Risk Management (ICH Q9) is used to identify risk elements. Regarding product quality, strict specifications based on the originator's quality profile are defined for biosimilars, which have to be met accordingly. As the production process of the originator product is undisclosed, no process development and manufacturing knowledge is available for follow-on biologics producers. These differences should be considered to fit risk management to the purposes of biosimilar process development. The risk assessment process as described in ICH Q9 should be reviewed and developed accordingly.

6.3 The risk assessment process

The three-step model initiates risk assessment with the identification of risk by understanding the linkage between the analyzed steps of product development, for example, between CQA and critical process parameter (CPP) selection (Figure 6.5). To visualize the logical linkage and to sort

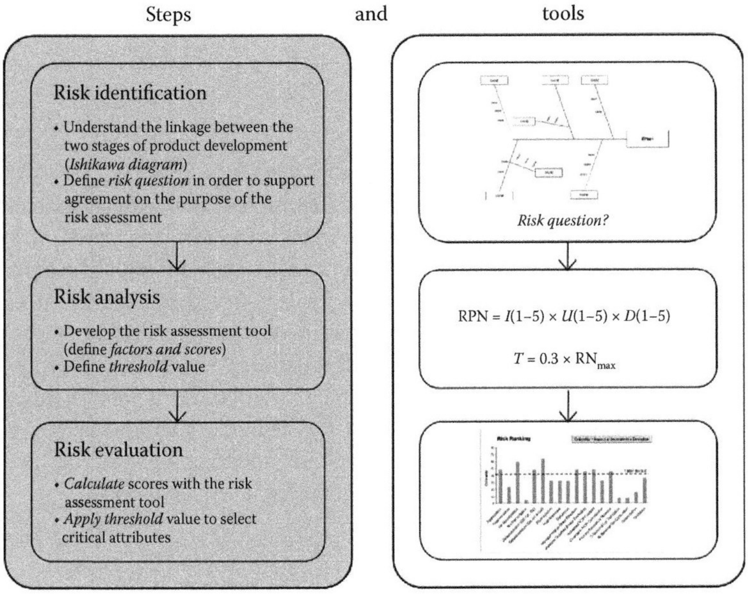

Figure 6.5 The general risk assessment process. The box on the left traces the three steps of risk assessment as described in ICH Q9, whereas the box on the right represents essential tools supporting the risk assessment process. (From Zalai, D. et al., *PDA J Pharm Sci Tech*, 67, 2013. With permission.)

all attributes by categories for the risk analysis, decision tools such as an Ishikawa diagram can be used. Afterward, the risk question—a clearly formulated sentence referring to the goal of the risk assessment—is defined. Risk question formulation supports the process to obtain an agreement on the purpose of the risk assessment. The progress of risk question formulation might be a challenging task due to the complex nature of biologics and the diverse concerns of interdisciplinary risk assessment teams.

The second step focuses on the assessment of criticality with the help of risk analysis tools. According to the ICH Q9 guidance, the risk is always defined as a function of the severity of potential harm. Consequently, a risk assessment tool always contains a factor that represents this severity. Additional factors can be chosen to optimize the tool for the exact purpose. After defining the score ranges for each factor, the maximal risk score can be calculated and subsequently the criticality threshold can be set. Although the threshold value has a great influence on the outcome of the risk assessment, there is no best practice reported for defining its value.

The last step of risk assessments is the calculation of risk scores and the subsequent ranking of the attributes. Finally, attributes receiving higher risk scores as the criticality threshold are designated as critical.

Eventually, the outcome of the risk assessment is dependent on the following elements of the process:

- Risk question definition
- Tailored risk assessment tool
- Criticality threshold definition

However, even very sophisticated risk assessment tools cannot extract valuable information from bad quality input data. In other words, risk assessment is a decision tool to identify criticality and does not replace the need for scientific knowledge. Accordingly, lack of information in early-stage process development was reported to be a major obstacle of risk assessment approaches. However, the growing experience of the pharmaceutical industry on the production of biologics will serve as a robust input for such purposes in the future. In order to integrate this knowledge in biopharmaceutical development, tailored risk assessment approaches are needed that are able to process prior knowledge in risk decisions.

6.3.1 Risk question definition and target linkages

In the QbD paradigm, risk assessments create junctions between successive stages of product development. Thereby, the understanding of linkages between these stages is initiated by a suitable risk assessment approach. First, visual and interactive tools can be used to organize data in accordance with the recommendations of the ICH Q9 guideline. The type of the visual tool can be selected based on the nature of the applied risk assessment technique. In early-stage process development, risk assessment is a deductive problem, answering the question, What can cause a failure in the clinical performance of the product? In order to trace back this problem to possible causes, visual tools such as Ishikawa diagrams are appropriate. In contrast, when the risk assessment addresses inductive problems answering the question, What can go wrong in the production process?, other types of visual tools such as flow charts or process mapping might be more suitable.

Ishikawa diagrams help to identify logical connections between different types of product or process-related attributes and thus support a better understanding of linkages between clinical performance, product, and process. This enhanced understanding can then be condensed into risk questions in order to support the identification of critical attributes via targeted risk assessments. Although the formulation of risk questions has not yet been a routine task in risk assessments, their use can facilitate the development of tailored risk assessment tools. In this contribution, risk questions are used to tighten the focus of risk assessments by enhancing the logical background of the linkages (Figure 6.6). A well-defined risk question already denominates some factors of the risk assessment tool. For example, the risk question for CQA selection contains the word *deviation*, which is also the third factor in the CQA risk assessment tool.

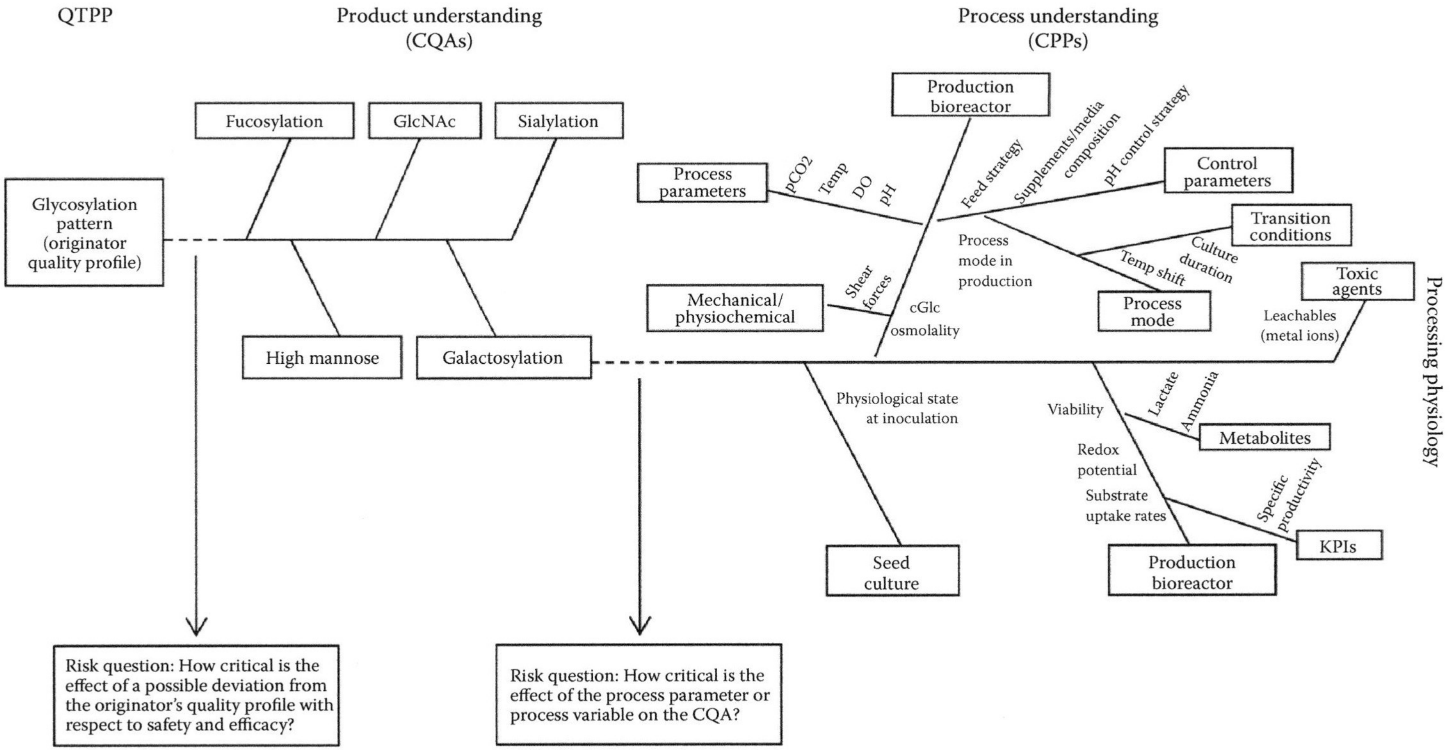

Figure 6.6 Multilevel Ishikawa diagram depicting the connection between process parameters, CQAs, and targeted quality profile. A data set of a selected QTPP specification (glycosylation pattern) and a selected CQA (galactosylation) is shown as an example. Dashed lines represent the logical linkage between consecutive stages of process development, condensed in risk questions. (From Zalai, D. et al., *PDA J Pharm Sci Tech*, 67, 2013. With permission.)

After the definition of CQAs, process parameters with a possible effect on these quality attributes are collected. Another benefit of Ishikawa diagrams is the possibility to structure the high number of parameters that influence cell culture performance. In Figure 6.7, process variables are divided into two groups and several subgroups in order to classify potential CPPs. This structure supported the understanding of the MOA as to how different variables might affect product quality and served as a roadmap for the assessment of criticality. Accordingly, process variables are divided into two main groups: processing and physiology. The latter group was defined after the identification of cell physiology as a complex variable with major effect on product quality in cell culture

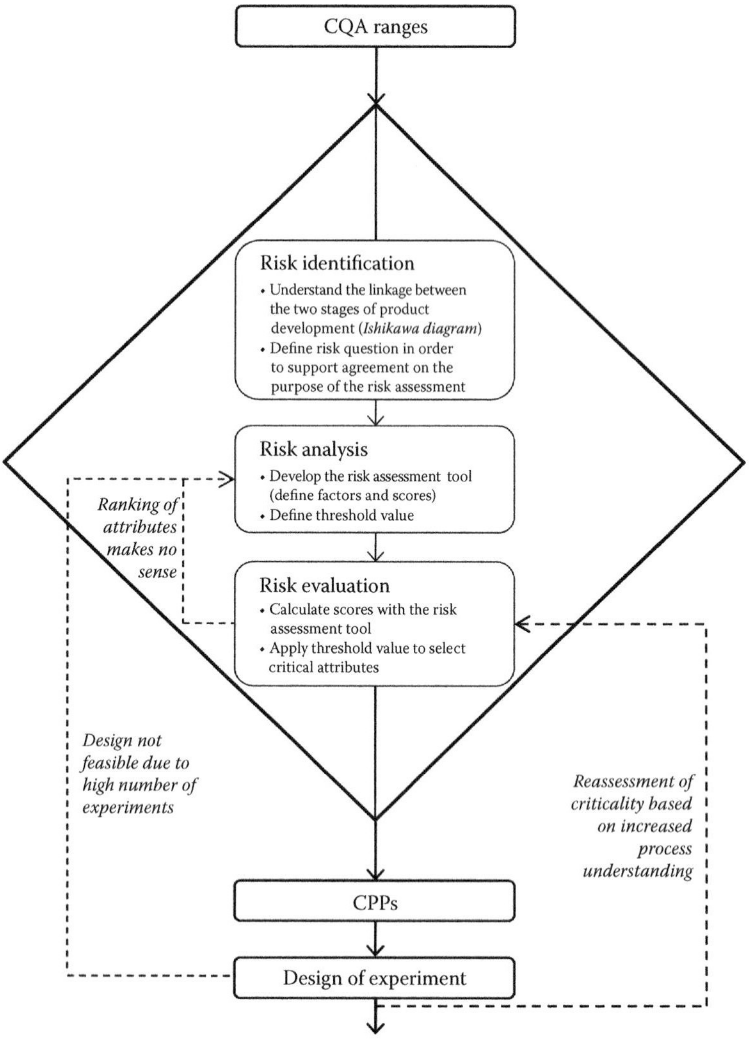

Figure 6.7 Iteration processes in CPP risk assessment. Dashed lines represent possible iteration reasons and paths.

processes. Although the complex physiology of mammalian cells (e.g., CHO) has been investigated in many studies, little is known about how this information can be coupled to product quality. Therefore, physiological parameters such as specific rates have to be defined to support the extraction of scalable and science-based information on physiology–product quality interactions in bioprocess development. The identification of such physiological parameters in early-stage development has to be facilitated by structured risk assessment approaches.

Ishikawa diagrams and risk questions support the proper understanding of linkages targeted by risk assessments. With the help of these tools, interdisciplinary team members can come to an agreement on the scope of risk assessments. Due to the high complexity of targeted bioprocesses, the approach depicts a promising tool for more efficient process development, especially in its early stages.

6.3.2 Development of tailored risk assessment tools

Risk assessment tools convert subject knowledge into quantitative information in order to assess criticality. The outcome is the risk number (RN), which is calculated by multiplying two or more factors. Although the ICH Q9 guideline lists a variety of risk assessment tools, it does not provide a clear definition as how to select the most appropriate one for the specific purpose. Some studies have reported the use of these tools during biopharmaceutical product development, but they did not provide extensive information on the reasons for selection. As already discussed, the factor severity is always included in the risk assessment tool to express the potential harm to pharmaceutical quality as the basis for the determination of criticality. Additional factors are used to improve the risk assessment tool by breaking up the risk into multiple components. For example, uncertainty is often used as a second factor besides severity to include the quality of input data as a possible source of risk. This is especially relevant in early-stage process development, where scientific knowledge is often lacking to fully understand the linkage between product- and process-related parameters. The two factors severity and uncertainty are included in both CQA and CPP risk assessment tools within this study.

If additional information is available that can increase the selectivity of the risk assessment, the tool has to be appended to process all the information at hand. An example is the original product's quality profile for biosimilars. Biosimilar guidelines in the EU and the United States put emphasis on analytical comparability with the original product. Consequently, the quality profile of biosimilars is highly determined by the originator product. In order to involve this additional information in biosimilar development, a third factor called deviation was added to the here-described risk assessment tool for CQA selection (Table 6.1). This factor incorporates the extent of acceptable deviations from the

Table 6.1 Overview of the Risk Assessment Tools for CQA and CPP Selection

	CQA Risk Assessment	CPP Risk Assessment
Linkage	CQAs–QTPP specification	CPPs–CQA ranges
Risk question	How critical is the effect of a possible deviation from the innovator's quality profile with respect to safety and efficacy?	How critical is the effect of the process parameter or process variable on CQAs?
Risk assessment tool	RN = severity × uncertainty × deviation	RN = severity × uncertainty × complexity
Scores for the third factor	Deviation (from the quality profile of the reference material): 1. No deviation in the quality profile 2. The low deviation in the quality profile or robust purification method deviation, limited purification efficiency 3. The severe deviation in the quality profile limited purification efficiency 4. The severe deviation in the quality profile, a variant cannot be purified	Complexity (of the mechanism responsible for the CPP–CQA effect): 1. The mechanism described by physical law 2. Simple mechanism with well-known characteristics 3. Complex mechanism with previously reported quantitative interactions 4. Complex mechanism without quantified characteristics 5. Very complex mechanism

originator product's quality profile. Quality attributes with minor importance would receive a low deviation score, indicating a higher acceptable deviation. Thus, this factor helps to prioritize the quality attributes for product development based on their effect on biosimilarity. However, as communicated by regulatory bodies, the effect of a deviation from the originator in attributes with low relevance has to be justified as well in biological assays. The factor deviation can also contain information about the purification capacity of downstream process steps if the risk assessment is conducted for the determination of CQAs in upstream process development (see Table 6.1).

Another example to incorporate additional information into the risk assessment in this study was, considering the complexity of the mechanisms, how process parameters can affect the investigated quality attributes. Accordingly, besides the factors severity and uncertainty, a third factor called complexity was added to the risk assessment tool of CPP selection. This factor quantifies as to which extent the mechanism of the CPP–CQA interaction can be described by a scientifically developed formula (Table 6.1). The higher the score, the more complex the mechanism and the less information available for its quantification. As the lack of reliable information on CPP–CQA interactions raises the uncertainty score of almost each process parameters and variables in early-stage process development, including complexity as a third factor, helped to differentiate CPP candidates based on scientific considerations. Introducing this factor also emphasizes the scope of CPP risk assessment at this stage of process development, which is not to select critical parameters for a finalized manufacturing process but rather to rank parameters in order to prioritize experiments for process development. These considerations justify the development of novel tools as described earlier instead of

Table 6.2 Decreased Number of Critical Attributes with Risk Assessment Tools Using Three Factors

	CQA Risk Assessment	CPP Risk Assessment
Two factors	67%	53%
Three factors	50%	39%

Note: The values represent the percentage of critical attributes with respect to all attributes involved in the risk assessment. The threshold values for the selection of criticality are defined based on the rule of $T = (1/n)RN_{max}$, where n is the number of factors.

failure mode and effects analysis, which is commonly used to assess the criticality of process parameters in manufacturing processes.

To demonstrate the effect of factor selection on the result of risk assessment, the ratio of critical attributes was calculated for the case of two or three factors. As shown in Table 6.2, the addition of a third factor decreased the ratio both in CQA and in CPP risk assessment. This observation suggests that the integration of additional knowledge with an appropriate factor in the risk assessment tool leads to the reduction of critical attributes and hence simplifies the experimental design for early process development. The lower number of critical attributes does not mean higher risk acceptance, but rather risk reduction by enhanced integration of prior knowledge into product development via efficient risk assessment tools.

6.3.3 Threshold definition for risk assessment

The criticality threshold expresses the level of risk that is accepted for a product or a process. As already stated earlier, its value has a great influence on the outcome of the risk assessment. The threshold value is always determined based on the acceptable level of risk. In the literature, threshold values around $0.2RN_{max}$ are commonly reported, resulting in an average of 70% of critical attributes. However, applying a static formula for criticality threshold calculation leads to variable outcomes when the number of factors is changed in the risk assessment tool. Thus, general formulas should be developed in order to deliver comparable results when adjustments in the risk assessment tool are made (Table 6.3). Such a formula is $(1/n)RN_{max}$, which calculates the criticality threshold based on the number of factors (n) involved in the risk assessment tool.

The final goal of criticality threshold selection in early-stage process development is to identify factors for the design of experiments along what is executable in the very strict development timeline of biosimilars. In this respect, the number of critical parameters is an important indicator of factor selection because it has a major effect on the experimental design. Table 6.3 shows how the threshold selection affects the number of critical attributes and demonstrates the need for threshold selection strategies that take the number of factors applied in the risk assessment

Table 6.3 Critical Attribute Selection Using Different Threshold Calculation Formulas

Threshold Calculation Formula	CQA Risk Assessment		CPP Risk Assessment	
	Two Factors	Three Factors	Two Factors	Three Factors
$(1/5)RN_{max}$	89%	78%	99%	72%
$(1/3)RN_{max}$	89%	50%	81%	39%
$(1/2)RN_{max}$	67%	11%	53%	6%

Note: The values represent the percentage of critical attributes with respect to all attributes. Criticality can be assessed with tools using two or three factors as described above. RN_{max} represents the maximal value of the risk score (all factors at the maximum score). Values in bold represent criticality corresponding to the $T = (1/n)RN_{max}$ rule.

tool into account. Accordingly, the results suggest that $(1/n)RN_{max}$ is an appropriate formula for threshold calculation.

6.4 Iteration of risk assessment

Risk assessments deliver a rank of attributes based on the calculated RN. Moreover, attributes with a higher RN than a predefined threshold are designated as critical. Thus, the outcome of the risk assessment is the rank and the number of critical attributes. Based on these results, the most critical tasks for process development are prioritized, and the first process characterization studies are designed. The knowledge gained in these experiments can result in increased process understanding and subsequent variation in the criticality of some attributes. Therefore, the risk assessment can be revised to integrate the obtained knowledge in process development decisions (see Figure 6.7).

The use of inappropriate factors in the risk assessment tool can lead to an unexpected rank of the attributes. In such cases, the risk assessment tool itself has to be revised and the factors modified.

Although the outcome of risk assessments can be modified by iterative processes shown in Figure 6.7, the predefined goal has to be considered to avoid missing the aim of the risk assessment. In other words, the revisions and subsequent adjustments in the threshold value or the risk assessment tool should not compromise patient safety for the simplification of product development.

Another interesting issue in risk management is the handling of noncritical data. Variables with a lower score than the risk threshold are designated as noncritical and do not have to be included further in the description of design space. However, the assessment of criticality is not static and it might change with the increase of product and process understanding. Consequently, noncritical variables can become critical throughout product development. Therefore, handling of noncritical data is a major question of QbD approaches. Well-developed risk assessment tools enable a more accurate determination of criticality and reduce the possibility of underestimated risk. Moreover, scheduled iterations in the QbD workflow support the revision of previously taken incorrect decisions. All these conclusions highlight the key role of risk management in early-stage biosimilar process development.

6.5 Development exercise

Development exercise is an example of creating CQAs for a filgrastim product and an mAb product. The exercise begins with first understanding the MoA, the mode of immunogenicity and safety outcomes, and the effectiveness. In most instances, all these aspects about the biological drug developed are well known. The main sources of information are the European public assessment reports, the FDA reports, the research publications, the customer promotional materials, the clinical promotional materials, the labels approved, and as amended, the corporate financial reports, etc. Once we have a good understanding of all these factors, the risk management is built as follows:

1. Quality attributes associated with the MoA; these include primary, secondary, and tertiary structures
2. Quality attributes associated with immunogenicity and safety; these include both chemical and physical (aggregation) modifications
3. Quality attributes altering effectiveness such as protein content, bioassay, receptor binding, immunoblotting
4. Quality attributes related to product- and process-related impurities that might impinge on some or all of the above quality attributes
5. Quality attributes supporting the dosage form performance such as pH, osmolality, concentration of surfactants

6.5.1 CQA assessments

1. What is the potential impact on patients when high or low levels of a variant or impurity are present?
   - Impact 2–20 points
   - Four impacts to consider: biological activity, immunogenicity, PK, and safety
2. How certain are we about Question 1?
   - Uncertain: 1–7 points
3. Combine as a risk ranking and filtering assessment.
4. The assessment will need to reflect route of administration, patient class, therapeutic window, etc.

5. Assigning CQAs independent of
   - Historical ranges and
   - Ability to control their level

The CQAs are defined in terms of *very high* to *none* for reach of the critical attribute and assigned the same level of rating scale as shown in Table 6.4; besides these attributes, there is an uncertainty scale—what if you find a peak in a chromatogram that is not present in the originator product or other such experiences. The uncertainty scale is described in Table 6.4.

The final calculation of CQA is given in Table 6.5.

The list of QTPP used for a biosimilar candidate filgrastim product is provided in Table 6.6. This list was created from literature and understanding of the molecule. The criticality level is determined by the impact of the attribute as measured by analytical techniques and their resulting clinical outcomes. This is specifically measured as it relates to the impact on efficacy (biological activity), PK/PD, immunogenicity, and safety. As the evaluated product is a biosimilar, a knowledge-based score is assigned to establish the extent of certainty about the impact in the clinic as defined in Table 6.5.

Table 6.4 Uncertainty Scale of Attributes

Rating	Uncertainty	Description (Variants and Host Impurities)	Description (Process Raw Materials)
7	Very high	No information (new variant)	No information (new)
5	High	Published external literature for variant in a related molecule	
3	Moderate	Nonclinical or in vitro data with this molecule. Data (nonclinical, in vitro or clinical) from a similar molecule	Component found in other products of sponsor, such as a leachable
2	Low	Variants are present in material used in clinical trials (it will likely be the PK study)	
1	Very low	Impact of specific variant established in clinical studies with this molecule	Generally recognized as safe or studied in clinical trials

Table 6.5 CQAs Assigned Based on Severity Score

Low		**Low**	**Uncertainty**			**High**
Impact		1	2	3	5	7
	20	**20**	**40**	**60**	**100**	**140**
	16	**16**	**32**	**48**	**80**	**112**
	12	12	**24**	**36**	**60**	**84**
	4	4	8	12	**20**	**28**
High	2	2	4	6	10	**14**

Note: >13 = CQA, shown in bold.

Table 6.6 Definition of Impact

Impact and Rating	Biological Activity	PK/PD	Immunogenicity	Safety
Very high (20)	**>100% change**	**>40% change in PK**	**ATA detected and conferred limits on safety**	**Irreversible adverse events (AEs)**
High (16)	**40%–100% change**	**20%–40% change in PK with impact on PD**	**ATA detected and conferred limits on effectiveness**	**Reversible AEs**
Moderate (12)	20%–40% change	20%–40% change in PK with no impact on PD	ATA detected with manageable in vivo effect	Manageable AEs
Low (4)	<20% change	<20% change in PK with no impact on PD	ATA detected with minimal in vivo effect	Minor, transient AEs
None (2)	No change	No impact on PK or PD	ATA not detected or ATA detected with no in vivo effect	No AEs
Comments	Must consider the loss of potency for isolated forms as certain forms may be superpotent: afucosylated anti-CD20s or aggregates	Use PD if available; unlike many glycoproteins, common IgG1 Fc glycans do not affect clearance; the impact of charge variation on clearance well documented; do small differences in the pI matter? The AUC of acidic variants matches the main form for some IgG1	Variants also present on plasma-derived IgG may be presumed low risk: demained Fc, glycated, loss of C-terminal lysine	Safety effects linked to specific characteristics are race, e.g., CDC (infusion reaction), or Gal(α1-3Gal) on cetuximab Fab glycans (anaphylaxis)

Note: CQA shown in bold. AEs, adverse events; ATA, anti-therapeutic antibody.

A CQA score is determined by multiplying the clinical impact score by the knowledge-based score. Since the analytical characteristics of filgrastim correlate well with the expected clinical outcome, they therefore are sensitive and predictive of the MOA. These attributes have been proven by experience with innovator and known MOA. Table 6.7

Table 6.7 Statistical Rigor of CQA Testing Methods

CQA	Statistical Tier
Primary structure: Molecular weight, peptide map, WB identification, disulfide linkage, amino acid analysis	0
MOA-related attributes: Potency, receptor binding, protein content	1
Subvisible particles, DSC	2
Antibody binding, SDS-PAGE, 1D and 2D NMR, intrinsic fluorescence, CD	3

Table 6.8 Quality Attributes for Similarity Assessment of Filgrastim

Quality Attribute	Critical Relevance	Criticality Ranking	Test Method
Identity: Primary structure	Efficacy, safety, immunogenicity	Very high	Molecular weight by LC ESI MS
Identity: Primary structure	Efficacy, safety, immunogenicity		Identity by WB analysis
Identity: Primary structure	Efficacy, safety, immunogenicity		Disulfide linkage analysis by peptide mapping and MS
Identity: Primary structure	Efficacy, safety, immunogenicity		Confirmation of amino and carboxyl termini by MS/MS
Identity: Primary structure	Efficacy, safety, immunogenicity		AAA
Identity: Primary structure	Efficacy, safety, immunogenicity		Peptide map–RP-HPLC
Identity: pI	Efficacy, safety, immunogenicity		Capillary IEF
Potency: Receptor binding	Efficacy, safety		Receptor-binding characteristics by ELISA
Potency: Receptor binding	Efficacy, safety		Antibody-binding characteristics by ELISA
Potency: Bioactivity	Efficacy, safety		In vitro biological activity by M-NFS-60 cell proliferation assay
Effectiveness: Protein concentration	Effectiveness		Protein concentration by RP-HPLC
Safety: Subvisible particles	Immunogenicity	High	Light obfuscation for subvisible particles (USP <787>)
Safety: Clarity	Safety, immunogenicity		Appearance by visual inspection
Identity: 3D structure	Efficacy, immunogenicity		2D heteronuclear single quantum coherence NMR
Identity: 3D structure	Efficacy, immunogenicity		1D ^{1}H NMR
Identity: Tertiary structure	Efficacy, immunogenicity		Intrinsic fluorescence spectroscopy
Identity: Tertiary structure	Efficacy, immunogenicity		DSC
Identity: Secondary structure	Efficacy, immunogenicity		Far-UV CD spectropolarimetry
Identity: Secondary structure	Efficacy, immunogenicity		Near-UV CD spectropolarimetry
Identity: 4D structure	Efficacy, immunogenicity		Thermodynamic equilibrium state testing
Purity: Variants oxidized	Efficacy		RP-HPLC
Safety: Impurity, process-related impurities	Immunogenicity		Tungsten level
Safety: Impurity, process-related	Immunogenicity		Extractables

(*Continued*)

Table 6.8 (Continued) Quality Attributes for Similarity Assessment of Filgrastim

Quality Attribute	Critical Relevance	Criticality Ranking	Test Method
Safety: Impurity, process-related	Immunogenicity		Leachable
Safety: Impurity, process-related	Immunogenicity		Silicone oil level
Safety: HCPs	Immunogenicity		ELISA with 2D SDS-PAGE to establish test effectiveness
Safety: Host cell DNA	Immunogenicity		Fluorescence-based quantitation test
Safety: Aggregates, covalent dimers	Immunogenicity		SEC (STM-0085); AUC
Formulation: Inactive component	None		Sorbitol content
Formulation: Inactive component	None		Polysorbate 80 content
Formulation: Inactive component	None		Acetate content
Purity: Succinamide species	None	Low	LC–MS
Purity: fMet1 species	None		LC–MS
Purity: Variants, N-terminal truncated	None	Very low	LC–MS
Purity: Reduced, partially reduced species	None		LC–MS
Purity: Phosphogluconoylation	None		LC–MS
Purity: Norleucine	None		LC–MS
Purity: Variants, sequence (His → Gin), (Asp → Glu), (Thr → Asp)	None		RP-HPLC-MS
Purity: Acetylated species	None		LC–MS
Purity: Deamidated species	None		LC–MS IEX RP-HPLC cIEF
Formulation: Property	None		Refractive index
Formulation: Property	None		Osmolality determination by freezing point depression
Formulation: Properties	None		pH

represents the defined quality attributes and their potential impact on clinical outcome. The attributes are evaluated and given critical levels of *very high*, *high*, *low*, and *very low*, which indicate a known impact on clinical and/or MOA. This is based on a mathematical calculation.

The FDA recommends using a statistical approach to evaluating quality attributes for a biosimilar product that is consistent with the risk assessment principles set forth in ICH Quality Guidelines Q8, Q9, Q10, and Q11. Consistent with these principles, quality attributes for analytical similarity program are assessed by tiered system approaches of varying statistical rigor as listed in Table 6.7. The details of statistical modeling are given in Chapter 8.

Table 6.8 describes CQAs for filgrastim.

The methods described in Table 6.8 are also risk-ranked relative to the ability to detect with reliability and sensitivity of the attribute being

Table 6.9 Quality Attributes for mAbs

Category	Quality Attribute	Methods
Physicochemical Characterization		
Primary structure	Amino acid sequence	Reduced RP-HPLC-ESI-MS peptide mapping, intact mass of the whole mAbs, HC, and LC by RP-HPLC-ESI-MS, Red. RP-HPLC-UV peptide mapping
HOS	Disulfide bridging	Non-reduced RP-HPLC-ESI-MS peptide mapping
	Free thiols	Ellman's assay
	Secondary and tertiary structures	CD, FTIR, HDX-MS, X-ray
	Thermodynamic stability	DSC
General charge heterogeneity and amino acid modifications	OK variant, acidic variants, basic variant, Gin-variant, Lys-variant, amidated proline Glycation Oxidation/deamidation/C-terminal variants	CEX digested/undigested Boronate affinity RP-HPLC-UV/MS peptide mapping
Glycosylation	Galactosylation, sialylation, mannosylation, afucosylation, bisecting GlcNAc, NGNA, α-galactose, qualitative glycosylation pattern	Normal phase–HPLC-FL
Size heterogeneity	Monomer, low–molecular weight and high–molecular weight variants (aggregates)	SEC, assymmetrical flow FFF
	Heavy chain, light chain, aglycosylated HC, clipped variants	Reduced CE-SDS
	Monomer, low–molecular weight (e.g., half antibodies and HHL variant) and high–molecular weight variants	Non-reduced CE-SDS
	Subvisible particles	Light obscuration (Peru, ≥10 μm)
	Visible particles	Visual inspection (Peru)
Functional Characterization		
Target and receptor binding	Fern binding Facer binding (Curia, FcγRilla, FcγRIlb, FcγRIlla(F158), FcγRIlla(V158), FcγRIllb	SPR SPR
Bioactivity	CD20 target binding	Cell-based binding assay
	CDC potency	Cell-based CDC assay
	ADCC potency	Cell-based ADDC assay
	Apoptosis	Cell-based apoptosis assay

Note: HHL, heavy-heavy light chain; SPR, surface plasmon resonance.

measured. Since this exercise is highly dependent on the specific molecule, given below is a classification criterion for CQAs for mAbs:

- Critical: High mannose–type glycans (carbohydrate structures) are often a critical quality attribute. This attribute reduces the amount of time the drug stays in the body. This attribute can also be important for how a biological medicine functions and treats a particular disease. To have similar efficacy, safety, and immunogenicity to a reference product, a biosimilar needs to match all critical quality attributes.

- Criticality Unclear: Fucosylated type–glycans (carbohydrate structures) are sometimes CQAs. Depending on the biological medicine and the disease being treated, this attribute may be significant, not important, or of unknown importance to biological function.
- Not Critical: The last amino acid that a cell adds to an antibody remains there only temporarily and it is later removed by the cell. It is acceptable for a biosimilar to have differences in this amino acid, as it does not impact how the antibody functions or how it moves through the body.

Table 6.9 shows the quality attributes for mAbs.

Bibliography

Abu-Absi, S. F., Yang, L., Thompson, P., Jiang, C., Kandula, S., Schilling, B., and Shukla, A. A. (2010) Defining process design space for monoclonal antibody cell culture. *Biotechnol Bioeng* 106 (6): 894–905.

Amgen Inc., Critical quality attributes, http://www.amgenbiosimilars.com/the-science/critical-quality-attributes/.

del Val, I. J., Kontoravdi, C., and Nagy, J. M. (2010) Towards the implementation of quality by design to the production of therapeutic monoclonal antibodies with desired glycosylation patterns. *Biotechnol Prog* 26 (6): 1505–1527.

Duval, A. (2012) Application of quality by design to the characterization of the cell culture process of a Fc–Fusion protein. *Eur J Pharm Biopharm* 81 (2): 426–437.

EMA (2008 December) Guideline on development, production, characterization and specifications for monoclonal antibodies and related products: EMEA/CHMP/BWP/157653/2007. European Medicines Agency, London.

FDA—Biosimilar: An update, (2012) http://www.fda.gov/downloads/AdvisoryCommittees/CommitteesMeetingMaterials/Drugs/AdvisoryCommitteeforPharmaceuticalScienceandClinicalPharmacology/UCM315764.pdf.

Horvath, B., Mun, M., and Laird, M. (2010) Characterization of a monoclonal antibody cell culture production process using a quality by design approach. *Mol Biotechnol* 45 (3): 203–206.

ICH Q6B. Specifications: Test procedures and acceptance criteria for biotechnological/biological products. http://wwwichorg/LOB/media/MEDIA432pdf.

ICH (2011 September) ICH harmonized tripartite guideline Q11: Development and manufacture of drug substances (chemical entities and biotechnological/biological entities), Step 3 Version.

ICH (1999 September) ICH topic Q6B specifications: Test procedures and acceptance criteria for biotechnological/biological products, Step 5 Version.

Kozlowski, S. (2010) Implementation Activities for QbD: The FDA Office of Biotechnology Products. Presentation at 2010 WCBP CMC Strategy Forum, Bethesda, MD.

Kudrin, A. (2012) Overview of the biosimilars: Strategic considerations of various issues. *J Generic Med: Bus J Generic Med Sect* 9 (4): 187–206.

Mandenius, C. F., Graumann, K., Schultz, T. W., Premstaller, A., Olsson, I. M., Petiot, E., Clemens, C., and Welin, M. (2009) Quality-by-design for biotechnology-related pharmaceuticals. *Biotechnol J* 4 (5): 600–609.

Nosal, R., and Schultz, T. (2008) PQLI definition of criticality. *J Pharm Innov* 3 (2): 69–78.

Rathore, A. S., Branning, R., and Cecchini, D. (2007) Quality: Design space for biotech products. *BioPharm Int* 2007:36–40.
Rathore, A. S. (2009) Roadmap for implementation of quality by design (QbD) for biotechnology products. *Trends Biotechnol* 27: 546–553.
Rathore, A. S., and Winkle, H. (2009) Quality by design for biopharmaceuticals. *Nat Biotech* 27 (1): 26–34.
Robert, P. C., and James, K. D. (2008) Risk-based quality by design (QbD): A Taguchi perspective on the assessment of product quality and the quantitative linkage of drug product parameters and clinical performance. *J Pharm Innov* 3 (1): 23–29.
Sagmeister, P., Wechselberger, P., and Herwig, C. (2012) Information processing: Rate-based investigation of cell physiological changes along design space development. *PDA J Pharm Sci Technol* 66 (6): 526–541.
Schneider, C. K., Vleminckx, C., Gravanis, I., Ehmann, F., Trouvin, J. H., Weise, M., and Thirstrup, S. (2012) Setting the stage for monoclonal antibodies. *Nat Biotech* 30 (12): 1179–1185.
Seely, R. J., and Haury, J., Applications of failure modes and effects analysis to biotechnology manufacturing processes. A. S. Rathore and G. Sofer (Eds.), in *Process Validation in Manufacturing of Biopharmaceuticals*, Oxford, UK: Taylor & Francis; 2005. pp. 13–30.
Yu, L. (2008) Pharmaceutical quality by design: Product and process development, understanding, and control. *Pharm Res* 25 (4): 781–791.
Zalai, D. et al. (2013) Risk-based process development of biosimilars as part of the quality by design paradigm. *PDA J Pharm Sci Tech* 67 (6): 569–580.

Chapter 7 Safety similarity

Out of this nettle, danger, we pluck this flower, safety.

William Shakespeare

7.1 Background

The safety of biosimilar products has long been the topic of hot debate and incessantly used as a warning sign by the originator product companies to alert clinicians, public, and other stakeholders as biosimilars began to take roots in Europe and now in the United States. The major safety concern is the immunogenicity. A therapeutic protein, recombinant or otherwise, can be immunogenic because the human immune system categorizes it as nonself. A protein injected into patients will be taken up by antigen-presenting cells and processed into smaller peptides. The T cells generated in the thymus are able to bind to the peptides presented in the grooves of major histocompatibility complex molecules on the surface of antigen-presenting cells. When the T cells recognize these peptides as foreign, they induce B cell proliferation. The B and T cells are both part of the adaptive immune system; however, B cells directly interact with the protein owing to the immunoglobulins present on their cell surfaces. After binding to the specific 3D structure of the protein, activated B cells recruit the complement system and the macrophages from the innate immune system to destroy and remove the antigen. Such an immune response against a foreign protein is called a classical immune response, which typically leads to the production of high-affinity antibodies of different isotypes, as well as memory cells responsible for an enhanced response to repeated challenge with the antigen (the principle of vaccination).

This immune response may have more or less serious consequences, from a simple tolerance reaction to antibodies, up to therapeutic inefficiency when the antibodies are neutralizing. Antibodies produced against therapeutic proteins like EPO, hematopoietic growth factors (GM-CSF), and thrombopoietin/megakaryocyte growth and development factor (TPO/MGDF) may have big consequences to the point of blocking not only the exogenous protein's activity but also the endogenous protein with the serious complications inherent in these actions.

The production of antibodies against biotechnology-derived proteins, like insulin, factor VIII or IX, or interferons, does not have the same serious consequences and treatments continue in the presence of the antibodies, adapting the doses of therapeutic protein.

The consequences of antibodies produced against mAbs have been observed since their first use, particularly, when these proteins are derived from animal or bacterial proteins. The reactions observed could be of a general order such as systemic reactions, during these products' injection, local reactions, or reactions of acute hypersensitivity (generally not due to the antibodies). The immune reactions of anaphylactic-type or allergic reactions are rare because of the better purification of proteins produced by recombinant DNA technology and the humanization of protein skeletons of mAbs. The production of neutralizing antibodies may correspond to several types of mechanisms like the direct bonding to a biological activity site or to a site that is not in direct relation but impedes its activity by a changed structural conformation. The nonneutralizing antibodies bind to the therapeutic protein site without affecting the biological activity site. If they do not directly neutralize the biological target, they may change the drug's bioavailability by an increase in the clearance of the bonding complex made with a result identical to that of biological activity neutralization.

When a biopharmaceutical product is immunogenic, its repeated administration to patients over an extended period generally enhances the risk of raising antibodies that can induce anaphylaxis, alter the PK properties of the protein, or inhibit binding of the drug to its target receptor rendering the protein ineffective. Anaphylaxis is caused by an immediate allergic reaction mediated by immunoglobulin E (IgE) antibodies against the product during an immune response with high titers of neutralizing IgG antibodies strongly decreasing the therapeutic activity of the protein. Another possible life-threatening clinical consequence of antibody formation is cross-reactivity with the endogenous protein produced by the patient.

Whatever the nature of the antibodies produced, the immune responses generated by therapeutic proteins pose a significant problem of safety and efficacy for the authorities in charge of evaluating and approving the marketing of biological medicinal products. Recommendations concerning the evaluation of the immunogenic profile of biosimilars compared to the references have been widely published. These recommendations are based on a multifactor approach taking into account the mechanisms involved: the different factors that may be part of the immune response, the level of expression of antibodies, and the possible rarity of the response observed. It is suggested that developers of biosimilar products evaluate the immunogenic risk, case by case, to ensure that it is safe to use. No specific method is recommended, taking into account the variability and the multiplicity of factors involved, but actions to take must be identified before clinical trials start, as well as evaluations that will be performed during pivotal clinical trials and evaluations that will be done after marketing of the product, notably within the framework of a risk management plan.

To measure the consequences of the risk linked to immunogenicity during the therapeutic use of biosimilar, immune mechanisms at play must be examined as well as factors having an influence on immunogenicity such as the disease state wherein the immune systems may be compromised such as in the use in patients undergoing chemotherapy.

Immunogenicity is a problem only when it is clinically relevant—when it has an effect on the safety or the efficacy of the therapeutic protein. Clinically relevant immunogenicity includes when antibodies change how the drug reacts in the body, when antibodies make the protein less therapeutically effective, when antibodies change natural proteins in the body, or when antibodies trigger a severe allergic reaction, which is very rare. Clinically relevant immunogenicity is not common but must be monitored for all therapies.

7.2 Immunogenicity

It is well established that repeated injection of even native human proteins can result in a break in immune tolerance to selfantigens in some patients leading to a humoral response against the protein that is enhanced when the protein is aggregated or partially denatured. Although in most cases an immune response to a biopharmaceutical has little or no clinical impact, ADAs do, however, pose a number of potential risks for the patient, particularly in the case of a neutralizing antibody response. Firstly, an ADA response can adversely affect the PK and the bioavailability of a drug thereby reducing the efficacy of treatment and necessitating either escalating the dose or switching to alternative therapy if such therapy is available. An ADA response can also adversely affect the safety of treatment and cause immune complex disease, allergic reactions and, in some cases, severe autoimmune reactions. Serious and lifethreatening adverse events can occur when ADAs cross-react with an essential, nonredundant endogenous protein such as EPO or TPO. Thus, several cases of PRCA were associated with the development of antibodies to recombinant EPO following a change in formulation. Similarly, the development of antibodies to PEGylated MGDF cross-reacted with endogenous MGDF, resulting in several cases of severe thrombocytopenia.

All biosimilar products are evaluated based on the regulatory guidelines such as the FDA guidance for binding antibodies and neutralizing antibodies. Binding antibodies bind to the protein but usually have no effect. Neutralizing antibodies can inhibit the function of the protein in the body. The FDA is more concerned with neutralizing antibodies because they are more likely to have clinical consequences. Because older products may have limited immunogenicity data based on tests with inadequate sensitivity, immunogenicity between a biosimilar and its reference product cannot be compared using data from the package insert of the reference product. Any comparison of immunogenicity will need a side-by-side clinical test of the biosimilar and its reference to ensure valid comparison. Without a side-by-side comparison, more sensitive tests may get higher antibody-positive results with the biosimilar.

Animal models do not predict immunogenicity in humans. Most animals (even primates) can develop a strong antibody response to human proteins. Immunogenicity testing in animals may be useful to evaluate drug functioning or toxicity changes that might result because of antibodies to the human protein, or to see if responses are the same to two different products. Aggregation, which is when proteins clump together, is the most common factor associated with increased immunogenicity. Aggregation should be a key part of analytical testing, but other product changes (e.g., impurities) have not been associated with increased immunogenicity.

The amount of premarket and postmarket immunogenicity data needed for the approval of a potential biosimilar product will depend on an analytical assessment of similarity between the biosimilar and its reference product, as well as the rate of clinical consequences of immunogenicity observed with the reference product. If an immune response to the reference is rare, two separate studies may be sufficient to evaluate immunogenicity: (a) premarket study to detect major differences in immune responses between biosimilar and reference and (b) postmarket study to detect subtle differences in immunogenicity. The FDA recommends that immunogenicity tests use the patient population that is most likely to show an immunological response for these studies.

Product changes associated with increased immunogenicity can be assessed using analytical tests. Protein aggregation is the primary product change associated with increased immunogenicity. Rigorous analytical testing comparing the biosimilar candidate to the originator reference product in head-to-head studies is the most sensitive way to test for likely immunogenicity in patients. These tests include the measurement of protein aggregates in the drug product and over its shelf life. Thus, analytical testing may be the best way to minimize immunogenicity of a biosimilar. While such tests also need to be done for originator biologics, it is much more difficult to anticipate likely immunological responses with a brand new product.

Most clinical comparator trials cannot detect true differences in clinically significant immunogenicity because the frequency of events is so low. With current statistical methods, very large clinical studies, with over 3000 patients each, would be needed to evaluate meaningful differences in immunogenicity. Consequently, a robust pharmacovigilance program, able to capture clinically relevant immunological responses during real-world use of the biologics, may be a better method to detect clinically relevant immunogenicity problems.

Differences in antibodies may not be relevant if there are no clinical consequences for patients. It is not expected that the possibly reduced immunogenicity of a biosimilar, through more modern manufacturing and better control of aggregation, will cause the FDA to remove the reference product from the market.

Eprex immunogenicity is often cited as a reason to demand clinical immunogenicity testing in biosimilars. Johnson & Johnson made a manufacturing change to Eprex (recombinant EPO) and removed a protein, human albumin, from the formulation of their product marketed in Europe. This change was overseen by regulators using the standard process of demonstrating high similarity with comparability studies of the pre- and postmanufacturing-changed products. The "new" Eprex induced antibodies to Eprex and to natural EPO found in the body, causing PRCA. Although the individual cases of PRCA were very serious, the actual incidence was low (2/10,000). Clinical studies could not have detected PRCA at such a low incidence. A clinical study to determine a difference in the rate of PRCA would have to have involved a very large number of patients. Instead, a robust pharmacovigilance system with analytical investigations eventually resolved the issue.

The predominant immune mechanisms leading to drug hypersensitivity may include from no effect to endogenous cross-reactivity (Table 7.1).

The risk of drug hypersensitivity can be increased by some patient-related factors, which include female gender, specific genetic polymorphism, as well as by some drug-related factors, which include the chemical properties, the molecular weight of the drug, and the route of administration. It is known that drugs with great structural complexity are more likely to be immunogenic. However, drugs with a small molecular weight (less than 1000 Da) may become immunogenic by coupling with carrier proteins, such as albumin, forming complexes. Moreover, the route of administration affects the immunogenicity, the subcutaneous route being more immunogenic than the intramuscular and intravenous routes.

Table 7.2 lists the incidence of immunogenicity of recombinant drugs.

It is noteworthy that about 5% of the U.S. population is allergic to food, and or recombinant proteins and antibodies, many fall within or below this incidence rate. Compounds like sargramostim, aldesleukin, and

Table 7.1 Listed Effects of Immune Responses from Various Drugs

Result of Immune Response	**Drug**
No effect	rh-GH
PK alteration	rh-Insulin
Reduced efficacy	GN-CSF, interferon alpha, interferon beta (the majority of patients become neutralizing antibody positive (NAbs+) within 6–18 months of treatment, while clinical impact of NAbs is delayed and is not seen until 24 months of therapy, abolishing activity
Loss of efficacy	Natalizumab (persistent antibodies)
Cross-reaction with endogenous	Factors VIII and IX, rh-EPO, rh-MDGF

Table 7.2 Immunogenicity of Recombinant Drugs

Incidence	Brand Product	Drug Substance
95%	Leukine	Sargramostim
74%	Proleukin	Aldesleukin
25%–45%	Betaferon	Interferon-beta-1b
12%–28%	Rebif	Interferon-beta-1a
14%–24%	Remicade (and its other biosimilars)	Infliximab
12%	Humira	Adalimumab
0%–26%	Rituxan	Rituximab
3.5%–5%	Erbitux	Cetuximab
2%–6%	Avonex	Interferon-beta-1a
0%–2%	Neupogen (and other biosimilars), Procrit, Neorecormon, Aranesp, Avastin, Neulasta, Genotropin (and other biosimilars), Herceptin	Filgrastim, EPO alpha, EPO beta, darbopoietin alpha, bevacizumab, pegfilgrastim, somatropin, trastuzumab

Source: Wadhwa, M., *Immunogenicity: What Do We Know and What Can We Measure?* EPAR 1, National Institute for Biological Standards and Control—Health Protection Agency, 2011. With permission.

interferon alfa 2a (a particular brand) show high incidence, some of which can be attributed to the formulation and manufacturing factors listed in Section 7.2.2.

7.2.1 Regulatory guidance

The assessment of immunogenicity is an important component of drug safety evaluation in preclinical, clinical, and postmarketing studies.

Draft Guidance for Industry Assay Development for Immunogenicity Testing of Therapeutic Proteins has recently been published by the U.S. FDA (http://www.fed.gov/Drugs/GuidanceComplianceRegulatoryInformation/Guidances/UCM192750.pdf). Similarly, guidelines on the immunogenicity assessment of biotechnologyderived therapeutic proteins established by the Committee for Medicinal Products for Human Use of the EMA came into effect in April 2008 (http://www.emea.europa.ed/pdfs/human/biosimilar/1432706en.pdf). These guidelines provide a general framework for a systematic and comprehensive evaluation of immunogenicity that should be modified, as appropriate, on a casebycase basis.

The approach to test immunogenicity is a risk-based approach that is clinically driven and takes into account PK data. Thus, biopharmaceuticals with no endogenous counterpart are considered to be of relatively low risk while drugs with a nonredundant endogenous counterpart are considered to present a high risk. A multitier approach to testing samples is also recommended. This consists of an appropriate screening assay capable of detecting both immunoglobulin M (IgM) and IgG ADAs, the sensitivity of which is such that a percentage of false-positive samples would be detected. The specificity of the samples that test positive in the screening assay are then reassayed in a confirmatory assay usually by competition with an unlabelled drug using the same assay format as that used for the screening assay. Samples that test positive for screening and confirmatory assays are then tested for the presence of neutralizing ADAs using a cellbased assay whenever possible. Although it may be appropriate to use ligandbinding assays for certain mAbs that target soluble antigens, some ADAs may not be detected using a ligandbinding assay. Thus, antibodies have been described to inhibit the antiviral activity of type I interferons by inducing hyperphosphorylation of a receptorassociated tyrosine kinase without inhibiting binding of the interferon to its receptor.

It is necessary to develop validation and standardization criteria that would be appropriate for the antibody assays being developed in various laboratories. It should be realized that the parameters (requiring validation) are unique to each method and its intended use and, therefore, must be carefully determined on a case-by-case basis.

7.2.2 Factors influencing immunogenicity of biosimilars

Therapeutic protein immunogenicity is influenced by different factors. Some concern the protein's very structure, how to produce it with its purification degree, its formulation, the treatment type, and the patients' characteristics, plus other factors possibly not known.

7.2.2.1 Molecule-specific factors

- The presence of nonhuman sequences
- Novel epitopes generated by amino acid substitution designed to enhance stability
- Novel epitopes created at the junction of fusion proteins
- Changes in glycosylation exposing cryptic B cell and T cell epitopes in the protein, or cause the protein to appear foreign to the immune system
- Carbohydrate moieties present eliciting the production of IgE antibodies; preexisting antibodies against galactoseα1,3-galactose have been shown to be responsible for IgEmediated anaphylactic reactions in patients treated with cetuximab
- PEGylation can reduce the immunogenicity of some proteins
- Patients producing antibodies to the PEG residue adversely affecting the efficacy
- Repeated administration causing a break in immune tolerance
- The presence of degradation products resulting from oxidation or deamination of the protein
- Aggregates, although the mechanism is not clearly understood
- Intrinsic immunomodulatory effects

7.2.2.1.1 Intrinsic immunomodulatory effects The duration of treatment and the route of administration also influence the immune response; for example, if administration of a protein in a single dose results in the production of lowaffinity IgM antibodies, the repeated dosing might result in the production of highaffinity and hightiter IgG antibodies, which may be neutralizing.

The conditions promoting an immune tolerance breakdown include

- Chronic treatment with repeated doses for months, even years;
- Absence of concomitant immunosuppressant treatment; and
- Route of administration (the subcutaneous injection is more immunogenic than intramuscular, itself more immunogenic than an intravenous injection).

7.2.2.2 Structural factors Proteins are complex molecules with primary, secondary, and tertiary structures. Changes in the primary structure may be the cause of an immunogenic reaction. Several cases are well known and published in the literature:

- Changing an insulin amino acid is enough to lead to a strong immunogenic response, whereas two amino acids inversion only leads to a PK change
- The homology degree of a recombinant protein with the natural protein may explain an immunogenic reaction
- Reactions of oxidation or deamidation of amino acids are known for triggering an immunogenic reaction by forming new epitopes. It is the example of human recombinant an interferon with one methionine, oxidized because of a modification of the purification process, that has led to nonneutralizing antibodies formation and which, returning to the initial process, has stopped being immunogenic
- The modification of stability characteristics of a protein with aggregates formation may have significant consequences in terms of immunogenicity by tolerance breakdown of the immune system

The significance of protein spatial conformation is well known for its biological activity as well as its stability. Partial modification of spatial conformation may occur after shear, by shaking, or by temperature modification (for example, temperature rise or freeze/thaw cycles).

7.2.2.2.1 Glycosylation Almost half of the therapeutic proteins that are approved or in clinical trials are glycosylated. Glycosylation is one of the most common and complex PTMs, which leads to the enzymatic addition of glycans on proteins. Glycans can influence the physicochemical (e.g., solubility, electrical charge, mass, size, folding, stability) as well as the biological (e.g., activity, half-life, cell surface receptor function) properties of proteins. The glycosylation profile of a protein is species specific and depends on the cell line and the culture conditions that are used for production. The presence and the structure of carbohydrate moieties can have a direct or indirect impact on the immunogenicity of therapeutic proteins, that is, the glycan structure itself can induce an immune response, or its presence can affect protein structure in such a way that the protein becomes immunogenic.

Glycosylation is an important factor in therapeutic protein immunogenicity. Glycans may impact the immunogenicity of therapeutic proteins in an indirect manner through their influence on folding, solubility, and structural stability of proteins. Besides making a protein more soluble, a carbohydrate moiety is sometimes able to cover an antigenic epitope.

7.2.2.3 Expression-related factors Fully functional mAbs also can be efficiently synthesized in transgenic plants. A major drawback of plant-derived glycoproteins is the presence of complex N-glycans with core xylose and core α1,3-fucose structures. These two glycoepitopes are foreign to humans due to differences in plant and mammalian glycosyltransferase repertoires.

The nonhuman glycan structures present on biopharmaceuticals can induce IgE-mediated reactions and/or anaphylaxis in allergic patients. Moreover, those glycoepitopes may enhance clearance and decrease therapeutic effect of biopharmaceuticals due to preexisting IgA, IgM, and IgG antibodies in certain patients. Neutralization of the therapeutic protein or cross-reactivity with the endogenous protein resulting from the presence of glycoepitopes is less likely, due to lack of reactivity toward the underlying protein backbone.

7.2.2.3.1 PEGylation Biopharmaceuticals can be chemically modified with the purpose of extending half-life or facilitating uptake by target receptors. An increasingly common type of engineering is the covalent attachment of polyethylene glycol (PEG) polymers to the peptide backbone. PEGylation adds additional molecular weight and lowers renal filtration resulting in the protection of proteins from proteolytic degradation. Similar to glycosylation, PEGylation may decrease immunogenicity by shielding the immunogenic epitopes while maintaining the native conformation of the protein. PEG polymers ranging in molecular weight from 12 to 40 kDa attached to different sites on the hydrophobic and immunogenic therapeutic proteins reduce the aggregation propensity and immunogenicity.

Some recombinant proteins are PEGylated in order to modify their PK. PEGylation of a protein is the process of attachment of PEG chains to the skeleton of the protein. The result is a decreased total half-life of the protein, protected proteolytic enzymes, and sometimes masked immunogenic sites. The new proteins so obtained differ by their conjugated structure, their molecular size, and their spatial conformation (linear, branched, or multibranched chains). Often does PEGylation lower the protein's immunogenicity, probably through multiple mechanisms related to blocked antigenic sites, improved solubility, and lower administration frequency of the therapeutic protein. In general, a branched PEG-protein is more efficient than a linear PEG-protein because of improved immunological properties.

7.2.3 Chemical degradation

Chemical modifications of proteins may include deamidation, oxidation, isomerization, hydrolysis, glycation, and C/N terminal heterogeneity of the protein, sometimes leading to aggregation. The susceptibility of an individual amino acid residue to chemical modification is dependent on the neighboring residues, the tertiary structure of the protein, and the solution conditions such as temperature, pH, and ionic strength. Chemical modification may give rise to a less favorable charge of the protein, thus leading to structural changes or even the formation of new covalent cross-links. Covalent aggregation is also a form of chemical degradation.

The deamidation of proteins accelerates at high temperature and high pH, and can occur during bioprocessing and storage. Moreover, deamidation can be accompanied by some degree of oxidation, conformational changes, fragmentation, and aggregation, posing serious risks for immunogenicity. Oxidation, another major chemical modification, can also reduce conformational stability and may cause the protein to aggregate. The oxidation of human serum albumin with hydroxyl radicals resulted in structural alterations and exposure of hydrophobic patches, causing increased immunogenicity.

7.2.3.1 Aggregation Aggregation phenomena may expose new epitopes to the protein's surface for which the immune system is intolerant. That leads to a standard immune response. In other conditions, protein aggregation may lead to presenting a multimeric antibody, which is known for not triggering B lymphocyte tolerance breakdown. This is why, in a therapeutic protein's analysis, it is important to look for the presence of aggregates and to limit their presence to a low level of the formulated drug.

Since aggregation is often accompanied by other structural changes in the protein, it is difficult to distinguish the individual impact of each factor on immunogenicity. Since the information on the nature of immunogenic aggregates from clinical studies is generally limited, animal models are used to provide insight into the link between aggregation and immunogenicity.

Nonnative aggregation can trigger structural changes in the protein leading to the creation of new epitopes or the exposure of existing epitopes. Native-like aggregates, however, are more likely to elicit ADAs that cross-react with the native protein and thus pose a greater risk to the patient. Native-like aggregates may resemble haptens on the surface of pathogens that form organized and repetitive structures that can cross-link B cell receptors in a multivalent manner.

Aggregates can be classified according to size, reversibility, secondary or tertiary structure, covalent modification, and morphology. One class of aggregates that are of particular concern includes subvisible particles or, more specifically, aggregates ranging from 0.1 to 10 μm in size. The current United States Pharmacopeia light obscuration test for drug approval requires that the number of particulates over 10 μm is ≤6000 per container, while the number of particulates over 25 μm is ≤600 per container. Industrial researchers agree that additional analysis of subvisible particles smaller than 10 μm would support product characterization and development. Subvisible particles are too large to be analyzed by standard quality control methods such as SEC and SDS-PAGE, but too small to be visually detected. Therefore, the use of additional, less routine methods such as asymmetrical flow FFF and microflow imaging (MFI) has been recommended for extended characterization following a risk-based approach.

Product characterization should not only be limited to monitoring protein particles, but also focus on nonprotein particles. Foreign micro- and nanoparticles, for example, shed from filling pumps or product containers, are able to induce protein aggregation or nucleate the formation of heterogeneous aggregates.

7.2.3.2 Manufacturing and processing factors In addition to intended modifications, a biopharmaceutical may be chemically modified through accidental degradation in one of the many bioprocessing steps: fermentation, virus inactivation, purification, polishing, formulation, filtration, filling, storage, transport, and administration. Chemical stresses during manufacturing and storage can be caused by exposure to light or elevated temperatures and presence of oxygen, metal ions, or peroxide impurities from excipients in the formulation. Trace amounts of iron, chromium, and nickel can leach into the formulation buffer via contact with stainless steel surfaces typically used during bioprocessing and catalyze the degradation reactions.

7.2.3.3 Impurities and other production contaminants Therapeutic proteins obtained through recombinant DNA technology are produced in various cellular systems where production-linked protein impurities originate. These proteins are called HCPs, considered endogenous proteins by the immune system, and may lead to antibody formation by the standard immune mechanism. If the anti-HCP antibodies do not neutralize the biological activity of the therapeutic protein of interest, they can nevertheless have consequences in terms of general effects including skin reactions, allergies, anaphylaxis, or serum sickness. Other contaminants, such as impurities, coming from chromatographic column resins or from enzymes used for refining therapeutic proteins' purification, may be found as traces in the finished product. Some impurities may be released by some compounds used for the capping process. These impurities may play the role of the amplifier for the immune response, even if they are not able to initiate an immune response themselves.

Process-related impurities, including traces of residual DNA or proteins from the expression system, or contaminants that leach from the product container, can also influence the immunogenicity of recombinant biopharmaceuticals. Several examples exist in the modification of the recombinant protein's immunogenicity with time, involving production of bacterial cells' endotoxin level. DNA G-C patterns from bacteria or degraded proteins are able to activate toll-like receptors and act as adjuvants. (Toll-like receptors are a class of proteins playing a key role in the innate immune response. They are *trans*-membrane proteins containing receptors that detect danger signals located in the extracellular milieu, a *trans*-membrane medium, and an intracellular medium allowing the activation signal transduction.) However, the action of these impurities is limited to nonhuman proteins with a pseudovaccination activity. The adjuvants are unable to stimulate an immune response based on a T lymphocyte's response independent of the tolerance breakdown of B lymphocytes.

7.2.3.4 Formulation changes Changes in formulations have been associated with ADAs. Two particularly interesting cases could illustrate how important the formulation and conservation conditions are. The first case concerns EPO. Cases of PRCA after treatment with EPO are known, but rare. Anti-EPO antibodies are formed exogenously as well as endogenously, after administration of recombinant human EPO (rHuEPO). These cases have occurred after a changed in the formulation of the finished product, with human albumin used as a stabilizer replaced by polysorbate 80. Different hypotheses to explain the immune system tolerance breakdown after administration of rHuEPO lead, among other things, to the impurities' extraction from the syringe's plunger rod stopper, playing booster in the presence of EPO. During the analysis of batches called into question, no increase in the level of aggregates or in the level of truncated or degraded EPO has been evidenced. In that case, there must have been several factors having fostered the immune system's tolerance breakdown. In particular, the subcutaneous route of administration may be incriminated, as it is known to produce a pseudovaccination effect.

The second case involves the conservation conditions of a freeze-dried formulation of interferon a-2a (rHuINF a-2a) that has been stabilized by human albumin. At room temperature, a partial oxidation of rHuINF a-2a has made the formation of aggregates easier with intact interferon and albumin. These aggregates led to the therapeutic preparation's immunogenicity.

These cases illustrate how important the finished product formulation study and the evaluation that has to be done of the possible consequences of a change compared to the initial formulation or its conservation conditions are. It is also particularly important to rigorously analyze the levels of impurities issued from the therapeutic protein's system of production.

The adverse response resulted from antibodies that neutralized endogenously produced protein and also caused the discontinuation of the MGDF.

7.3 Immunogenicity testing

The current most practical and commonly used approach for testing unwanted immunogenicity is the detection, measurement, and characterization of antibodies specifically generated for the product. It is anticipated that better models of evaluating immunogenicity will become available in the future that may include DNA microarrays. Generally, no single assay can provide all the necessary information on the immunogenicity profile of a biological product and as a result, a panel of carefully selected and validated assays for detection and measurement of antibodies is used. These antibody responses are then correlated with the PK/PD and clinical effects when evaluated to determine if the antibodies create a "meaningful difference" in determining the safety and the efficacy of these products.

7.3.1 Testing protocols

Development of biosimilars requires studies to measure ADAs and comparison of relative immunogenicity rates of the biosimilar and the reference products. Even though there exist guidelines from the FDA for the development of biosimilars, details on executing these with reference to antibody assays and their validation are not clear.

The development of an immunogenicity assay for a biosimilar program should be preceded by sufficient in vitro analytical results to establish analytical and pharmacological similarities on multiple lots. The comparison of the immunogenicity potential becomes more relevant if there are unknown or trivial analytical differences, such as relative levels of aggregation, or impurities, between the products that might contribute to differences in immunogenicity. Immunogenicity testing alone is not adequate to establish structural similarity of the products.

Many of the immunogenicity assays used to test the originator molecules were developed over a decade ago and thus had limitations inherent to the platforms and the reagents utilized at that time. The current guidance on immunogenicity assay development and validation provides more sensitive and drug-tolerant assays, making it difficult to compare the results with data available in approved BLA documents for the reference listed product.

The platforms that are typically utilized for these assays are ligand-binding assays via ELISA and electrochemiluminescence methods; however, several emerging technologies can also be utilized, such as BiaCore or Octet, Luminex, and Gyrolab.

Another critical component of all immunogenicity assays is the production of an appropriate PC and may include the use of commercially available polyclonal or antiidiotypic antibodies to the reference product, affinity-purified ADAs to the biosimilar and/or reference product, as well as immune serum from hyperimmunized animals dosed with the biosimilar and/or the reference product. It is important to collect serum from any animals evaluated during preclinical testing that could potentially provide an ADA PC for the immunogenicity assay in order to limit the number of animals required to procure this necessary reagent. The need for one or more PCs may also be influenced by the strategy that will be used for the assay(s) and the overall development.

There are two predominant strategies for proceeding through an immunogenicity testing plan based on the utilization of a single assay or two separate assays. Using either strategy, the assays must have a high level of similarity for all parameters evaluated. A typical ELISA-based immunogenicity assay consists of the drug bound to a 96-well plate, which is used to capture any ADAs that are present in the serum or plasma samples when they are applied to the plate. This complex is then detected using an enzyme-labeled form of the drug in the case of a bridging assay. The levels of colorimetric or relative light units that are detected in the assay correspond to the level of ADAs present in the serum or plasma samples. The assay is evaluated based on sensitivity (the lowest amount of antibody that can be detected in the assay), precision, drug tolerance, specificity, selectivity, prozone, and accuracy of titration.

7.3.2 A single assay

The single assay is developed for both products, and a limited set of parameters should be evaluated during validation including screening cut-point, specificity cut-point, precision, and drug tolerance for both products in order to ensure that the assay is capable of detecting antibodies from both the biosimilar and the reference product. This may involve the conjugation of a reporter molecule such as biotin or ruthenium to both the biosimilar and the reference product to facilitate the detection of antibodies when a bridging assay format is utilized. It is critical to ensure that the method of conjugation is tightly controlled and that these reagents are labeled in a reproducible manner in order to obtain comparable signals between the two reagents. Although the assay is essentially developed as two assays with respect to screening cut-point and precision, all other parameters should be evaluated on the background of the biosimilar assay (a plate coated with the biosimilar and detected with an enzyme-labeled biosimilar) where the biosimilar will be used to capture all potential antibodies from the biosimilar or the reference product in the serum or plasma samples. When this strategy is used, it is essential to determine the specificity cut-point by immune depletion with both the test and the reference product, as well as to test each positive sample for specificity to both products. Likewise, the drug tolerance of the assay must be defined for both molecules to ensure that the assay is tolerant to similar levels of circulating drug. The major limitation of using a single-assay approach is that the approach will allow the evaluation of only similar or enhanced levels of biosimilar immunogenicity in relation to the reference product. If there are unique antibodies that are generated to the reference product, they will not be detected by this assay. This is not a good strategy for those seeking a designation of interchangeability.

7.3.3 Two assays

The use of the two-assay approach entails a full validation of two separate assays, one for the detection of antibodies generated to the biosimilar and one for the detection of antibodies generated to the reference product. This strategy is most useful when looking for an interchangeability designation, as the approach will allow a direct comparison of the immunogenicity rates of each molecule. The limitation of this approach is generally cost, as each serum or plasma sample would need to be run in each assay in order to truly assess if the immunogenicity potential of the two products is the same and to control for any variability observed between the two assays. This approach is also suitable for defining decreased immunogenicity rates for the biosimilar in comparison with the reference product, which could be potentially due to differences in production.

7.3.4 Testing strategy

Immunogenicity testing should be done on the basis of a risk assessment and is usually done in several stages:

- Screening assay that detects all antibodies binding to the biopharmaceutical (ADAs) in serum samples from animals or patients
- Confirmatory assay to eliminate false-positive samples and assay for neutralizing antibodies that detects those serum samples that contain neutralizing antibodies
- Characterization of ADAs detected in serum samples

Screening for ADA is usually done using suitable ELISA formats or radioimmuneprecipitation (RIPA), e.g., with 125I-labeled antibodies or SPR. The same assays are used for the confirmation step, e.g., by demonstrating inhibition of binding by an excess of the drug. Bridging ELISA formats are particularly useful in early project stages and for different animal species when project-specific immunological reagents are not available. To run a bridging ELISA, a labeled drug is needed, however. The label may be detected directly (e.g., fluorescein) or indirectly via an amplification system.

7.3.5 Assays for detection of antibodies

Common methods available include binding assays based on immunochemical procedures such as solid or liquid phase immunoassays, RIPA, and biophysical methods such as SPR. These assays determine the presence (or the absence) of antibodies based on the ability of the antibodies to recognize the relevant antigenic determinants in the therapeutic protein. These assays have their own advantages and disadvantages as described in the following:

- Direct-format binding assays (coating with antigen and detecting with labeled anti-Ig) are rapid and relatively easy to use but prone to spurious binding or matrix effects and antigen mobilization may mask or alter epitopes.
- Indirect-format binding assays (coating with a specific mAb or biotin, etc. followed by antigen) have high throughput, excellent sensitivity, and coating with a specific mAb keeping the antigen in oriented position and provide consistent coating and maintains antigen conformation, species specificity, and isotype detection determined by secondary reagent; however, the detection reagent may differ between control and sample and extensive studies are required to demonstrate that the coating mAb does not mask or alter epitopes. The test may also fail to detect low-affinity antibodies and has species specificity, and its isotype detection requires determination by secondary reagents.
- Bridging-format electrochemiluminescence offers high throughput and use of high concentrations of matrix but requires two antigen conjugates (biotin and TAG) and antigen labeling may alter/denature antigen, or mask/alter epitopes.
- RIPA (SPR) is tolerant to interference from antigen, provides signal detection consistent during life of TAG conjugate, has moderate to high throughput, good sensitivity, and can be concrete and automated; it contains information on specificity, isotypes, relative binding affinity, and relative concentration and enables detection of both low-affinity and high-affinity antibodies, and detection reagents are not required. However, it requires dedicated equipment; reagents are costly and vendor specific. It can be isotype specific, may fail to detect rapidly dissociating antibodies, and requires radiolabeled antigens that may alter or denature the antigen; decay of radiolabel may affect antigen stability. Also, it may require immobilization of the antigen, which may alter the conformation of the native protein and the regeneration step may degrade the antigen; the sensitivity is less than that found in binding assays.

None of these assays can assess the ability of the antibodies to neutralize the biological activity of the therapeutic proteins that is an important element in the assessment of immunogenicity. For the evaluation of the neutralizing ability, the use of an appropriate noncell-based competitive ligand-binding assay or a cell-based neutralization assay is required.

Testing for immunogenicity is performed during the preclinical and clinical phases. The U.S. FDA *Guidance for Industry: Assay Development for Immunogenicity Testing of Therapeutic Proteins* states that an immunogenicity assay should, in addition to being sensitive, also be able to detect all isotypes, in particular, IgM and all IgG isotypes. The recommended sensitivity is 250 to 500 ng/mL. Studies are performed in three steps: screening, confirmation, and characterization of positives. Initial screening can result in false positives, and, therefore, the initial screening assay is usually followed by a confirmatory assay. After identification and confirmation of positive samples, a full characterization of ADAs in terms of assessment of isotype (class or subclass), binding stability, epitope specificity, and neutralizing capacity gives valuable information of the nature of the studied immune response. The IgG4 is second to IgG1 as the major isotype in ADAs developed for therapeutic mAbs. IgG4 has been associated with immune responses generated under conditions of high doses and prolonged exposure to therapeutic proteins. IgG4 ADAs can be difficult to detect in traditional bridging or homogenous ELISA and ECL™ (enhanced chemiluminescent) assays due to their bispecific nature.

7.3.6 Cell-based neutralization assays

The development of improved assays, particularly cell-based assays for the detection of neutralizing antibodies that allow immunogenicity to be determined with precision and the comparison of immunogenicity data between biopharmaceuticals, are critical for the development of less immunogenic and safer biopharmaceuticals.

The biological activity of a therapeutic is often evaluated using an in vitro cell-based assay based on a functional aspect of the protein or the MOA. These assays can be categorized into those that detect signaling responses soon after the protein-receptor interaction has occurred (early stage) or those that provide a measurable readout after the culmination of a cellular response (late stage). Since these assays assess the cellular response in vitro to a protein, they constitute an ideal and appropriate logical approach for the development of a cell-based neutralization assay. It should be realized that different types of bioassay procedures can be used as the basis of a neutralization assay for a biological.

A cell-based neutralization assay can be defined as an in vitro assay utilizing cells that interact with or respond to the therapeutic either directly or indirectly in a measurable manner in the presence of a test sample for the detection of antiproduct neutralizing antibodies. The detection of neutralizing antibodies is based on the principle that any sample containing an antibody (of a neutralizing nature) would reduce or abolish the biological activity induced by a known concentration of the therapeutic in a cell-based assay.

Most biological therapeutics can be broadly categorized into agonists or antagonists based on their desired effect in vivo. While agonists (e.g., cytokines, growth factors, hormones, agonistic mAbs) induce a response by directly binding to receptors on the target cell surface, therapeutics with antagonistic properties (e.g., soluble receptors, antagonistic mAbs) act by blocking the binding of a ligand to the target receptor expressed on the cell surface. As a result, assay formats and designs of neutralizing antibody assays can vary depending on the biological and the type of assay being used.

Although regulatory authorities recommend the use of cellbased assays for the detection and the quantification of neutralizing antibodies, cell-based assays often give variable results and are difficult to standardize. Conventional cell-based assays for neutralizing antibodies are based upon the assessment of a drug-induced response in a drug-sensitive cell line, and the ability of an antibody to inhibit that response. The form of the assay can considerably vary, however, reflecting the diversity of the biopharmaceuticals currently employed in the clinic. Drug-induced responses vary from stimulation of cell proliferation in the presence of a growth factor, such as EPO or GMCSF, or induction of apoptosis in the presence of TNFα to inhibition of virus replication in interferon-treated cells. Such druginduced responses are complex events involving the transcriptional activation or modulation of numerous genes. Drug-induced biological responses also often take several days to develop and are influenced by a number of factors that are difficult to control.

A series of engineered reporter cell lines has been developed for the quantification of the activity and the neutralizing antibody response to biopharmaceuticals that eliminate many of the limitations of conventional cellbased assays.

In order to improve the performance of conventional cell-based assays and to develop assays that allow more direct comparisons of immunogenicity data, reporter cell lines were established based on transfection of cells with the firefly luciferase reporter gene regulated by a drug-responsive chimeric promoter. These assays allow the drug activity, and the neutralization of drug activity, to be determined selectively and with a high degree of precision within a few hours by measuring light emission. In addition, the use of a single common druginduced response for a variety of different drugs facilitates comparisons of immunogenicity data.

Conventional cell-based assays are difficult to standardize due in part to assay variation resulting from changes in culture conditions and genetic and epigenetic changes that can occur, as cells are continuously cultivated in the laboratory. Assay variation can be minimized by the use of cell banks and the preparation of each lot of assay cells under standardized conditions from an individually frozen vial. Each lot of assay cells is thus in an identical physiological condition. Assay-ready cells can be manufactured under conditions of current GMPs, and stored frozen for several years without loss of drug sensitivity.

For neutralization assays, a recommended approach for expressing data is to report results as the amount of serum required to neutralize the biological activity induced by a constant quantity of the antigen. In some instances, however, it may be necessary to use an antibody standard or a reference preparation for expressing the levels of neutralizing antibodies in the test samples relative to the amounts of the neutralizing antibodies in the reference antibody preparation. It may also be possible to express antibody levels using arbitrary units provided that the unit has been well defined for the reference material. Although this approach is not ideal (the heterogeneous nature of polyclonal antibodies is particularly problematical for this), the use of this strategy may provide relatively precise estimates of antibody levels in the test samples and can reduce variability. This situation is most likely to occur when a number of sequential samples from the same animal or patient are available, and it is hard to include all samples from all patients in the same assays for establishing a valid comparison of antibody levels between different samples/patients.

7.3.7 Biosensor-based immunoassays

This method, unlike most other platforms, does not require the use of a labeled secondary reagent. Although several types of biosensors are available, the vast majority of published biosensor data cites the use of Biacore instruments (https://www.biacore.com/lifesciences/index.html) for monitoring the immune response in preclinical phases and clinical trials. Several models of Biacore are automated and also compliant with the 21 CFR part 11 requirement, which facilitates the use of this instrument for regulatory submissions.

The Biacore utilizes SPR to detect the increase in mass on the surface of the sensor chip following binding of an antibody to the antigen immobilized on the sensor chip. This increase in mass is directly proportional to the amount of antigen-binding antibody present in the serum sample being tested. The ability of the instrument to monitor the interaction in real-time and provide a continuous signal of the events occurring on the sensor surface enables the detection of rapidly dissociating or low-affinity antibodies if these are present in the sample. The detection of low-affinity antibodies is necessary as these antibodies have the potential to neutralize the therapeutic product and may predict the generation of a later mature immune response. Furthermore, characterization of the antibodies in terms of affinities, antibody class, and subclass can also be easily performed. These attributes have contributed to the increased use and popularity of this platform in studies on immunogenicity.

While the assays described are useful for identifying antibody-positive samples, it is important to include an additional confirmatory step in the assessment strategy to ensure that the generated antibodies are specifically targeted to the therapeutic.

7.3.8 Confirmation of antibody positive samples

A confirmatory approach can include the use of different methods (ELISAs, competitive immunoassays, SPR, etc.), although an assay based on a different scientific principle from that used for the screening assay should usually be considered. It is also necessary to select a confirmatory assay taking into account the limitations and the characteristics of the screening assay. In most cases, assay specificity can be demonstrated by the addition of free antigen to a serum sample spiked with known amounts of antibody and by looking for inhibition of the expected signal. This approach itself can form the basis of a confirmatory assay.

The use of the immunoblotting procedure, which provides information concerning the specificity of the antibodies detected, is valuable as the antibodies may have specificity for other components (e.g., contaminants) in the product and can cause data to be misinterpreted. For example, very small levels of expression system–derived bacterial proteins in rDNA products can cause significant antibody development, whereas the human sequence major protein present (the active principle) may be much less immunogenic. However, other procedures, e.g., analytical radioimmunoprecipitation assays, can also be used for specificity studies.

The use of assays described earlier does not obviate the requirement for a functional cell-based neutralization assay. The latter should be incorporated into the strategy for immunogenicity assessment as it has been shown that results from bioassays can often be correlated with the effect of antibodies on clinical response. Some developers conduct neutralization assays at both preclinical and clinical levels as part of their product development program, while others implement these assays at the clinical stage after considering whether the therapeutic is low or high risk.

Overall, the decision to put a biosimilar on the market is made if its effectiveness is similar, and its immunogenic profile is at least comparable or improved in comparison to the first licensed product. However, this decision is made on limited data. The similarity testing program may disclose substantial differences in terms of immunogenic profiles, but is probably unable to detect minor differences and rare events. For that reason, clinical trials complemented by a pharmacovigilance program are often required for evaluating a recombinant protein's safety in patients. Undesirable effects of these drugs are very rare, yet require a follow-up during the life of the product.

This includes testing all those attributes that can trigger a side effect such as immunogenicity; included here are aggregates, dimers, subvisible and visible particles, HCP, host cell DNA, etc. The nonclinical studies are generally required to establish overall toxicology, such as in an animal model; however, in several situations, an animal model may not be readily available, such as in the case of mAbs. Several creative models have recently been proposed including transgenic mice, etc. Also included here are safety assessments at the toxicological level and in the clinical pharmacology of the product, such as PK and PD data.

This is perhaps one of the most difficult areas of biosimilar product development. All protein therapeutic contain particles, and these can be immunogenic.

Subvisible and submicron particles and aggregates of various sizes can be tested using methods such as HIAC, MFI, dynamic light scattering (DLS), FFF, AUC-sedimentation velocity, and SEC-HPLC-LS. It is most important to determine if a higher level of subvisible particles is nonproteinaceous.

All protein therapeutics contain (higher or lower levels of) aggregates and particulate matter and most of these products are immunogenic. Aggregation results from fermentation/expression, purification, formulation, filling, transport, and storage administration. Some of the factors influencing protein aggregation include temperature, interfaces, freeze–thaw, container, pH, excipients, ionic strength, and concentration. Protein aggregates are assemblies of protein molecules that are highly heterogeneous regarding their size, reversibility, protein conformation, covalent modifications, and morphology. It is hard to predict which form will be more immunogenic. It is because even a simple dimer can adopt various shapes and characteristics based on pH, process stress, light, osmolality, etc. The micronsized IgG aggregates induced by shaking remain at subcutaneous injection site for longer than a month and how it affects the long-term immunogenicity remains unknown.

The particles have different size ranges and the methods used to detect them are limited in their ability to detect them (Table 7.3). Most monomers are less than 10 nm and oligomers less than 100 nm.

Table 7.3 Methods Used to Analyze Different Particle Sizes

Methodology	Range of Detection
HP-SEC	1 to 90 nm (does not differentiate other particles)
SDS-PAGE	1 to 100 nm
DLS	1 nm to 2 μm
Nanoparticle tracking analysis	30 nm to 2 μm
FFF	5 nm to 9 μm
MFI	0.8 to 200 μm
Light obscuration	1 to 200 μm
Microscopy	5 to 200 μm
Visible	500 μm to 5 mm+

New insights from quantifying subvisible particles show that beyond potential immunogenicity, particle sizes and levels are important product quality attributes; a mass of protein (e.g., <0.1%) in particles may not be detectable as loss of monomer; subvisible particle analysis provides very sensitive early detection of protein aggregation and new insights into aggregation pathways, manufacturing, and formulation development. Even trace levels of particles can impact the subsequent stability of protein solutions.

Beyond protein particles, these include glass particles from containers, glass cartridges, and syringes, are siliconized, and free silicone oil droplets can be generated; in syringes, there may be tungsten particles and salts from needle insertion process, and rubber or silicone particles can come from stoppers; stainless steel and other particles from filling pumps and particles shed from filters during prefilling sterile filtration. These particles can adsorb onto proteins and make them more immunogenic.

Aggregates, including subvisible particles, are critical quality attributes and the removal of these reduces immunogenicity; a good example is that of Betaferon that contains a lot of aggregates and particulate matter and is one of the most immunogenic therapeutic protein product.

7.3.9 Stability

Degradation over time can significantly change the safety profile of a biological product more than it can affect potency. Aggregation over time is a significant concern. As a result, the FDA requires side-by-side stability testing of the reference product. Additionally, tests include forced degradation, accelerated stability, and stressed stability. Following are the highlights of the required stability testing plan:

- Demonstrate that the drug product is stable during the period of PK/PD study; this applies to both the drug substance as well as the drug product
- Conduct real-time, stressed and accelerated stability studies side by side with the reference product

Comparative stability studies under long-term storage conditions, accelerated conditions, and stress conditions, including mechanical stress and photostability, are conducted as well. Real-time accelerated conditions are used as recommended by ICH Q5C and ICH Q1A to evaluate the stability profiles of the proposed biosimilar and the U.S.-licensed reference product.

7.4 Nonclinical testing

Nonclinical or preclinical studies in animal models allow connecting activity with the PK effect relevant to the clinical application. Measurements in toxicokinetics including the determination of the level of antibodies with the study of crossed reactions and of the neutralization capacity are necessary; the studies must last long enough to show any difference relevant in terms of toxicity and/or immune response between the biosimilar and the first licensed product. However, these studies are not intended to establish toxic dose ranges. Where required, local tolerance studies are also conducted but other routine toxicological tests (safety pharmacology, reproductive tests, mutagenicity, carcinogenicity) are not necessary. The preclinical study program is a limited program due to the fact that the toxicology data are known for the first licensed reference product, and it is not necessary to repeat all the studies to know the biosimilar.

There are several key measures in conducting nonclinical studies. For example, the dose chosen should be such to elicit some side effects; this is analogous to studying dose response in the linear range and not within the plateau ranges. There is a general consensus to reduce the animal studies where possible, and the biosimilar product developer is encouraged to hold meetings with regulatory agencies and develop a clear understanding of what would be considered minimally required. Generally, if these studies are required, then an IND will not be approved unless these data are available.

Understanding the limitations of nonclinical testing is important. This raises certain scientific and logistic questions. First, the high variability in animal toxicity PK/PD data most often makes comparisons between products superfluous. Second, there are a large number of products for which there exists no viable toxicity model in animals, such as mAbs and fusion proteins. Testing them in animals does not establish safety profile. When a new molecule is developed, the emphasis is on examining gross toxicity responses; all of these concerns are resolved when the product is approved for use in humans.

Even the assessment of immunogenicity in animal models does not provide any useful projection of immunogenicity in humans. All of these understandings have begun to be discussed at the regulatory agency level. In all likelihood, both the FDA and the EMA will be amenable to waiver or reduce preclinical testing when the analytical similarity data are impressive, more particularly for mAbs and fusion proteins. Biosimilar product developers need to challenge preclinical testing for all products to make this a more accepted practice. Unfortunately, many developers of biosimilar products with large resources take a more conservative path and conduct these superfluous studies anyway, raising the bar for smaller developers. The licensed reference product companies have refused to accept analytical similarity data in lieu of preclinical and clinical testings and keep pushing the need for these studies, to raise both the financial and the time burden against biosimilars.

The safety of new compounds is tested in preclinical testing in animals prior to introducing them into humans. When the agencies began developing guidelines to demonstrate the safety of biosimilar products, preclinical testing was made part of the safety demonstration with one difference, that the sponsor was to show these safety profiles compared with the licensed reference product.

7.5 Conclusion

While some recombinant products like filgrastim have almost no immunogenicity, other glycosylated products many show a very high level of immune response–triggering ability. The developers of biosimilar products will face the greatest challenge in providing data that show comparable immunogenicity against the reference product; in some instances, this may raise the question of appropriateness when tested in humans. A large number of surrogate tests are available today, and many more will become available in the future that will give the sponsors an opportunity to model the immunogenic response without exposing patients or healthy subjects. A keen understanding of what makes a product more or less immunogenic, as described in this chapter is an important step in establishing biosimilarity as the FDA expects.

Bibliography

Abraham, I., and MacDonald, K. (2012 September) Clinical safety of biosimilar recombinant human erythropoietins. *Expert Opin Drug Saf* 11 (5): 819–840.

Abraham, I., Tharmarajah, S., and MacDonald, K. (2103 March) Clinical safety of biosimilar recombinant human granulocyte colony–stimulating factors. *Expert Opin Drug Saf* 12 (2): 235–246.

Alten, R., and Cronstein, B. N. (2015 June) Clinical trial development for biosimilars. *Semin Arthritis Rheum* 44 6 Suppl: S2–S8.

Barbosa, M. D., Kumar, S., Loughrey, H., and Singh, S. K. (2012 December) Biosimilars and biobetters as tools for understanding and mitigating the immunogenicity of biotherapeutics. *Drug Discov Today* 17 (23–24): 1282–1288.

Bennett, C. L. et al. (2014 December) Regulatory and clinical considerations for biosimilar oncology drugs. *Lancet Oncol* 15 (13): e594–e605.

Biggioggero, M., Danova, M., Genovese, U., Locatelli, F., Meroni, P. L., Pane, F., and Scaglione, F. (2015 June) The challenging definition of naïve patient for biological drug use. *Autoimmun Rev* 14 (6): 543–546.

Cai, X. Y., Gouty, D., Baughman, S., Ramakrishnan, M., and Cullen, C. (2011 March) Recommendations and requirements for the design of bioanalytical testing used in comparability studies for biosimilar drug development. *Bioanalysis* 3 (5): 535–540.

Cai, X. Y., Thomas, J., Cullen, C., and Gouty, D. (2012 September) Challenges of developing and validating immunogenicity assays to support comparability studies for biosimilar drug development. *Bioanalysis* 4 (17): 2169–2177. Review. PubMed PMID: 23013399.

Camacho, L. H., Frost, C. P., Abella, E., Morrow, P. K., and Whittaker, S. (2014 August) Biosimilars 101: Considerations for U. S. oncologists in clinical practice. *Cancer Med* 3 (4): 889–899.

Castañeda-Hernández, G., Szekanecz, Z., Mysler, E., Azevedo, V. F., Guzman, R., Gutierrez, M., Rodríguez, W., and Karateev, D. (2014 December) Biopharmaceuticals for rheumatic diseases in Latin America, Europe, Russia, and India: Innovators, biosimilars, and intended copies. *Joint Bone Spine* 81 (6): 471–477.

Chamberlain, P. (2013 March) Assessing immunogenicity of biosimilar therapeutic monoclonal antibodies: Regulatory and bioanalytical considerations. *Bioanalysis* 5 (5): 561–574.

Dörner, T., and Kay, J. (2015) Biosimilars in rheumatology: Current perspectives and lessons learnt. *Nat Rev Rheumatol* 11 (13): 713–724.

Dörner, T., Strand, V., Castañeda-Hernández, G., Ferraccioli, G., Isaacs, J. D., Kvien, T. K., Martin-Mola, E., Mittendorf, T., Smolen, J. S., and Burmester, G. R. (2013 March) The role of biosimilars in the treatment of rheumatic diseases. *Ann Rheum Dis* 72 (3): 322–328.

Dranitsaris, G., Amir, E., and Dorward, K. (2011 August 20) Biosimilars of biological drug therapies: Regulatory, clinical and commercial considerations. *Drugs* 71 (12): 1527–1536.

Dranitsaris, G., Dorward, K., Hatzimichael, E., and Amir, E. (2013 April) Clinical trial design in biosimilar drug development. *Invest New Drugs* 31 (2): 479–487.

El-Baky, N. A., and Redwan, E. M. (2015) Therapeutic alpha-interferons protein: Structure, production, and biosimilar. *Prep Biochem Biotechnol* 45 (2): 109–127.

Feagan, B. G. et al. (2014 July) The challenge of indication extrapolation for infliximab biosimilars. *Biologicals* 42 (4): 177–183.

Fiorino, G., and Danese, S. (2014 June) The biosimilar road in inflammatory bowel disease: The right way? *Best Pract Res Clin Gastroenterol* 28 (3): 465–471.

Fiorino, G., Girolomoni, G., Lapadula, G., Orlando, A., Danese, S., and Olivieri, I., SIR, SIDeMaST, and IG-IBD (2014 July) The use of biosimilars in immune-mediated disease: A joint Italian Society of Rheumatology (SIR), Italian Society of Dermatology (SIDeMaST), and Italian Group of Inflammatory Bowel Disease (IG-IBD) position paper. *Autoimmun Rev* 13 (7): 751–755.

Fonseca, J. E. et al. (2014 January–March) The Portuguese Society of Rheumatology position paper on the use of biosimilars. *Acta Reumatol Port* 39 (1): 60–71. Review. PubMed PMID: 24811463.

Girault, D. (2015 January–February) Biosimilars: From technical to pharmacoeconomic considerations. 30th Rencontres Nationales de Pharmacologie etRecherche clinique pour l'Innovation et l'Evaluation des Technologies de Santé. Tables rondes. *Therapie* 70 (1): 37–55.

Heinemann, L., Home, P. D., and Hompesch, M. (2015 October) Biosimilar insulins: Guidance for data interpretation by clinicians and users. *Diabetes Obes Metab* 17 (10): 911–918.

Hlavaty, T., and Letkovsky, J. (2014 June) Biosimilars in the therapy of inflammatory bowel diseases. *Eur J Gastroenterol Hepatol* 26 (6): 581–587.

Isaacs, J. D., Cutolo, M., Keystone, E. C., Park, W., and Braun, J. (2016) Biosimilars in immune-mediated inflammatory diseases: Initial lessons from the first approved biosimilar anti-tumour necrosis factor monoclonal antibody. *J Intern Med* 279 (1): 41–59.

Jelkmann, W. (2012 May) Biosimilar recombinant human erythropoietins ("epoetins") and future erythropoiesis-stimulating treatments. *Expert Opin Biol Ther* 12 (5): 581–592.

Kálmán-Szekeres, Z., Olajos, M., and Ganzler, K. (2012 October) Analytical aspects of biosimilarity issues of protein drugs. *J Pharm Biomed Anal* 69: 185–195.

Kes, P., Mesar, I., Bašić-Jukić, N., and Rački, S. (2014 April) What doctors need to know about biosimilar medicinal products? *Acta Med Croatica* 68 (2): 201–205. Review. Croatian. PubMed PMID: 26012160.

McKeage, K. (2014 June) A review of CT-P: An infliximab biosimilar. *BioDrugs* 28 (3): 313–321.

Mendes de Abreu, M., Strand, V., Levy, R. A., and Araujo, D. V. (2014 June) Putting the value into biosimilar decision making: The judgment value criteria. *Autoimmun Rev* 13 (6): 678–684.

Milchert, M., Fliciński, J., Brzosko, M. (2014 July 22) Biosimilars in rheumatology and other fields of medicine. *Postepy Hig Med Dosw (Online)* 68: 970–975.

Morfini, M. (2014 November) Innovative approach for improved rFVIII concentrate. *Eur J Haematol* 93 (5): 361–368.

Nandurkar, H., Chong, B., Salem, H., Gallus, A., Ferro, V., and McKinnon, R., (2014 May) Low-molecular-weight heparin biosimilars: Potential implications for clinical practice. *Intern Med J* 44 (5): 497–500.

Niederwieser, D., and Schmitz, S. (2011 April) Biosimilar agents in oncology/haematology: From approval to practice. *Eur J Haematol* 86 (4): 277–288.

Papamichael, K. et al. (2015 November) Review article: Pharmacological aspects of anti-TNF biosimilars in inflammatory bowel diseases. *Aliment Pharmacol Ther* 42 (10): 1158–1169.

Ranjan, N., Mahajan, V. K., and Misra, M. (2011 December) Biosimilars: The "future" of biologic therapy? *J Dermatolog Treat* 22 (6): 319–322.

Rinaudo-Gaujous, M., Paul, S., Tedesco, E. D., Genin, C., Roblin, X., and Peyrin-Biroulet, L. (2013 October) Review article: Biosimilars are the next generation of drugs for liver and gastrointestinal diseases. *Aliment Pharmacol Ther* 38 (8): 914–924.

Rudick, R. A., and Goelz, S. E. (2011 May 15) Beta-interferon for multiple sclerosis. *Exp Cell Res* 317 (9): 1301–1311.

Swierkot, J. (2013) Biosimilars—Opportunity or threat? *Wiad Lek* 66 (2 Pt 2): 200–205. Review. Polish. PubMed PMID: 25775818.

Wadhwa, M. (2011) *Immunogenicity: What Do We Know and What Can We Measure?* EPAR 1, National Institute for Biological Standards and Control—Health Protection Agency.

Weise, M. et al. (2012 December 20) Biosimilars: What clinicians should know. *Blood* 120 (26): 5111–5117.

Willrich, M. A., Murray, D. L., and Snyder, M. R. (2015 February) Tumor necrosis factor inhibitors: Clinical utility in autoimmune diseases. *Transl Res* 165 (2): 270–282.

Woroń, J., and Kocić, I. (2014 November) The story of biosimilars—Chance or threat? *Pol Merkur Lekarski* 37 (221): 311–315. Review. Polish. PubMed PMID: 25546996.

Yoo, D. H. (2014 August) The rise of biosimilars: Potential benefits and drawbacks in rheumatoid arthritis. *Expert Rev Clin Immunol* 10 (8): 981–983.

Chapter 8 Formulation similarity

The formula "two and two make five" is not without its attractions.
Fyodor Dostoevsky

8.1 Background

Biosimilarity means "the (a) biological product is highly similar to the reference product notwithstanding *minor differences in clinically inactive components*; and there are no clinically meaningful differences between the biological product and the reference product in terms of the safety, purity, and potency of the product" [emphasis added]. The clinically inactive components are formulation related. As an example, the first biosimilar product approved in the United States, Zarxio, had a different buffer system (glutamate versus acetate in the originator) and a different pH (4.5 versus 4.0) for a filgrastim product. While differences in the pH and the buffer composition of a subcutaneous product may affect the absorption profile, the FDA concluded that these differences are not "clinically meaningful."

By way of background, the FDA's regulations implementing FDCA § 505(j)(4)(H), which concerns abbreviated NDA approval and inactive ingredient composition and safety, provide that, for certain types of drug products, generic drug formulations may deviate from the reference licensed drug formulation only in certain respects. For example, the FDA's regulations for parenteral drug products at 21 CFR § 314.94(a)(9)(iii) state:

> Generally, a drug product intended for parenteral use shall contain the same inactive ingredients and in the same concentration as the [RLD] identified by the applicant under paragraph (a)(3) of this section. However, an applicant may seek approval of a drug product that *differs from the [RLD] in preservative, buffer, or antioxidant* provided that the applicant identifies and characterizes the differences and provides information demonstrating that the differences do not affect the safety or efficacy of the proposed drug product [emphasis added].

Preservative, buffer, and antioxidant changes in generic parenteral drug products are referred to as *exception excipients*, which may qualitatively or quantitatively differ from the reference product formulation.

There are several scenarios wherein a biosimilar developer may choose a different formulation than what is approved for the reference-licensed drug. First, the reference product formulation may be protected under a patent; as the composition patents for biological drugs have come off patent, the originators have embarked on an aggressive strategy to patent all other components of the product, including the formulations; although many of these patents will eventually be challenged and in all likelihood be taken down, the biosimilar developer faces a choice, when sharing its dossier with the originator, how far to go to obviate any IP, regardless of this robustness. In other instances, the formulation change may be required to improve the product. An interesting example is that of Humira.

> The current commercial formulation of HUMIRA (each 0.8 mL) contains adalimumab 40 mg, citric acid monohydrate 1.04 mg, dibasic sodium phosphate dihydrate 1.22 mg, mannitol 9.6 mg, monobasic sodium phosphate dihydrate 0.69 mg, polysorbate 80 0.8 mg, sodium chloride 4.93 mg, sodium citrate 0.24 mg and Water for Injection, USP. Sodium hydroxide is added as necessary to adjust pH.

The PCT/US2013/0586181 (Coherus) provides a claim that states:

> An aqueous, buffered pharmaceutical composition comprising adalimumab and a buffer, wherein (i) the composition is free or substantially free of a buffer combination that comprises both a citrate buffer and a phosphate buffer; and (ii) the composition exhibits long-term stability. So if both citrate and phosphate are used then, this IP does not apply.

Citrate is well known to cause significant discomfort and as a result, Humira has been proposed to be reformulated as a high-concentration buffer-free formulation, for which a new patent (8,821,865) has been issued claiming the following:

A liquid aqueous formulation comprising:

> (1) 100 mg/mL of adalimumab; (2) 1.0 mg/mL of polysorbate 80; and (3) 42 mg/mL of mannitol; wherein the formulation has a pH of 4.7 to 5.7 and does not contain a buffer or a salt, and wherein injection of the formulation into a human subject results in a Pain Visual Analog Scale (VAS) score of less than 1.0.

Obviously, the issue of discomfort using citrate was well known to the originator, but the change is proposed only when the composition patent is about to expire—this will not keep the competition out but provide the originator an opportunity to differentiate their product as safer. Whether these considerations borderline on ethical grounds or not remains to be seen.

U.S. Patent 8,795,670 states:

> A stable liquid aqueous pharmaceutical formulation comprising (a) a human IgG1 anti-human Tumor Necrosis Factor alpha (TNFα) antibody, or an antigen-binding portion thereof, at a concentration of 45 to 105 mg/mL,

(b) a polyol, (c) a polysorbate at a concentration of 0.1 to 10 mg/mL, and (d) a buffer system comprising histidine and having a pH of 4.5 to 7.0, wherein the antibody comprises the light chain variable region and the heavy chain variable region of D2E7.

The example provided above should serve as a warning to biosimilar product developers of the challenges they will face in establishing formulation similarity.

The native structure of a protein molecule is the result of balancing effects such as covalent linkages, hydrophobic interactions, electrostatic interactions, hydrogen bonding, and van der Waals forces. Protein stability is controlled by innumerable intrinsic and extrinsic factors, but the major ones are primary sequence, 3D structure, subunit associations, and PTMs. Extrinsic contributing factors include pH, osmolarity, protein concentration, formulation excipients, and exposure of a product to physical stress from temperature, light, and/or agitation. Leachables from container-closure systems and contamination from the environment (e.g., metals and proteases) also exacerbate product degradation. All these features make protein degradation a very complex physiochemical phenomenon, so formulation optimization is a core aspect of biotechnology product development.

8.2 Drug substance and drug product stability

A biosimilar developer has access to the exact formulation used by the originator because of the nature of the product being an injectable. In almost all instances, unless otherwise dictated by IP, safety improvement and constraints related to the availability of inert components of the correct specification, the formulation of a biosimilar should be the same as that of the originator product. However, in developing a QTPP, the biosimilar developer must analyze multiple lots of the originator product since the labeling of inactive components gives no indication of the acceptance ranges; for example, it is not uncommon for a product to contain a surfactant with a range of ±50% to 80%.

The formulation of biopharmaceuticals is a vast field of study with two peculiarities compared to small-molecule drugs. First, most protein drugs are administered by parenteral routes, and, as a result, most of the science of protein drug formulation deals with the art of injectable formulations. Second, there are several common structural features of all proteins, such as functional groups like methionine, cysteine, histidine, tryptophan, and tyrosine, all of which are subject to oxidation, requiring some common approaches to establishing stable products. On the other hand, conformational changes and aggregation are properties peculiar to large molecules that require the inclusion of formulation components that can be highly specific. The quality of inactive components can have a far greater impact on the formulation than those found in pharmaceuticals,

Table 8.1 Impact of Various Formulation and Environmental Factors on the Degradation of Proteins

Factor	Impact
pH	Hydrolysis, deamidation
Buffer species	Deamidation
Other excipients	Maillard reaction
Light	Photodecomposition
Oxygen	Oxidation
Metal ions	Hydrolysis, oxidation
Temperature	Most routes

and it requires detailed studies, particularly those components that can enhance oxidation of proteins. Also significant for proteins is the physical degradation that can lead to significant safety issues.

Varieties of formulation factors that can induce instability are shown in Table 8.1. These factors are well studied and anticipated from the knowledge of the chemistry of all types of molecules. However, the impact on safety and efficacy is peculiar to biopharmaceuticals.

Compared to small-molecule drugs, biopharmaceuticals are typically more sensitive to slight changes in solution chemistry. They remain compositionally and conformationally stable only within a relatively narrow range of pH and osmolarity, and many require additionally supportive formulation components to stay in solution, particularly over time. Even lyophilized protein products are subject to significant degradation,

Table 8.2 Typical Stability Problems Observed in Protein Pharmaceuticals

Problems	Potential Causes	Possible Solutions
Noncovalent aggregation	Solubility, structural changes, heat, shear, surface, denaturants, impurities	pH, ionic additives, amino acids, surfactants, protein concentration, raw material purity
Covalent aggregation	Disulfide scrambling, other unknown mechanisms	pH, inhibit noncovalent aggregation
Deamidation	pH <5.0 or pH >6.0	pH optimization
Cyclic imide	pH around 5	pH optimization
Cleavages	Protease impurity, other unknown mechanisms	pH, product purity, inhibitors
Oxidation	Active oxygen species, free radicals, metals, light, impurity	Excipient purity, free-radical scavenger, active oxygen scavengers, methionine
Surface denaturation, adsorption	Low-protein concentration, specific affinity, protein hydrophobicity	Surfactants, protein concentration, pH

unlike the small-molecule drugs that would be highly stable in most lyophilized formulations.

Table 8.2 summarizes typical stability problems observed during protein formulation development and potential methods to solve each problem. The list does not represent the complexity of multiple problems that can be experienced with a given protein; as a result, the formulation research should be designed to handle each protein based on its unique stability profile.

8.3 Physical degradation

Proteins degrade upon physical stresses of many types including hydrophobic surfaces, heating, lyophilization, reconstitution, contact with organic solvents, shaking and many other permutations, and combinations of physical and chemical factors. The final result of physical stress can be denaturation, adsorption on the container walls, precipitation, or aggregation.

Aggregation is a common problem encountered during manufacture and storage of proteins. The potential for aggregated forms is often enhanced by exposure to a protein to liquid–air, liquid–solid, and even liquid–liquid interfaces. Mechanical stresses of agitation (shaking, stirring, pipetting, or pumping through tubes) can cause protein aggregation. Freezing and thawing can promote it as well. Solution conditions such as temperature, protein concentration, pH, and ionic strength can affect the rate and the amount of aggregates observed.

Aggregated proteins are a significant concern for biopharmaceutical products because they may be associated with decreased bioactivity and increased immunogenicity. Macromolecular protein complexes can trigger a patient's immune system to recognize the protein as nonself and mount an antigenic response.

Protein aggregates are formed by mechanisms such as domain swapping, strand association, edge–edge association, or beta strand stacking. The term *aggregation* usually refers to multimers of proteins, e.g., dimers, trimers, tetramers, all the way to large polymers. The aggregates can be noncovalent or covalent (disulfide-linked), and these can be present as fully soluble in a clear solution, partially insoluble in a turbid solution, or mostly insoluble as a precipitate that collects in the bottom of the container. Nonspecific protein-to-protein association resulting from interactions among solvent-exposed hydrophobic groups can also form aggregates. The covalent aggregation is not reversible. The weakly associated noncovalent aggregate can be reversible, and it usually follows the path of dimers to multimers; the strongly associated noncovalent aggregates are not reversible by dilution and may result in precipitation. Based on the size range, aggregates have been classified into the following categories: (a) submicron (<1 μm in size) particles, which are conventionally referred to as soluble particles; (b) subvisible particles (1–100 μm in size); and (c) visible particles (>100 μm in size).

There are several models of aggregation. In the native-to-unfolded-to-aggregate model, denatured or unfolded molecules aggregate due to hydrophobic interactions. Aggregate formation driven by hydrophobic effect happen when the normally buried hydrophobic regions are exposed. The rate of reaction in this model increases with temperature since unfolding increases with temperature and reactions generally follow first-order kinetics.

In the model native-to-unfolded-to-aggregate wherein the intermediate yields the aggregate, the misfolded intermediates are often thermodynamically stable and can be part of the native-state ensemble. Therefore, aggregation is not an unnatural state of a protein and can occur even under conditions favoring the native state.

The mechanism of protein aggregation involves two stages: a nucleation process which is followed by growth of the nuclei in a critical mass. The level of aggregation can be monitored by the turbidity measurement. However, turbidity is not necessarily an indicator of aggregation. The assembly of initially native and folded proteins can result in irreversible nonnative structures that may contain high levels of nonnative intermolecular β-sheet structures. The onset, rate, and final morphology of the aggregate depend on solution conditions such as pH, salt species, salt concentration, cosolutes, excipients, and surfactants. The exact nature of an aggregate is a function of the relative intrinsic thermodynamic stability of the native state.

Because of the many physical and chemical manipulations required in upstream production and downstream processing, followed by formulation and filling operations, the aggregation of protein biopharmaceuticals can be induced during nearly every step of the process including at hold points, shipping, and long-term storage. Agitation (e.g., shaking, stirring, and shearing) of protein solutions, can promote aggregation at the air–liquid interfaces, where protein molecules may align and unfold, exposing their hydrophobic regions for the charge-based association. Agitation-induced aggregation has been observed in numerous protein products, including recombinant factor XIII, human growth hormone, hemoglobin, and insulin. Minimizing foaming caused by agitation during manufacture (as well as during product use) may be critical to preventing significant loss of protein activity or generation of visible particulate matter. The antimicrobial preservatives used in multidose formulations can also induce protein aggregation. For example, benzyl alcohol accelerates the aggregation of rhGCSF because it favors partially unfolded conformations of the protein. Increasing antimicrobial preservative levels may enhance the hydrophobicity of a formulation and could affect a protein's aqueous solubility. Phenol and *m*-cresol can considerably destabilize a protein: Phenol promotes the formation of both soluble and insoluble aggregates, whereas *m*-cresol can precipitate protein.

Freezing and thawing that can occur multiple times throughout production and use of protein therapeutics can dramatically affect protein aggregation. Generation of water-ice crystals at a container's periphery (where heat transfer is greatest) can produce a "salting out" effect, whereby the protein and the excipients become increasingly concentrated at the slowly freezing center of a container.

The high-salt and/or high-protein concentrations can result in precipitation and aggregation during freezing, which is not completely reversible upon thawing. The effect can be seen with thyroid-stimulating hormone: When stored at −80°C, 4°C, or 24°C for up to 90 days, it remained stable, but when frozen to −20°C, it lost >40% potency in that period, which was attributed to subunit dissociation. Multiple freezing and thawing cycles can exacerbate that effect and lead to a cumulative impact on the generation and the growth of subvisible and visible particulates. A change in pH can come from crystallization of buffer components during freezing. In one study, potassium phosphate buffers demonstrated a much smaller pH change on freezing than did sodium phosphate buffers.

The causes of aggregation that are related to the process are summarized as follows:

- Fermentation/Expression: Inclusion bodies
- Purification: Shear, pH, ionic strength
- Filtration: Surface interaction, shear
- Fill/Finish: Surface interaction, shear, contamination (e.g., silicone oil)
- Freeze/Thaw: Cryoconcentration, pH changes, ice–solution interfaces
- Shipping: Agitation, temperature cycling
- Lyophilization: Cryoconcentration, pH changes, ice–solution interfaces, dehydration
- Administration: Diluents, component materials and surfaces, leachables

Protein aggregation upon oxidation can result in a faster reaction and may show precipitates within a few minutes; it is also highly pH dependent.

One of the most difficult parts of formulating proteins comes when they are dispensed in prefilled syringes that have silicone oil lubrication. A 10-fold variability in absorbance at 350 nm in proteins packaged in various brands of syringes is not uncommon. It depends on the quantity and the type of silicone used. A properly folded mAb, for example, can form an intermediate upon hydrophobic interaction with silicone in the syringe resulting in partial unfolding that will first yield to a soluble aggregate followed by a visible precipitation depending on the concentration of silicone to which the mAb is exposed. Subvisible and visible particles together are referred to as insoluble particles. Particles that belong to the size range of 0.1–1 μm are at times referred to as small subvisible particles.

The formulation in sucrose can also increase aggregation over time because of protein glycation when sucrose is hydrolyzed. The presence of certain ligands—including certain ions—may enhance aggregation. Interactions with metal surfaces can lead to epitaxic denaturation, which triggers aggregate formation. Foreign particles from the environment, manufacturing processes, or container-closure systems (e.g., silicone oil) can also induce aggregation. Even handling protein products at compounding pharmacies can induce aggregation 10-fold above initially observed amounts.

8.4 Chemical degradation

Chemical instability refers to the formation or destruction of covalent bonds within a polypeptide or protein structures. Chemical modifications of protein include mainly oxidation, deamidation, reduction, and hydrolysis. Unfolding, dissociation, denaturation, aggregation, and precipitation are known as conformational or physical instabilities. In some cases, protein degradation pathways are synergistic: A chemical event may trigger a physical event, such as when oxidation is followed by aggregation. Generally, physical changes may not bring any significant clinical risk in small molecule drugs, except in the PK profile; in the case of biosimilars, these are crucial in determining the safety of these drugs.

Chemical degradation may occur in a number of different ways. This type of degradation affects the primary sequence and may also lead to significant changes in the HOS. Examples of chemical degradation include deamidation, oxidation, isomerization, clipping/fragmentation, and cross-linking. Deamidation is probably the most common type of chemical degradation encountered in mAb-based biotherapeutics. The reaction is favored at neutral and basic pH. There are examples of deamidation occurring at lower pH. However, that has been reported to occur primarily through a mechanism independent of succinimide formation; for instance, deamidation of Asn in the A chain of insulin is favored at pH <5, which is mediated via the formation of cyclic anhydride intermediate. There are factors other than pH that influence the rate of deamidation, e.g., sequence and local structure (steric effect). Amino acids present at the carboxyl end of Asn have been reported to influence the rate of deamidation; the decrease in rate has been correlated with an increase in size and branching of the side chain.

Isomerization is another common method of chemical degradation that shares the common outcome with deamidation. It can directly occur from Asp residue or from the succinimide intermediate. Similar to deamidation, isomerization is favored at neutral and basic pH, and the rate has been reported to be influenced by the steric effect.

Hydrolysis of a peptide bond leads to fragmentation of the protein. Some peptide bonds, such as Asp–Gly and Asp–Pro, are sensitive to hydrolysis. Asp–Y sequence has been reported to be 100 times more sensitive to hydrolysis than any other peptide bonds. At times, hydrolysis is the natural, subsequent reaction following deamidation of Asn residue, as is observed with insulin.

Furthermore, mAbs may contain certain residues that are sensitive to oxidation, such as Met, Tyr, Trp, His, and Cys. Although not as prevalent as deamidation and isomerization, oxidation has been reported to be the major pathway of degradation for certain proteins, e.g., OKT3 (IgG2), which demonstrated oxidation at several Met residues and free Cys under 5°C storage condition.

Several external factors induce oxidation, including exposure to light, contamination with a trace amount of transition metal ion, and presence of degradation product of an excipient (e.g., hydrogen peroxide from polysorbate degradation). The consequence of oxidation may include an increase in the aggregation. Oxidation is most commonly observed with the Met residue, and the major by-product of such reaction is the formation of sulfoxide and sulfone. Two factors that affect the rate of oxidation are the local structure around the oxidation-sensitive group (e.g., surface exposure and steric hindrance) and the solution pH. In some cases, an increase in solution pH has been found to increase the rate of oxidation, but the pH-dependent increase in oxidation is not a general phenomenon.

Protein oxidation is a covalent modification induced by reactive oxygen intermediates or other oxidants such as chemicals such as hydrogen peroxide (which often appears in formulations as a contaminant of polysorbates, leaching from disposable tubing, etc.), oxygen, metal ions, and other excipients. UV light is another major factor requiring proteins to be protected from light. Oxidation results in the modification of Met, Cys, Trp, His, and Tyr residues, which are primary formulation development relevant residues.

Photooxidation can change the primary, secondary, and tertiary structures of proteins and can lead to differences in long-term stability, bioactivity, or immunogenicity. Exposure to light can trigger a chain of biochemical events that continue to affect a protein even after the light source is turned off. These effects depend on the amount of energy imparted to a protein and the presence of environmental oxygen. Photooxidation is initiated when a compound absorbs a certain wavelength of light, which provides enough energy to raise the molecule to an excited state. The excited molecule can then transfer that energy to the molecular oxygen, converting it to reactive singlet oxygen atoms. This is how tryptophan, histidine, and tyrosine can be modified by light in the presence of oxygen. Tyrosine photooxidation can produce mono-, di-, tri-, and tetrahydroxy tyrosine as by-products. Aggregation is observed in some proteins due to cross-linking between oxidized tyrosine residues. Metal ion–catalyzed oxidation depends on the concentration of metal ions in the environment. The presence of 0.15 ppm chloride salts of Fe^{3+}, Ca^{2+}, Cu^{2+}, Mg^{2+}, or Zn^{2+} does not affect the rate of oxidation for human insulin–like growth factor-1, but when the metal concentration is increased to 1 ppm, a significant increase in oxidation is observed.

Oxidation can be induced during protein processing and storage by peroxide contamination resulting from polysorbates and PEGs, both commonly used as pharmaceutical excipients. A correlation has been observed between the peroxide content in Tween 80 and the degree of oxidation in rhG-CSF, and peroxide-induced oxidation appeared more severe than that from atmospheric oxygen. Peroxide can also leach from plastic or elastomeric materials used in the primary packaging container-closure systems, including prefilled syringes.

The removal of headspace oxygen by degassing may be effective for preventing oxidation in some cases. Filling steps are carried out under nitrogen pressure, and vial headspace oxygen is replaced with an inert gas such as nitrogen to prevent oxidation. With some oxidation-sensitive proteins, processing is carried out in the presence of an inert gas such as nitrogen or argon. For multidose drug preparations, the use of cartridges with negligible headspace overcomes oxidation and related consequences.

Chemical degradation may also result from cross-linking, which may or may not be mediated by the formation of a disulfide bond. When cross-linking is disulfide bond mediated, the reaction occurs either by the formation of a new disulfide bond or by disulfide bond exchange. Intramolecular disulfide linkage may lead to a change in tertiary structure, whereas intermolecular (or interdomain) disulfide linkage may result in change in quaternary structure or formation of covalent aggregates. At higher pH, the formation of reactive thiolate ion (S^-), from the thiol group (–SH) of Cys residue, is favored, which may increase the probability of disulfide linkage formation. There are instances of covalent cross-linking that may occur between different amino acid residues besides Cys, which, unlike disulfide linkage, are nonreducible.

While the specific effects of various chemical reactions remain difficult to predict, the general impact of these reactions on the acidity is universally observed in protein products as shown in Table 8.3.

Table 8.3 Effect of Chemical Modifications of Proteins on Acidity Function and Charge Heterogeneity

Chemical Modification	**Acidity/Charge Heterogeneity**
Deamidation	More acidic ($z = -1$)
Succinimide formation	More basic or neutral
Glycation	More acidic
Pyroglutamate formation	More acidic ($z = -1$)
Peptide bond hydrolysis	Either acidic or basic

The most common routes of chemical and physical degradations of biopharmaceuticals are shown in Figure 8.1.

Multimeric proteins with two or more subunits can become dissociated into monomers, and monomers (or single peptide chain proteins) can degrade into peptide fragments. Nonenzymatic fragmentation usually proceeds by hydrolysis of peptide bonds by amino acids, releasing polypeptides of lower molecular weight than the intact parent protein. Peptide bonds of Asp–Gly and Asp–Pro is most susceptible to hydrolytic protein cleavage. Antibody hydrolysis often occurs in the hinge region, which is the most flexible domain of an antibody. However, decreasing the pH from 9 to 5 can shift the peptide hydrolysis sites of a recombinant mAb, showing increased cleavage outside that region.

The presence and the position of oligosaccharides also affect the rate of peptide hydrolysis at low pH levels. Depending on location, the hinge region cleavage is not affected, although fragmentation in the CH2 domain decreases. Hydrolytic cleavage of peptide bonds by acidic and basic hydrolyses do not necessarily have the same effects. Recombinant human macrophage colony–stimulating factor yields different peptide fragments in solutions with acidic and basic pH. Enzymatic protein fragmentation can be caused by the proteolytic activity of residual or contaminating proteases—or in select cases, autoproteolysis of an enzymatic protein.

Appropriately buffering formulations to maintain their solution pH in a suitable range for each protein type is the key to minimizing hydrolytic fragmentation. For example, calcitonin undergoes hydrolysis at basic pH, but no such degradation is observed at pH 7 even at room temperature. Buffer composition may also affect hydrolysis. Recombinant human macrophage colony–stimulating factor fragmentation was observed in

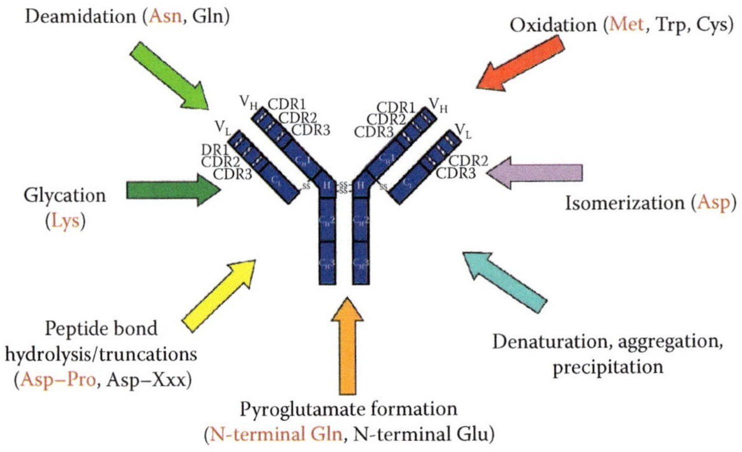

Figure 8.1 Common routes of protein degradation.

phosphate-buffered solutions but not in histidine-buffered solutions at identical pH and ionic strengths. It is also important to minimize the potential presence of proteases in protein purification, either from sources intrinsic to the production process (e.g., HCPs) or from extrinsic sources of contamination (e.g., adventitious microbes).

8.5 Higher-concentration formulations

Treatments with high doses of more than 1 mg/kg or 100 mg per dose often require the development of formulations at concentrations exceeding 100 mg/mL because of the small volume (<1.5 mL) that can be given by the subcutaneous routes. For proteins that have the propensity to aggregate at higher concentrations, achieving such high-concentration formulations is a developmental challenge. Even for the intravenous delivery route where large volumes can be administered, protein concentrations of tens of milligrams per milliliter may be needed for high dosing regimens, and this may pose stability challenges for some proteins.

Protein–protein interaction in a high-concentration formulation may result in reversible self-association, which may further progress toward the formation of insoluble aggregates. At a higher concentration, the probability of one molecule bumping into another increases, enhancing the probabililty of formation of reversible oligomers such as a dimer, tetramers, etc. The formation of aggregates occurs through multiple mechanisms, including the formation of covalent linkages (e.g., disulfide exchange). Even minor conformational change in the native structure may lead to the formation of aggregates. The probability of such occurrence is greater in higher concentration.

High concentration is defined by the solution, in which a significant portion of the solution volume (≥0.1) is occupied by the solutes. Another definition of a high-concentration solution is the situation in which the molecular size and the distance between the van der Waals surfaces are on the same order of magnitude. Irrespective of the definition, high concentration refers to intermolecular distance or molecular proximity. The primary challenge in achieving high-concentration formulation is the solubility of the target protein. Solubility is controlled by its molecular property (sequence, charge distribution, etc.), as well as by the solution condition, such as pH, ionic strength, excipient concentration, etc. The solubility of a protein is defined by the maximum amount of the protein that can be present in a solution, without the appearance of any visible aggregates, precipitates, etc. A more technical definition will be the maximum amount of protein that remains in solution, following 30 min of centrifugation at 30,000*g* in the presence of cosolute. Besides solubility, there are other issues associated with the development of high-concentration mAb formulation. These include opalescence, viscosity, and aggregation. Opalescence is commonly expressed by nephelometric turbidity unit. However, opalescence is not necessarily equivalent to turbidity. Typically, a solution becomes turbid due to the presence of particulates. However, opalescence may result even if the solution is free of any particulates as a result of Raleigh scattering. Although opalescence is not a major issue, and may occur independent of aggregation, it remains a major concern as it may fail to satisfy patient compliance due to its appearance. Reversible protein–protein and liquid–liquid phase separations may also lead to opalescence. Protein–protein interaction at high concentration is a major factor that may influence opalescence and viscosity. When molecules are in close proximity, they can interact with each other, resulting in reversible self-association, and increase in viscosity, opalescence, and even aggregation. Protein–protein interaction has been explained by various theories, including molecular crowding, or excluded volume effect, and proximity energy effect, etc.

The increase in viscosity at high concentration has a major impact on manufacturability and injectability. Tangential flow filtration (TFF) is one of the main technologies used for buffer exchange and concentrating proteins during large-scale manufacture (clinical as well as commercial). The increase in viscosity at high concentration may create back pressure high enough to exceed the capacity of the pump. The TFF process itself is considerably stressful to the mAb, as rapid pumping and continuous circulation through the narrow tubing create significant cavitation and shear stress. The increase in back pressure, due to the increase in viscosity, may further retard the process which can be even more destabilizing to the protein. At a minimum, this increases the processing time, and in turn, the cost of manufacture. The increase in viscosity has a significant impact on the administration of subcutaneous dosage form. The ease of subcutaneous injection is described by the glide force, or the extrusion force, which refers to the force required to push the liquid through the syringe. While there are various factors including needle gauge and length of the needle that are associated with glide force, one of the main contributing factors is solution viscosity. Viscosity has been reported to be directly correlated to glide force for subcutaneous injection. The increase in viscosity increases the time of injection, and also the pain at the injection site, which may lead to a decrease in patient compliance.

8.6 Formulation considerations

The optimization of formulation variables for product stability is the most critical part of protein formulation development. Various formulation excipients and buffers (Table 8.4) can be utilized and must, therefore, be chosen to maximize the pharmaceutical quality of the product (i.e., stability and activity) without introducing significant side effects. Among the listed formulation variables, the most powerful one is pH. Problems associated with the physical properties of a protein, e.g., precipitation due to solubility and/or stability, are generally very difficult to

Table 8.4 Important Components of Protein Formulations

Formulation Variables	Desired Attributes	Examples
pH	Provides good physical properties of protein, minimizes degradations	
Stabilizer	Inhibits degradations, effective at low concentrations	Surfactants, sugars, salts, antioxidants
Solubilizer	Improves the solubility, effective at low concentrations	Salts, amino acids, surfactants
Buffer	Good buffering capacity, stable to temperature change, stable to freezing, good safety record	Phosphate, acetate, histidine, glutamate
Tonicity modifier; bulking agent	Inert, good safety record	Sodium chloride, sorbitol, mannitol, glycine

manage by other formulation means. The optimization of pH is a simple but very useful solution for such problems. Most chemical reactions are also affected by pH, e.g., deamidation, cyclic imide formation, disulfide scrambling, peptide bond cleavage, and oxidation. Other functional excipients should also be carefully evaluated for the benefit of the product (e.g., use of sucrose to stabilize protein during lyophilization and storage in the dried solid).

A protein solution can typically be stabilized against aggregation and precipitation by optimizing solution pH and ionic strength; adding sugars, amino acids, and/or polyols; and using surfactants. Comprehensive evaluation of optimal pH and osmotic conditions is a key element of formulation development to prevent protein aggregation or precipitation. Irreversible aggregation due to denaturation can be prevented with surfactants, polyols, or sugars.

In many cases, nonionic detergents (surfactants) are added to increase stability and to prevent aggregation. The protein–surfactant interaction is hydrophobic, so these compounds stabilize proteins by lowering the surface tension of their solution and binding to hydrophobic sites on their surfaces, thus reducing the possibility of protein–protein interactions that could lead to aggregate formation. The nonionic detergents Tween 20 and Tween 80 can prevent the formation of soluble protein aggregates with surfactant concentrations below the critical micelle concentrations. Polysorbate (Tween) 80 added to IgG solutions stabilizes small aggregates and prevents them from growing into larger particles. Chelating agents can also be used to prevent metal-induced protein aggregation.

An analysis of common components of biological drugs formulations shows that most ingredients are used as the following:

1. Buffering agents to assure that the pH is maintained at the most stable level, and these include phosphates, citrates, and acetates

2. Stabilizers such as surfactants and sugars contain polysorbates, albumin, mannitol, sucrose and sorbitol
3. Tonicity- and conductivity-adjusting ingredients including some sugars and electrolytes like sodium chloride

Of the approximately 200 biological injectable drugs, the percentage of most prevalent components is given in Figure 8.2.

The science of stabilizing drugs through formulation efforts is well studied and understood, but the uncertainties arise when formulating large protein molecules for there is no definite way to predict the behavior of these molecules. A case in point is the change in the formulation of EPO. A change from albumin stabilizer to polysorbate, which would have otherwise been a logical choice, resulted in PRCA and deaths because the surfactants caused the leaching out from rubber stoppers that produced a structural change in the structure of EPO that triggered the toxic response. It is for this reason that the sponsor of biosimilar products too has to fully understand the dynamic of protein drug degradation.

An isotonic formulation is one that essentially has the same osmotic pressure as the human blood. Isotonic formulations will generally have an osmotic pressure from about 250 to 350 mOsmol/kg H_2O. Buffering agents are one or more components that, when added to an aqueous solution, are able to protect the solution against variations in pH that can result when adding acid or alkali, or upon dilution with a solvent. In

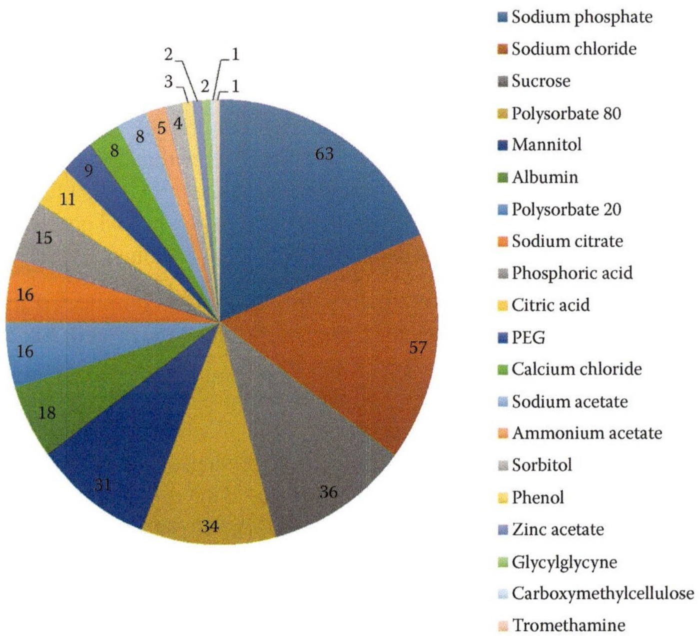

Figure 8.2 Percentage of occurrences of common formulation components in biological drugs. (Clockwise begin with sodium phosphate = 63.)

addition to phosphate buffers, glycinate, carbonate, and citrate buffers can be used, in which case, sodium, potassium, or ammonium ions can serve as a counterion.

Lyoprotectants include molecules, which, when combined with a protein of interest, prevent or reduce chemical and/or physical instability of the protein upon lyophilization and subsequent storage. Preservatives include an agent that reduces bacterial action and that may be optionally added to the formulations herein. The addition of a preservative may, for example, facilitate the production of a multiuse (multiple-dose) formulation. Examples of potential preservatives include octadecyldimethylbenzyl ammonium chloride, hexamethonium chloride, benzalkonium chloride (a mixture of alkyl benzyl dimethylammonium chlorides in which the alkyl groups are long-chain compounds), and benzethonium chloride. Other types of preservatives include aromatic alcohols such as phenol, butyl, and benzyl alcohol, alkyl parabens such as methyl or propyl paraben, catechol, resorcinol, cyclohexanol, 3-pentanol, and m-cresol.

Surfactants are surface-active molecules containing both a hydrophobic portion (e.g., alkyl chain) and a hydrophilic portion (e.g., carboxyl and carboxylate groups). The surfactant may be added to the formulations of the invention. Surfactants suitable for use in the formulations of the present invention include, but are not limited to, polysorbates (e.g., polysorbates 20 or 80); poloxamers (e.g., poloxamer 188); sorbitan esters and derivatives; Triton; sodium lauryl sulfate; sodium octyl glycoside; lauryl, myristyl, linoleyl, or stearyl sulfobetadine; lauryl, linoleyl, or stearyl sarcosine; linoleyl, myristyl, or cetyl betaine; lauramidopropyl, cocamidopropyl, linoleamidopropyl, myristamidopropyl, palmidopropyl, or isostearamidopropyl betaine (e.g., lauroamidopropyl); myristamidopropyl, palmidopropyl, or isostearamidopropyl dimethylamine; sodium methyl cocoyl or disodium methyl oleyl taurate; and the MONAQUAT™ series (Mona Industries, Inc., Paterson, NJ), PEG, polypropyl glycol, and copolymers of ethylene and propylene glycol (e.g., Pluronics, PF68).

The principles governing protein solubility are more complicated than those for synthetic small molecules, thus overcoming the protein solubility issue takes different strategies. Operationally, solubility for proteins could be described by the maximum amount of protein in the presence of cosolutes whereby the solution remains visibly clear (i.e., does not show protein precipitates, crystals, or gels). The dependence of protein solubility on ionic strength, salt form, pH, temperature, and certain excipients is well demonstrated by changes in bulk water surface tension and protein binding to water and ions versus self-association. The binding of proteins to specific excipients or salts influences solubility through changes in protein conformation or masking of certain amino acids involved in self-interaction. Proteins are also preferentially hydrated (and stabilized as more compact conformations) by certain salts, amino acids, and sugars, leading to their altered solubility.

Aggregation, which requires bimolecular collision, is expected to be the primary degradation pathway in protein solutions. The relationship of concentration to aggregate formation depends on the size of the aggregates as well as the mechanism of association. A typical approach to minimize aggregation is to restrict the mobility of proteins in order to reduce the number of collisions.

Lyophilization with appropriate excipients may improve protein stability against aggregation by decreasing protein mobility and by restricting conformational flexibility with the added benefit of minimizing hydrolytic reactions consequent to the removal of water. The addition of appropriate excipients, including lyoprotectants, can prevent the formation of aggregates during the lyophilization process as well as during storage of the final product. A key parameter for effective protection is the molar ratio of the lyoprotectant to the protein. Generally, molar ratios of 300:1 or greater are required to provide suitable stability, especially for room temperature storage. Such ratios can also, however, lead to an undesirable increase in viscosity.

Lyophilization allows for designing a formulation with appropriate stability and tonicity. Although isotonicity is not necessarily required for subcutaneous administration, it may be desirable for minimizing pain upon administration. The isotonicity of a lyophile is difficult to achieve because both the protein and the excipients are concentrated during the reconstitution process. Excipients with protein molar ratios of 500:1 will result in hypertonic preparations if the final protein concentration is targeted for >100 mg/mL. If the desire is to achieve an isotonic formulation, then a choice of the lower molar ratio of excipient is necessary.

Determining the highest protein concentration achievable remains an empirical exercise due to the labile nature of protein conformation and the propensity to interact with itself, with surfaces, and with specific solutes.

8.7 Demonstrating equivalence of formulations

To demonstrate the similarity of formulation, the sponsor needs to show the equivalent stability of the active ingredient; this may require demonstrating the stability of the originator formulation and the stability of the originator drug substance (extracted from originator product) in the proposed biosimilar formulation.

To predict potential stability problems within a short period and to develop appropriate analytical methods, proteins are exposed to stronger-than-real stresses and various degradation products induced by the stresses are examined. The results obtained from these so-called accelerated stability studies might also be useful to predict the kinetics of the degradation processes under real handling conditions, when there are no sufficient

Table 8.5 Common Conditions Used to Accelerate Protein Degradation

Stresses	Routine Ranges	Practical Applications	Problems to Monitor
Temperature	0°C–50°C	Storage, shipping, handling, delivery	Structural changes (precipitation, aggregation, recovery loss), solubility, increased reaction rates for all degradations
Light	>1.2 million lux h illumination, >200 W h/m^2 UV energy	Light exposure, container, package	Oxidation, cleavage
Freezing	Multiple freeze–thaw, liquid nitrogen freeze	Frozen storage, accidental freezing, lyophilization	Precipitation, aggregation, pH change, crystallization of excipients
Oxidation	Oxygen purge, peroxide spike	Storage, excipient stability, impurity	Oxidations, inactivation
Humidity	0%–100% RH	Storage, container integrity, powder	Moisture content, moisture related degradations
Mechanical stresses	Vortex, agitation, shear stress (3000 s^{-1})	Manufacturing, filling, shipping, handling, delivery	Precipitation, aggregation, recovery loss
Other denaturants	–	Impurities, pH, denaturing excipients	Precipitation, aggregation, recovery loss, structural changes

real-time results available because of time and resource constraints. However, the accelerated stability study is not acceptable to determine the expiry of the product, so it is best used to rank order the importance of different degradation pathways. Approaches and cautions in the extrapolation of data from accelerated stability testing to real-time stability and normal handling conditions are later discussed in detail.

Conditions that accelerate various degradation reactions in protein products and potential problems to monitor are listed in Table 8.5. Proteins contain numerous amino acid side chains and delicate 3D structures, which can be susceptible to different stresses. Therefore, it is important to test the protein under a variety of physical and chemical stresses in order to provide a good simulation of the degradation products that can be generated.

8.7.1 Standard studies

8.7.1.1 Storage stability study Documenting that the formulation will keep the protein stable until the desired expiry can be the most time-consuming part of formulation development. The expiry requirements are determined by distribution, not regulatory requirements. One year is probably too short for effective manufacturing and distribution through normal channels. In general, a shelf life of 18 months is considered acceptable for commercialization. The results obtained from accelerated stability studies are useful for predicting potential degradation products and appropriate analytical methods, but whatever the actual shelf life, it must be supported by sufficient real-time storage data to obtain regulatory approval. Thus, it is important to establish a final formulation and

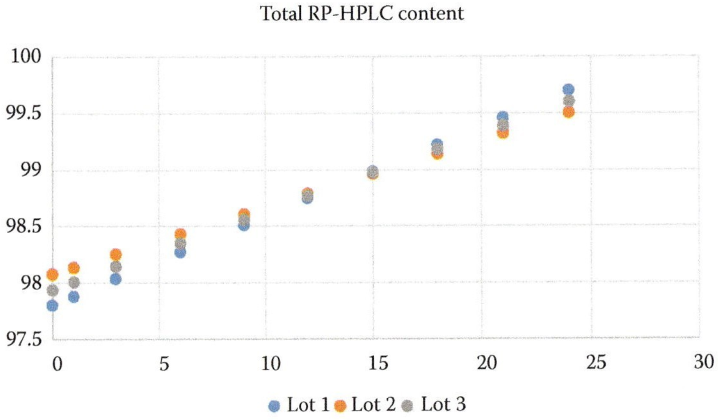

Figure 8.3 Stability data presentation for three lots of a biosimilar product: Lot 1 had a start content of 99.7 and a degradation rate of 0.08% per month, Lot 2 had a start content of 99.5 and a degradation rate of 0.06% per month, and Lot 3 had a start content of 99.6 and a degradation rate of 0.07% per month. The *y* axis is the protein content, and the *x* axis is the time left to expiry, assuming shelf life of 24 months at 5°C.

start the real-time storage studies as early as possible during product development. Figure 8.3 shows how a typical stability profile would be presented to FDA.

8.7.1.2 Process development Formulations that can be prepared on a small scale without experiencing any problems may encounter significant problems during the scale-up of the process. For example, mixing solutions in a large stainless steel tank, pumping solutions through stainless steel tubing, and filtering and filling through a high-speed filling machine can introduce unexpected stresses to the protein. An increase in the formation of particulates, along with a loss of proteins due to surface adsorption and aggregation, has been routinely observed. It is important to expose the formulation to equivalent stresses and make sure that no formulation adjustment is necessary to accommodate the manufacturing processes. Again, this testing should be done as early in the development process as possible.

8.7.1.3 Transportation, handling, and delivery study Unexpected environmental changes can be encountered during the distribution and the handling of products (e.g., accidental freezing, exposure to temperatures different from the recommended conditions, vigorous agitation). It is critical to develop formulation with these stresses in mind because they can compromise the quality of the product.

Also, during administration to the patient, proteins can be exposed to different types of stresses introduced by the device and the routes of delivery. Examples include incompatibility with the delivery device (e.g., protein aggregation induced by exposure to tubing surfaces) and/or concomitant medication (e.g., protein aggregation induced by coadministered antibiotics).

8.7.1.4 Preclinical and clinical studies Results documenting the maintenance of the biophysical and biochemical properties of the protein are essential for a final formulation decision. Before finalizing the formulation, it is also important to confirm that it does not affect critical in vivo biological properties of the protein (e.g., activity, PK profile, and toxicity profile). The maintenance of a protein's biophysical properties can be examined using various structural analyses (e.g., CD, fluorescence, and infrared spectroscopies). It is possible to determine the biochemical equivalence of the protein pharmaceutical by in vitro activity and/or preclinical in vivo bioassays. Results supporting the toxicity profile of the formulation can be generated by both preclinical and clinical studies.

8.8 Conclusion

Establishing biosimilarity becomes more complex when the biosimilar developer is forced to adopt a formulation different from that used by the originator. Demonstrating the stability of biosimilar drug substance in the originator buffer, and vice versa, becomes a difficult task; also, there are greater risks of leaving any residual uncertainty that might require the FDA to ask for clinical studies. A deep understanding of the formulation of proteins is required to overcome this great hurdle and satisfy the FDA requirements of "no clinically meaningful difference."

Bibliography

Ahern, T. J. and Manning, M. C. *Stability of Protein Pharmaceuticals: Part A—Chemical and Physical Pathways of Protein Degradation.* Pharmaceutical Biotechnology Series, Volume 7, New York: Plenum Press; 1992.

Ahern, T. J. and Manning, M. C. *Stability of Protein Pharmaceuticals: Part B—In Vivo Pathways of Degradation and Strategies for Protein Stabilization.* Pharmaceutical Biotechnology Series, Volume 7, New York: Plenum Press; 1992.

Arakawa, T., Prestrelski, S., Kinney, W., and Carpenter, J. F. (1993) Factors affecting short-term and long-term stabilities of proteins. *Adv Drug Delivery Rev* 10: 1.

Berghout, A. (2011 September) Clinical programs in the development of similar biotherapeutic products: Rationale and general principles. *Biologicals* 39 (5): 293–296.

Berkowitz, S. A., Engen, J. R., Mazzeo, J. R., and Jones, G. B. (2012 June 29) Analytical tools for characterizing biopharmaceuticals and the implications for biosimilars. *Nat Rev Drug Discov* 11 (7): 527–540.

Brewster, M. E., Hora, M. S., Simpkins, J. W., and Bodor, J. (1991) Use of 2-hydroxy propyl-beta-cyclodextrin as a solubilizing and stabilizing excipient for protein drugs. *Pharm Res* 8: 792.
Cai, X. Y., Gouty, D., Baughman, S., Ramakrishnan, M., and Cullen, C. (2011 March) Recommendations and requirements for the design of bioanalytical testing used in comparability studies for biosimilar drug development. *Bioanalysis* 3 (5): 535–540.
Chen, T. (1992) Formulation concerns of protein drugs. *Drug Dev Ind Pharmacy* 18: 1311.
Cleland, J. L., Powell, M. F., and Shire, S. J. (1993) The development of stable protein formulations—A close look at protein aggregation, deamidation and oxidation. *Crit Rev Ther Drug* 11: 60.
Combe, C., Tredree, R. L., and Schellekens, H. (2005 July) Biosimilar epoetins: An analysis based on recently implemented European medicines evaluation agency guidelines on comparability of biopharmaceutical proteins. *Pharmacotherapy* 25 (7): 954–962.
Connolly, B. D. et al. (2012) Weak interactions govern the viscosity of concentrated antibody solutions: High-throughput analysis using the diffusion interaction parameter. *Biophys J* 103 (1): 69–78.
Covic, A. and Kuhlmann, M. K. (2007) Biosimilars: Recent developments. *Int Urol Nephrol* 39 (1): 261–266.
Desanvicente-Celis, Z., Gomez-Lopez, A., and Anaya, J. M. (2012 December) Similar biotherapeutic products: Overview and reflections. *Immunotherapy* 4 (12): 1841–1857.
Drouet, L. (2012 March) Low molecular weight heparin biosimilars: How much similarity for how much clinical benefit? *Target Oncol* 7 Suppl 1: S35–S42.
EMEA (1999 October) Development pharmaceutics for biotechnological and biological products: Annex to note for guidance on development pharmaceutics (CPMP/QWP/155/96). EMEA, London, UK.
EMEA (1998 January) Note for guidance on development of pharmaceutics (CPMP/BWP/328/99). EMEA, London, UK.
Fagain, C. O. (1995) Understanding and increasing protein stability. *Biochim Biophys Acta* 1252: 1
Francis, G. E., Fisher, D., Delgado, C., Malik, F., Gardiner, A., and Neale, D. (1998) PEGylation of cytokines and other therapeutic proteins and peptides. *Int J Hematol* 68 (1): 1–18.
FDA (1995 November) Content and format of investigational new drug applications (INDs) for phase 1 studies of drugs, including well-characterized, therapeutic, biotechnology-derived products. FDA, Silver Spring, MD.
FDA (1996 April) Demonstration of Comparability of human biological products, including Therapeutic Biotechnology-Derived Products. http://www.fda.gov/Drugs/GuidanceComplianceRegulatoryInformation/Guidances/UCM122879.htm.
FDA (2010 November)—Guidance for Industry. ANDAs: Impurities in Drug Products (Draft Guidance). http://www.fda.gov/downloads/Drugs/GuidanceComplianceRegulatoryInformation/Guidances/UCM072861.pdf (OGD).
FDA (2015 May)—Guidance for Industry: Biosimilars: Additional Questions and Answers regarding Implementation of the Biologics Price Competition and Innovation Act of 2009 (Draft Guidance). http://www.fda.gov/downloads/Drugs/GuidanceComplianceRegulatoryInformation/Guidances/UCM273001.pdf (Biosimilarity Revision 1).
FDA (1997 July 24)—Guidance for Industry: Changes to an Approved Application: For Specified Biotechnology and Specified Synthetic Biological Products. 21 CFR 601.12, 314.70; Vol 62. No. 142. http://www.fda.gov/downloads/Drugs/GuidancecomplianceRegulatoryInformation/Guidances/UCM124805.pdf.

FDA (2014 May)—Guidance for Industry: Clinical Pharmacology Data to Support a Demonstration of Biosimilarity to a Reference Product. http://www.fda.gov/downloads/Drugs/GuidanceComplianceRegulatoryInformation/Guidances/UCM397017.pdf (Biosimilars).

FDA (2014 May)—Guidance for Industry: Clinical Pharmacology Data to Support a Demonstration of Biosimilarity to a Reference Product (Draft Guidance). http://www.fda.gov/downloads/Drugs/GuidanceComplianceRegulatoryInformation/Guidances/UCM397017.pdf (Biosimilar).

FDA (2015 April)—Guidance for Industry: Demonstrating Biosimilarity of a Therapeutic Protein Product to a Reference Product. U.S. Department of Health and Human Services, Food and Drug Administration, Center for Drug Evaluation and Research (CDER), Center for Biologics Evaluation and Research (CBER). http://www.fda.gov/downloads/Drugs/GuidanceCompliance RegulatoryInformation/Guidances/UCM291134.pdf.

FDA (1999 February)—Guidance for Industry: For the Submission of Chemistry, Manufacturing and Controls and Establishment Description Information for Human Plasma-Derived Biological Products, Animal Plasma or Serum-Derived Products. http://www.fda.gov/downloads/BiologicsBloodVaccines/Guidance ComplianceRegulatoryInformation/Guidances/Blood/ucm080825.pdf.

FDA (2013 March)—Guidance for Industry: Formal Meetings between the FDA and Biosimilar Biological Product Sponsors or Applicants (Draft Guidance). http://www.fda.gov/downloads/Drugs/GuidanceComplianceRegulatoryInformation/Guidances/UCM345649.pdf (Procedural).

FDA (2003 May)—Guidance for Industry: INDs for Phase 2 and 3 Studies of Drugs, including Specified Therapeutic Biotechnology-Derived Products Chemistry, Manufacturing, and Controls Content and Format (Draft Guidance). http://www.fda.gov/downloads/Drugs/GuidanceComplianceRegulatoryInformation/Guidances/UCM070567.pdf.

FDA (2015 April)—Guidance for Industry: Quality Considerations in Demonstrating Biosimilarity of a Therapeutic Protein Product to a Reference Product. http://www.fda.gov/downloads/Drugs/GuidanceComplianceRegulatoryInformation/Guidances/UCM291134.pdf (Biosimilarity).

FDA (2014 August)—Guidance for Industry: Reference Product Exclusivity for Biological Products Filed under Section 351(a) of the PHS Act (Draft Guidance). http://www.fda.gov/downloads/Drugs/GuidanceComplianceRegulatory Information/Guidances/UCM407844.pdf (Procedural).

FDA (2015 April)—Guidance for Industry: Scientific Considerations in Demonstrating Biosimilarity to a Reference Product. http://www.fda.gov/downloads/Drugs/GuidanceComplianceRegulatoryInformation/Guidances/UCM291128.pdf (Biosimilarity).

FDA (1998 June)—Guidance for Industry: Stability Testing for Drug Substances and Drug Products (Draft Guidances). http://www.fda.gov/ohrms/dockets/98fr/980362gd.pdf.

FDA (1987 February)—Guideline for Submitting Documentation for the Stability of Human Drugs and Biologics. http://www.rsihata.com/updateguidance/usfda2/2005-1/old028fn.pdf.

FDA. U.S. FDA—Biosimilars. http://www.fda.gov/drugs/developmentapprovalprocess/howdrugsaredevelopedandapproved/approvalapplications/therapeuticbiologic applications/biosimilars/default.htm.

Fransson, J., Hallen, D., and Florin-Robertsson, E. (1997) Solvent effects on the solubility and physical stability of human insulin-like growth factor I. *Pharm Res* 14: 606.

Freire, E., Schön, A., Hutchins, B. M., and Brown, R. K. (2013) Chemical denaturation as a tool in the formulation optimization of biologics. *Drug Discov Today* 18 (19–20): 1007–1013.

García Alfonso, P. (2010 March) Biosimilar filgrastim: From development to record. *Farm Hosp* 34 Suppl 1: 19–24.

Genazzani, A. A., Biggio, G., Caputi, A. P., Del Tacca, M., Drago, F., Fantozzi, R., and Canonico, P. L. (2007) Biosimilar drugs: Concerns and opportunities. *BioDrugs* 21 (6): 351–356.
Goswami, S., Wang, W., Arakawa, T., and Ohtake, S. (2013) Developments and challenges for mAb-based therapeutics, *Antibodies* 2: 452–500.
Guerra, P. I., Acklin, C., Kosky, A. A., Davis, J. M., Treuheit, M. J., and Brems, D. N. (1998) PEGylation prevents the N-terminal degradation of megakaryocyte growth and development factor *Pharm Res* 15: 1822.
Hadavand, N., Valadkhani, M., and Zarbakhsh A. (2011 September) Current regulatory and scientific considerations for approving biosimilars in Iran. *Biologicals* 39 (5): 325–327.
Herron, J. N., Jiskoot, W., and Crommelin, D. J. A. *Physical Methods to Characterize Pharmaceutical Proteins*. Pharmaceutical Biotechnology Series, Volume 7, New York: Plenum Press; 1995.
ICH (1996) Final guideline on stability testing of biotechnological/biological products. *Fed Regist* 61 (133): 36466–36469.
ICH (1997) Guidelines for the photostability testing of new drug substances and products. *Fed Regist* 62 (95): 27115–27122.
ICH (1999) Guidance on specifications: Test procedures and acceptance criteria for biotechnological/biological products. *Fed Regist* 64 (159): 44928–44935.
ICH (2006 November) Impurities in new drug products. The ICH. http://www.fda.gov/downloads/drugs/guidanceandcompliance-regulatoryinformation/guidances/ucm073389.pdf.
ICH (1994) Stability testing of new drug substances and products. *Fed Regist* 59 (183): 48754–48759.
Jones, A. J. S. (1993) Analysis of polypeptides and proteins. *Adv Drug Del Rev* 10: 29.
Kolvenbach, C. G., Narhi, L. O., Philo, J. S., Li, T., Zhang, M., and Arakawa, T. (1997) Granulocyte-colony stimulating factor maintains a thermally stable, compact, partially folded structure at pH 2. *J Pept Res* 50: 310.
Kresse, G. B. (2009 August) Biosimilars—Science, status, and strategic perspective. *Eur J Pharm Biopharm* 72 (3): 479–486.
Kuhlmann, M. and Covic, A. (2006 October) The protein science of biosimilars. *Nephrol Dial Transplant* 21 Suppl 5: v4–v8. Review. PubMed PMID: 16959791.
Lam, X. M., Patapoff, T. W., and Nguyen, T. H. (1997) The effect of benzyl alcohol on recombinant human interferon-gamma. *Pharm Res* 14: 725.
Lipiäinen, T., Peltoniemi, M., Sarkhel, S., Yrjönen, T., Vuorela, H., Urtti, A., and Juppo, A. (2015 February) Formulation and stability of cytokine therapeutics. *J Pharm Sci* 104 (2): 307–326.
Liu, J., Nguyen, M. D., Andya, J. D., and Shire, S. J. (2005) Reversible self-association increases the viscosity of a concentrated monoclonal antibody in aqueous solution. *J Pharm Sci* 94 (9): 1928–1948.
Maa, Y. F. and Hsu, C. C. (1996) Aggregation of recombinant human growth hormone induced by phenolic compounds. *Int J Pharm* 140: 155.
Manning, M. C., Matsuura, J. E., Kendrick, B. S., Meyer, J. D., Dormish, J. J., Vrkljan, M., Ruth, J. R., Carpenter, J. F., and Shefter, E. (1995) Approaches for increasing the solution stability of proteins. *Biotech Bioeng* 48: 506.
Matthews, B. R. (1999) Regulatory aspects of stability testing in Europe. *Drug Dev Indust Pharm* 25: 831.
Mellstedt, H., Niederwieser, D., and Ludwig, H. (2008 March) The challenge of biosimilars. *Ann Oncol* 19 (3): 411–419.
Müller, R., Renner, C., Gabay, C., Cassata, G., Lohri, A., and Hasler, P. (2014 July 1) The advent of biosimilars: Challenges and risks. *Swiss Med Wkly* 144: w13980.
Mysler, E. (2015 February) Biosimilars: Clinical interpretation and implications for drug development. *Curr Rheumatol Rep* 17 (2): 8.
Nema, S., Washkuhn, R. J., and Brendel, R. J. (1997) Excipients and their use in injectable products. *PDA J Pharm Sci Technol* 51: 166.

Pearlman, R. and Wang, Y. J. *Formulation, Characterization, and Stability of Protein Drugs: Case Histories*. Pharmaceutical Biotechnology Series, Volume 7, New York: Plenum Press; 1996.

Powell, M. F., Nguyen, T., and Baloian, L. (1998) Compendium of excipients for parenteral formulations. *PDA J Pharm Sci Technol* 52 (5): 238–311.

Price, W. N. 2nd, and Rai, A. K. (2015 April 10) Drug development: Are trade secrets delaying biosimilars? *Science* 348 (6231): 188–189.

Rais, I. (2012 November) When two do the same, it is not the same: Requirements for development and quality of biosimilars. *Pharm Unserer Zeit* 41 (6): 453–456.

Rak Tkaczuk, K. H. and Jacobs, I. A. (2014) Biosimilars in oncology: From development to clinical practice. *Semin Oncol* Suppl 3: S3–S12.

Reubsaet, J. L. E., Beijnen, J. H., Bult, A., Van-Maanen, R. J., Marchal, J. A. D., and Underberg, W. J. M. (1998) Analytical techniques used to study the degradation of proteins and peptides: Chemical instability. *J Pharm Biomed Anal* 17: 955.

Schön, A., Brown, R. K., Hutchins, B. M., and Freire, E. (2013) Ligand binding analysis and screening by chemical denaturation shift. *Anal Biochem* 443 (1): 52–57.

Tsiftsoglou, A. S., Ruiz, S., and Schneider, C. K. (2013 June) Development and regulation of biosimilars: Current status and future challenges. *BioDrugs* 27 (3): 203–211.

Volkin, D. B., Mach, H., and Middaugh, C. R. (1997) Degradative covalent reactions important to protein. *Stability Molec Biotech* 8: 5.

Wang, Y. J. and Hanson, M. A. (1988) Parenteral formulations of proteins and peptides: Stability and stabilizers. *J Parent Sci Technol* 42: S4.

Wang, Y. J. and Pearlman, R. *Stability and Characterization of Protein and Peptide Drugs: Case Histories*. Pharmaceutical Biotechnology Series, Volume 7, New York: Plenum Press; 1993.

Yamaguchi, T. and Arato, T. (2011 September) Quality, safety and efficacy of follow-on biologics in Japan. *Biologicals* 39 (5): 328–332.

Zelenetz, A. D. et al. (2011 September) NCCN biosimilars white paper: Regulatory, scientific, and patient safety perspectives. *J Natl Compr Canc Netw* 9 Suppl 4: S1–S22.

Chapter 9 Statistical Approach to Analytical Similarity

If your experiment needs a statistician, you need a better experiment.

Ernest Rutherford

9.1 Background

[Note: While most readers will be adequately informed of the basic vocabulary of statistical terms used in this chapter, some vocabulary is unique and other needs a fresh understanding. For this reason, I have provided a Glossary of Terms at the end of this chapter.]

The most significant step in establishing biosimilarity between a biosimilar candidate product and a reference product is the demonstration of analytical similarity to demonstrate that there is no clinically meaningful difference between the two products. This demonstration of similarity further extends to nonclinical pharmacology, clinical pharmacology, and clinical trials. In 2017, the FDA issued a draft guidance on statistical testing methodologies applicable to biosimilars, and it is highly recommended that any updates to this guidance be consulted by the developers. This guidance serves as a companion document to the guidance for industry *Quality Considerations in Demonstrating Biosimilarity of a Therapeutic Protein Product to a Reference Product.* (FDA: Guidance Compliance)

Section 351(i) of the PHS Act defines *biosimilarity* to mean "that the biological product is highly similar to the reference product notwithstanding minor differences in clinically inactive components" and that "there are no clinically meaningful differences between the biological product and the reference product in terms of the safety, purity and potency of the product." A 351(k) application for a proposed biosimilar product must include information demonstrating biosimilarity based on data derived from, among other things, "analytical studies that demonstrate that the biological product is highly similar to the reference product notwithstanding minor differences in clinically inactive components." Specifically, in the *Scientific Considerations in Demonstrating Biosimilarity to a*

Reference Product guidance for industry, the FDA described the totality-of-the-evidence approach that the FDA would use in the review of biosimilar applications. The results of statistical analyses conducted to support a demonstration that a proposed product is "highly similar" to U.S.-licensed reference product (hereinafter the *reference product* or the *U.S.-licensed reference product*) are considered within the context of totality-of-the-evidence in determining if a proposed product is biosimilar to a reference product. The *Quality Considerations in Demonstrating Biosimilarity of a Therapeutic Protein Product to a Reference Product* guidance for industry describes the FDA's recommendations to sponsors on the scientific and technical information (including analytical studies to support a demonstration that a proposed biosimilar is highly similar to the reference product), for the chemistry, manufacturing, and controls (CMC) section of a marketing application for a proposed product submitted under section 351(k) of the PHS Act (FDA: 2015). In general, an analytical similarity assessment involves a comparison of structural/physicochemical and functional attributes using multiple lots of the proposed biosimilar product and the reference product.

Conducting appropriate statistical analyses in the evaluation of analytical similarity can provide a high degree of confidence in the results and reduce the potential for bias. However, there are many challenges in designing the statistical analyses to be performed.

- First, there may be a limited number of reference product lots, and those obtained may be the result of biased sampling, leading to imprecise and possibly inaccurate estimates of the distributions of important quality attributes for the reference product.
- Second, there may also be a limited number of proposed biosimilar lots, and the available lots may not reflect the true variability of biosimilar product manufacturing.
- Third, there are a large number of potential quality attributes that can be compared in an evaluation of analytical similarity and subjecting all of these attributes to formal statistical tests in the context of limited lots could lead to concluding incorrectly that a large number of truly highly similar products are not highly similar.

To address these challenges, the FDA recommends using a risk-based approach in the analytical similarity assessment of quality attributes. This approach to the evaluation of analytical similarity consists of several steps. The first step is a determination of the quality attributes that characterize the reference product in terms of its structural/physicochemical and functional properties. In the second step, these quality attributes are then ranked according to their risk of potential clinical impact. Third, these attributes/assays are evaluated according to one of three tiers of statistical approaches based on a consideration of risk ranking as well as other factors. It should be noted, however, that some attributes may be important but not amenable to quantitative evaluation.

9.2 Reference and biosimilar products

The FDA recommends that the analytical similarity evaluation begin with an understanding of the structural/physicochemical and functional attributes of the reference product. Based on information obtained about these attributes during development of the proposed biosimilar, the sponsor should develop an analytical similarity assessment plan (see Section 9.3.1). A key component of this plan is the description of lots available for similarity testing. The following factors should be considered when selecting lots to be used in the analytical similarity assessment:

- *Number of reference product lots*—To establish meaningful similarity acceptance criteria, sponsors should acquire a sufficient number of reference product lots. We recommend a minimum of 10 reference product lots be sampled. In cases where limited numbers of reference product lots are available (e.g., for certain orphan drugs), alternate analytical similarity assessments should be proposed and discussed with the FDA.
- *Number of biosimilar product lots*—To allow for meaningful comparisons, the FDA recommends a minimum of 10 biosimilar lots be included in the analytical similarity assessment.
- *Variability in reference product lots*—The reference product lots selected should represent the variability of the reference product. Lots with remaining expiry spanning the reference product shelf life should be selected. The date of the analytical testing as well as the product expiration date should be provided in the application. Expired reference product should not be included in the similarity assessment to avoid bias.
- *Accounting for reference product and biosimilar product lots*—Sponsors should account for all of the reference product lots available to them. A list should be provided in the application of all lots that were evaluated in any manner even if a particular lot was not used in the final similarity assessment. The list should include the disposition of each lot and the specific physicochemical, functional, animal, and clinical studies for which a lot was used. When a lot is specifically selected to be included in or excluded from certain studies, a justification should be provided. Similar information on every manufactured drug substance and drug product lot of the proposed biosimilar product should also be provided.
- *U.S.-licensed reference product and other comparators*—The analytical similarity acceptance criteria should be derived using data from an analysis of the U.S.-licensed reference product, and the similarity assessment should be based on a direct comparison of the proposed biosimilar product to the U.S.-licensed reference product. As a scientific matter, combining data from the U.S.-licensed reference product and comparator products approved outside of the United States to determine

the acceptance criteria or to perform the analytical similarity assessment generally would not be expected to support a determination that the proposed biosimilar is highly similar to the U.S.-licensed reference product. For example, combining data from U.S.-licensed reference product and non–U.S.-licensed comparator products may result in broader similarity acceptance criteria than would be obtained by relying solely on U.S.-licensed reference product lots due to increased variability of the products. Sponsors are encouraged to discuss with the FDA, during drug development, any plans to use data derived from products approved outside of the United States.

- *Biosimilar lots manufactured with different processes*—It may be possible to combine data in the analytical similarity assessment from proposed biosimilar product lots manufactured with different processes and/or at different scales. However, data should be provided in the 351(k) biologics license application to support comparability of any materials manufactured with the different processes and/or scales.

9.3 General principles for evaluating analytical similarity

Analytical similarity should be assessed by using appropriate statistical methods to evaluate the analytical data. Methods of varying statistical rigor should be applied depending on the risk ranking of the quality attributes. Sponsors should develop an analytical similarity assessment plan that includes their proposed statistical approach to evaluation and then should discuss this approach with the FDA as early in the development program as feasible. The final analytical similarity report, which should include the analytical similarity assessment plan, should be included when a 351(k) biologics license application is submitted. The development of the analytical similarity assessment plan is the topic of Section 9.3.1, followed by a discussion of the FDA's current thinking on the statistical methods to be applied for evaluation.

9.3.1 Analytical similarity assessment plan

The FDA recommends that the analytical similarity assessment plan be carefully designed to identify and address all factors that could impact the determination about whether the proposed biosimilar is highly similar to the reference product. Some factors that may need to be considered include

- *Differences in age of the lots produced at testing*—It is recognized that differences in the age of the proposed biosimilar and reference product lots at the time of testing may result in analytical differences. There should, therefore, be a prespecified plan to address how changes in attributes over the shelf life will be incorporated into the determination of the similarity acceptance criteria.

- *Multiple testing results*—When there are multiple testing results for the same lot with a given quality attribute or assay, the biosimilar applicant should prespecify which results will be selected for analytical similarity assessment.
- *Assay performance*—The assay methodologies and assay designs used in the analytical similarity assessment should be carefully considered and optimized, as needed. Poor assay performance, including high assay variability, should not be used to justify selection of either a particular evaluation tier or an inappropriately broad similarity acceptance criterion.
- *Differences in attributes that will be considered acceptable*—It may be known in advance that a difference less than or equal to a certain amount for a particular quality attribute would not be expected to have a clinical impact. In this situation, supporting information and an adequate justification for the allowable differences should be provided in the application.

The FDA recommends that the analytical similarity assessment plan be developed in four stages, corresponding to the following activities:

- Development of the risk ranking of the reference product's quality attributes based on the potential impact on the clinical performance categories (i.e., the product's activity as well as pharmacokinetic/pharmacodynamic [PK/PD], safety, and immunogenicity profiles)
- Determination of the statistical methods to be used for evaluating each quality attribute based on the risk ranking and on other factors
- Development of the statistical analysis plan
- Finalization of the analytical similarity assessment plan

These four stages are described in more detail in the following subsections.

9.3.1.1 Development of risk ranking of attributes

The FDA recommends that biosimilar sponsors develop a risk assessment tool to evaluate and rank the reference product quality attributes in terms of potential clinical impact. (Certain quality evaluations of the reference product—e.g., its degradation rates, which are determined from stability or forced degradation studies—generally would not be included in the risk ranking. However, these evaluations will still factor into the assessment of the analytical similarity of the proposed biosimilar and reference product.) The risk assessment tool should be developed considering, at a minimum, the following two factors:

- *Potential impact of an attribute on clinical performance*—Specifically, the FDA recommends that sponsors consider the impact of an attribute on activity as well as on PK/PD, safety, and immunogenicity profiles. For example, sponsors should consider available public information, as well as the sponsor's characterization of the reference product, in determining the potential impact of an attribute on clinical performance.

- *The degree of uncertainty around a certain quality attribute*— For example, when there is limited understanding of the clinical impact of an attribute, the FDA recommends that that attribute be ranked as having higher risk because of the uncertainty involved.

The FDA recommends that an attribute that is a high risk for any one of the performance categories (i.e., activity, PK/PD, safety, or immunogenicity) should be classified as high risk. Ideally, the risk assessment tool should result in a list of attributes ordered by the risk to the patient. The risk scores for attributes should, therefore, be proportional to patient risk. Because there may be a limited number of attributes that can be evaluated with equivalence testing (see Section 9.3.1.2), attributes that are known to be of high risk to patients (i.e., high impact attributes) should be a priority over attributes with unknown but potentially high risk (i.e., attributes with a high-risk ranking due to uncertainty).
The scoring criteria used in the risk assessment should be clearly defined and justified in the analytical similarity assessment plan, and the risk ranking for each attribute should be justified with appropriate citations to the literature and data provided.

9.3.1.2 Determination of the statistical methods to be used

The FDA's current approach to evaluating analytical similarity is to define three tiers corresponding to the use of three different methods for comparing attributes. The FDA believes that the use of these three tiers with appropriate similarity acceptance criteria should help support a demonstration that the proposed biosimilar is highly similar to the reference product. Equivalence testing (Tier 1) is typically recommended for quality attributes with the highest risk ranking and should generally include assay(s) that evaluate clinically relevant mechanism(s) of action of the product for each indication for which approval is sought. The use of quality ranges (Tier 2) is recommended for quality attributes with a lower risk ranking, and an approach that uses visual comparisons (Tier 3) is recommended for quality attributes with the lowest risk ranking. The three methods are described in Section 9.3.2.

In addition to risk ranking, however, other factors should be considered in determining which tier of statistical evaluation should be applied to a particular attribute or assay. Although many attributes may be considered high risk, subjecting all of these attributes to Tier 1 testing may result in a false negative conclusion (i.e., a determination that a product is not highly similar when it truly is). Some additional factors, besides risk, that should be considered when determining the appropriate tier include

- *Level of the attribute*—An attribute of the reference product known to be of high risk but present at a level that is unlikely to have significant clinical impact could potentially be assessed at a lower tier. To justify placing a high risk attribute in a lower tier for this reason, the level of the attribute should be confirmed in both the reference product (as determined by the proposed biosimilar sponsor's analysis of the reference product) and the proposed biosimilar product. The selected limits regarding the level of an attribute should be defined and justified. The justification should also include consideration of how the level of the attribute changes over time.
- *Assays used for assessing the attribute*—Although multiple, orthogonal assays are encouraged for assessing a single attribute, not all assays need to be included in the same tier of assessment. The assay with the best performance characteristics for detecting product differences should be used for testing with the highest tier methods, while other assays should be used for testing with lower tier methods. A justification should be provided for the assays selected for testing at each tier.
- *Types of attributes/assays*—Some attributes or the assays used to assess the attribute will, by their nature, be excluded from certain statistical evaluations. For example, compendia assays, qualitative assays, or limit assays might be excluded from evaluation with Tier 1 and, in some cases, Tier 2 methods. The analytical similarity assessment plan should clearly define the conditions used to exclude assays from evaluation at any tier.

Applicable data and cited literature should be provided in the application to support the use of any additional factors in determining the appropriate tier of statistical assessment.

9.3.1.3 Development of the statistical analysis plan

A detailed statistical analysis plan should be developed and included in the analytical similarity assessment plan because the statistical aspects of the evaluation will impact whether or not the similarity acceptance criteria are ultimately met. The plan for the statistical evaluation of analytical similarity requires the selection of design features from among many possibilities. These design features include the following five factors:

- The choice and risk ranking of attributes
- The statistical approach (tier) for assessing each attribute
- The number of proposed biosimilar and reference product lots to be evaluated for each attribute, and the number of replicates to be evaluated per lot
- For each attribute, a determination of the largest acceptable difference between the proposed biosimilar and reference product that is considered to not have clinical impact
- The methods of statistical analysis for each tier, and the type of assay(s) used to evaluate each attribute

It is well known that bias may be introduced when there is an opportunity to select the most desirable result from a number of results obtained; consequently, the probability of a false positive result may be increased, and any estimated differences between the products are likely to be biased toward equivalence. Therefore, to minimize bias and the chance of erroneous conclusions, the statistical analysis plan should be prespecified to the fullest extent possible. In some cases, it may be necessary to first collect preliminary data (e.g., to get an initial estimate of the variability of the reference product's attribute or to select an assay at the outset before finalizing the statistical analysis plan).

9.3.1.4 Finalization of the analytical similarity assessment plan

The final analytical similarity assessment plan should include the risk ranking of attributes, the specification of tiers of evaluation to be used for each attribute/assay, and the final statistical analysis plan. The plan should specify the anticipated availability of both proposed biosimilar and reference product lots for evaluation of each attribute/assay and should include a rationale as to why the proposed number of lots will be sufficient for evaluation purposes. The analytical similarity assessment plan should be discussed with the FDA as early in the biosimilar development program as possible so that agreement can be reached on which attributes/assays should be evaluated in each tier. The final analytical similarity assessment plan should be submitted to the FDA prior to initiating the final analytical assessments; typically this would be done in connection with a meeting with the FDA.

9.3.2 Statistical methods for evaluation

The FDA's current thinking on the statistical evaluation of analytical similarity is described in this section. Sponsors that intend to propose alternative statistical approaches to the FDA should do so during the analysis planning stage.

9.3.2.1 Tier 1 (equivalence test)

9.3.2.1.1 Hypotheses and statistical tests

Analytical similarity of the quality attributes determined to have the highest potential clinical impact (based on the risk ranking and other factors, as described in Section 9.3.1) should be evaluated through formal statistical tests of equivalence. Equivalence of attributes measured on a continuous scale can be assessed by testing the difference in means between the proposed biosimilar and reference product.

In the following formulas, μT and μR denote the population means, and σ_T^2 and $\sigma_R^2\sigma$ denote the population variances of the proposed biosimilar and reference product, respectively. To test for equivalence in means, the null and alternative hypotheses are given by

$$H_0: \mu T - \mu R \leq -\delta \text{ or } \mu T - \mu R \geq \delta$$
$$H_a: -\delta < \mu T - \mu R < \delta$$

In these formulas, δ is a positive number denoting the largest acceptable difference between the proposed biosimilar and reference product that is considered to not have clinical impact (i.e., the "equivalence margin"). Analytical similarity is supported if the null hypothesis of non-equivalence, H_0, is rejected. In other words, the statistical equivalence in means is established if the results of the statistical analysis indicate, with high confidence, that

$$-\delta < \mu T - \mu R < \delta$$

A test of the equivalence hypothesis can be conducted by requiring the simultaneous rejection of the following two one-sided null hypotheses:

$$H_{01}: \mu T - \mu R \leq \delta \text{ vs. } H_{a1}: \mu T - \mu R > -\delta$$
$$H_{02}: \mu T - \mu R \geq \delta \text{ vs. } H_{a2}: \mu T - \mu R < \delta$$

The probability of making a Type I error (i.e., declaring incorrectly that a biosimilar product's particular attribute is equivalent to a reference product's particular attribute) for a test of the equivalence hypothesis is controlled at the prespecified level α, provided each of the two one-sided hypotheses, H_{01} and H_{02}, is tested at the same level α.

A convenient way to simultaneously test the two null hypotheses defining equivalence is through a confidence-interval-based test. If the (1–2α)100% two-sided confidence interval of the mean difference lies within (–δ, δ), then both null hypotheses are rejected, and the Type I error probability is controlled at level α for a conclusion of equivalence. For example, a 5% Type I error probability is obtained by requiring a 90% confidence interval to lie within (–δ, δ).

9.3.2.1.2 Margin determination

Determining an appropriate margin is a critical but challenging step for equivalence testing in any setting. Ideally, it would be possible to establish and prespecify a biologically or clinically meaningful equivalence margin based on scientific knowledge or past experience. Often, however, such a margin is not readily available for every quality attribute deemed important enough for Tier 1 testing in a biosimilar development program. With this limitation, the FDA currently recommends use of an equivalence margin that is a function of the reference product's variability for the attribute being tested. Specifically, the equivalence margin should be in the form of $f \times \sigma_R$, where f is a fixed constant, and σ_R is the standard deviation of the quality attribute of the reference product. This suggested form of the equivalence margin is based on three criteria:

- The goal of ensuring that values of the attribute being tested for the proposed biosimilar tend to fall within the reference product distribution
- The desire to have a unified representation of the margin for all Tier 1 quality attributes despite different levels of variability
- The goal of having sufficient power for practical sample sizes

After examining a range of possible values for the constant *f*, the FDA determined that a reasonable value should be 1.5. With $\delta = 1.5\ \sigma_R$, the test generally should support equivalence if the 90% confidence interval of the difference in means lies within the interval ($-1.5\ \sigma_R$, $1.5\ \sigma_R$) (i.e., the lower limit of the 90% confidence interval for the difference in means is greater than $-1.5\ \sigma_R$ and the upper limit is less than $1.5\ \sigma_R$). Use of this multiplier in computing the equivalence margin results in a test with reasonable properties under what the FDA considers are realistic conditions. For example, if 10 biosimilar and 10 reference product lots are available, and the variability of the attribute for the reference product (σ_R) is known and not estimated from the sponsor's data, this test has adequate power (i.e., at least 85%) to reject the null hypotheses in favor of equivalence when the true underlying mean difference between the proposed biosimilar and the reference products is small, namely, equal to $\sigma_R/8$, assuming a test of size $\alpha = 0.05$. If the true difference between products is less than $\sigma_R/8$, power will be increased.

A limitation of the proposed approach to setting the equivalence margin is that σ_R is usually not known and must be estimated from the current reference product lots available to the sponsor. If one uses a *t*-test and does not consider the uncertainty in the estimate of the margin, the Type I error probability may be inflated. Alternative tests can be constructed to account for this additional uncertainty, but additional research is needed to better understand the operating characteristics of these tests (such as the small sample size performance of a Wald test based on large-sample approximations; Bickel and Doksum 2007).

9.3.2.2 Tier 2 (quality range approach)

For Tier 2, the similarity acceptance criteria based on reference product results for a specific quality attribute should be defined as $(\hat{\mu}_R - X\hat{\sigma}_R, \hat{\mu}_R + X\hat{\sigma}_R)$, where $\hat{\mu}_R$ is the sample mean and $\hat{\sigma}_R$ is the sample standard deviation based on the reference product lots. The multiplier (X) should be scientifically justified for that attribute and discussed with the FDA. Based on our experience, methods such as the tolerance interval approach and the min-max approach are not recommended (Dong et al. 2015).

Analytical similarity generally should be demonstrated for a quality attribute if a sufficient percentage of test lot values (e.g., 90%) fall within the quality range defined above for that attribute. The lots used for Tier 2 testing should, if possible, be the same as those used for Tier 1 testing.

It is clear that for a given critical attribute, the quality range is set based on test results of available reference lots. If x=1.645, the FDA would expect 90% of the test results from reference lots lie within the quality range. If x is chosen to be 1.96, the FDA will expect that about 95% test results of reference lots will fall within the quality range. As a result, the selection of x could impact the quality range and consequently the percentage of test lot values that will fall within the quality range. Thus, the FDA indicates that the standard deviation multiplier (x) should be appropriately justified. For information, the FDA used a factor of 2 when evaluating the receptor binding data for EP2006 (FDA ODAC 2015). For the analytical similarity protocol, the developer may use an x value of 3, as suggested by the FDA, and then calculate the exact x value to meet the test; regardless of the number chosen, the developer provides a justification for selection. It allows approximately one standard deviation of reference for shifting, which may be adjusted based on biologist reviewers' recommendations. However, some sponsors propose using the concept of tolerance interval in order to ensure that there are a high percentage of test values for the lots from the test products that fall within the quality range. It, however, should be noted that the percentage decreases when the difference in mean between the reference product and the proposed biosimilar product increases. This is also true when $\sigma_T \ll \sigma_R$. Even the tolerance interval is used as the quality range. This problem is commonly encountered mainly because the quality range approach does not take into consideration

- The difference in means between the reference product and the proposed biosimilar product.
- The heterogeneity among lots within and between products. In practice, it is very likely that a biosimilar product with small variability but a mean response that is away from the reference mean (e.g., within the acceptance range of $\sigma_R/8$ as suggested by the FDA) will fall outside the quality range. In this case, a further evaluation of the data points that fall outside the quality range is necessary to rule out the possibility by chance alone.

9.3.2.3 Tier 3 (visual displays)

Attributes to be evaluated in Tier 3 should correspond either to those of lowest risk for potential clinical impact or those attributes that are important but not amenable to formal tests of hypotheses or quantitative evaluation. Various forms of visual displays may be used to compare the distribution of values from the proposed biosimilar and reference lots, and a subjective determination of the similarity should be made based on those displays. The lots used for the Tier 3 evaluation should be the same as, or a subset of, the lots used for Tier 1 and Tier 2 evaluations. The number of lots needed for the Tier 3 evaluation can depend upon a number of factors, including, for example, the expected lot-to-lot variability of the attribute. In cases where limited lot-to-lot variability is expected, a single lot of the proposed biosimilar and reference product for the Tier 3 evaluation may be acceptable.

9.3.2.4 Additional considerations

The FDA also recommends considering the following:

- The variance of an attribute (e.g., σ 2) encompasses both the within-lot and between-lot variance components. It is recommended that sponsors examine the contribution of the two variance components, as estimated from their lots, to help understand the performance of the assay. High assay variability generally is not an appropriate justification for a large value of δ. Instead, the assay should be optimized and/or the number of replicates per lot should be increased to reduce variability. We note that, in either case, lots of both the proposed biosimilar and the reference product should be assessed with the same number of replicates for that attribute, and the margin and all subsequent calculations should be defined using all lot values.
- For all quantitative quality attributes, including those subject to Tier 1 and 2 evaluations, descriptive statistics and visual displays should be used to present the reference and proposed biosimilar product distributions. In addition, the sponsor should submit sufficient data in its application to allow the FDA to conduct independent analyses.
- When the calculated equivalence margins or quality ranges are too wide or narrow, the FDA may adjust them to more appropriate levels.

It is important to note that the FDA's final assessment as to whether a proposed biosimilar is highly similar to the reference product is made upon the totality of the evidence, rather than the passing or failing of the analytical similarity criteria of any one tier or any one attribute. For example, the FDA generally will consider the impact of an enhanced manufacturing control strategy when making this final assessment.

In creating a statistical model, the FDA has made certain assumptions and certain assertions. First, the FDA assumes that any observed difference in clinical response between the reference product and the proposed biosimilar product is proportional to the variability of the critical quality attributes (CQAs). Some have criticized this strict correlation assumption based on the claim that the biological products are known to produce a nonlinear response. Secondly, the question of how much similarity must be demonstrated to assure that there is no clinically meaningful difference remains to be determined. To obviate this criticism, the FDA takes a case-by-case approach wherein molecule-dependent attributes are presented by the developer of the product to demonstrate similarity.

The FDA and all other highly regulated agencies agree that the biosimilar products need not be identical because they cannot be, but these differences should not produce any clinically meaningful difference. This requires identification of CQAs of the product based on the understanding of the mechanism of action (MOA) and the factors affecting the pharmacokinetics and pharmacodynamics of the biosimilar product to form a sound basis for demonstrating analytical similarity. Given below is a stepwise approach to developing a plan for analytical similarity demonstration:

- Evaluate quality attributes consistent with the risk assessment principles ICH Quality Guidelines Q8, Q9, Q10, and Q11.
- Consider criticality risk ranking of quality attributes with regard to their potential impact on activity, PK/PD, safety, and immunogenicity.
- Use a tiered approach for assessment as suggested by the FDA:
  - Equivalence interval testing for *some* high-risk attributes ($c*\sigma_R$; c=1.5 unless otherwise justified a higher number) (Tier 1).
  - Quality ranges (mean ± X*SD) for *other* high- to low-risk attributes; generally X=3 or lower (Tier 2).
  - Raw/graphical comparisons for *other* attributes (Tier 3); graphical output may come in the evaluation of high-risk attributes. Tier 3 refers to the presentation of data and does not necessarily mean an irrelevant attribute.

The regulatory agencies require that the biosimilar product developer create a risk-based model to identify the critical attributes, critical to safety, potency, and purity that can make a meaningful difference in *commercial supply* of the product. For identifying CQAs at various stages of the manufacturing process, most biosimilar product developers assign CQAs based on the MOA or PK, which are believed to be relevant to clinical outcomes. It is a reasonable assumption that change in the MOA or PK of a given quality attribute is predictive of clinical outcomes. However, the primary assumption that there is a well-established relationship between in vitro assays and in vivo testing (i.e., in vitro assays and in vivo testing correlation) needs to be validated. Under the validated in vitro assays and in vivo testing correlation relationship, the criticality (or risk ranking) can then be assessed based on the degree of the relationship. In practice, most biosimilar product developers provide clinical rationales for the assignment of the CQAs without using a statistical approach for the establishment of in vitro assays and in vivo testing correlation. The assignment of the CQAs without using a statistical approach is considered subjective and hence is somewhat misleading.

The biosimilar product developers face many challenges including a limited number of lots of reference product available, different testing methods resulting in different data types, and on deciding what difference is meaningful and what is not, finally establishing acceptable similarity margins and presenting the data in a convincing manner. "The plurality of candidates of critical quality attributes within specific developments, as well as the usually low number of drug lots available, had been identified as the most limiting factors, rendering the use of statistical routines usually performed on the basis of patient clinical data inappropriate most of the time" (EMA 2013).

9.3.3 Design and conduct of similarity testing

The analytical similarity testing forms the most critical stage of determining whether a biosimilar candidate is indeed a viable candidate. Just like the FDA evaluates a biosimilar candidate in a step-by-step basis, so are the analytical similarity testing protocols. In Chapter 6, I elaborated on what constitutes a CQAs, and in this chapter, I discussed how to demonstrate equivalence using the biopharmaceutical tools listed in Chapter 5. Figure 9.1 shows the tier-based approach from a different perspective—process of demonstration.

The salient features of this pyramid are given below:

1. *Critical quality attributes*—These are highly product specific and process dependent, and contain all elements of safety, purity, and potency considerations that can be clinically meaningful.
2. *Analytical methods*—The CQAs are rank-ordered, and suitable analytical methods are developed. Now that several pharmacopeia include monographs of several biosimilar products,

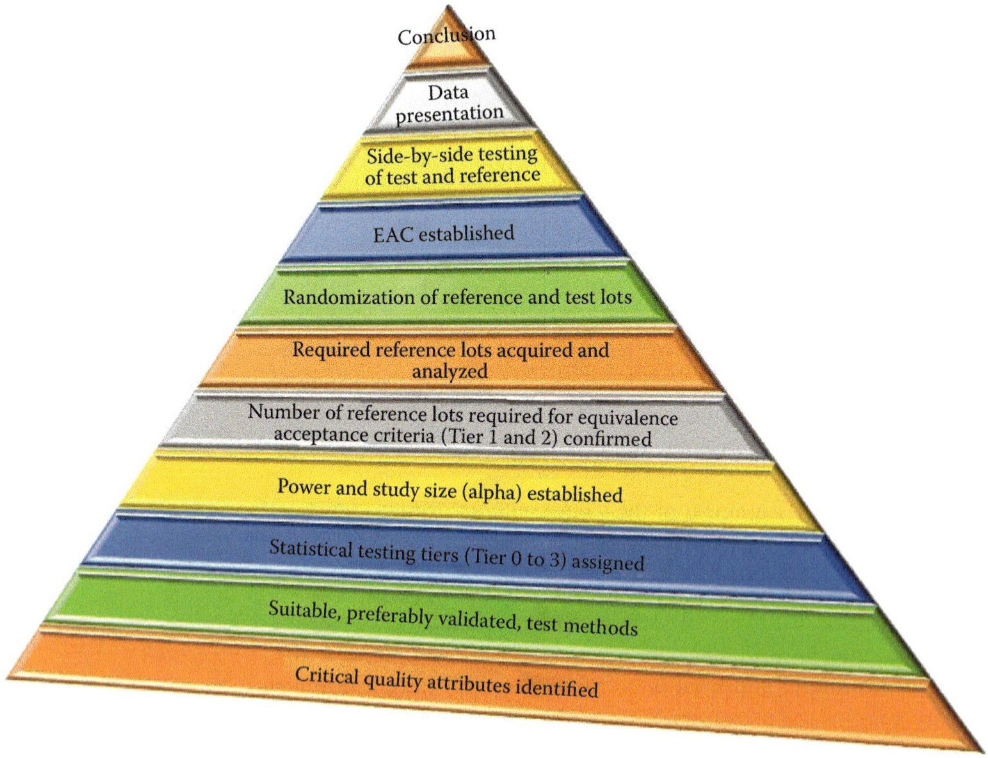

Figure 9.1 Stepwise approach to establishing analytical similarity.

this should be a starting point; however, it is well known that not all pharmacopeia methods are suitable for the purpose of demonstrating analytical similarity—the developer may want to explore cross pharmacopeia methods or other reported methods. Obviously, choosing a pharmacopeia method reduces the workload as only a verification step is involved, not the validation. This consideration is highly important for analytical methods to have provided a high degree of variability such as bioassays. The FDA expects the developer to choose and/or develop a method that has lower variability. What is low will depend on the nature of test, but the developer may want to conduct a literature search to establish to quote what is a generally accepted variability for the stated methods to justify its own coefficient of variation of the test method.

3. *A selection of statistical tiers*—As shown above, the FDA classifies all statistical testing into three categories depending on the relative impact of the testing on clinical efficacy and safety. At this stage, a test will be classified as Tier 1, 2, or 3.
4. *A number of lots tested side by side*—A common question asked by the biosimilar developer is, "how many lots should be tested?" While the FDA has not clearly described its expectations, except for Tier 1, wherein a difference equal to $\sigma/8$ should be detectable, this allows calculation of the power of testing as shown later in the chapter. Ideally, if 10 different lots of reference and test products are available, this should provide sufficient power, generally over 80%, which should be acceptable to the FDA.
5. *Selection of power and alpha*: The Type I error (based on alpha) is the FDA risk, and the Type 2 (based on beta) is the developer's risk; a proper selection of both is needed to establish an equivalence acceptance criterion. As we will see, the FDA can be flexible on Type I error if the developer can show that the attribute can be tightened in its limits through manufacturing controls.
6. The number of reference lots to establish acceptance criteria is based on the standard deviation of the reference lots. How many lots to use will depend on the degree of variability. In most instances, between 5 and 10 lots will be needed to establish a reasonably narrow standard deviation. Know that there are two ways of doing it—first by adopting less variable testing methods and second by increasing the number of test lots.
7. Randomization of lots is something that the FDA recommends, meaning that the lots of both the reference and the test are not picked out with bias—only good lots of the test and only bad lots of the reference. This expectation of the FDA can be very

difficult to manage because of the paucity of the number of reference lots generally available. To overcome this bias, the developer may develop an internal system wherein lots are assigned for testing prior to being manufactured, and the reference lots included without first testing them.

8. Depending on the tier of testing, an analytical acceptance criterion is established particularly for the Tier 1 testing where the interval would be $1.5*\sigma_R$ and for Tier 2 testing it will be $3*\sigma_R$. These values must be established prior to beginning the testing of the lots side by side.
9. Now the lots can be tested side by side, ideally blinded so the analytical laboratory will not know the identity of the lot tested. This can be challenging when the base formulations are different as it happened when the first product was approved by the FDA—in that case, a blinding is not possible since test methods would have to be adjusted for differences in the base buffer.
10. The data are presented in a form that makes it easier to judge analytical similarity. Generally, the developer would use a validated statistics program like SAS, MINITAB, JMP, or others. A typical presentation will include data display, summary statistics, and a graphical presentation of the basis of meeting acceptance criteria, such as a 90% CI plot and EAC or dispersion of values within $3*\sigma$. For Tier 3 testing, a graphical presentation is made to demonstrate the degree of super-imposability.
11. Conclusions are drawn whether a test met the predefined acceptance criteria.

9.4 Managing tiers

While approving its first biosimilar product, the FDA stated the following:

> *"In analyzing the EP2006 submission of analytical similarity, the following conclusions were made: '***Identical*** primary structure; highly similar secondary and tertiary structure; highly similar purity and stability profiles; and highly similar receptor binding and biological activity.'"*

This statement by the FDA is precise as to what is considered more or less important; the primary structure, regardless of which tiers are applied, must be identical, meaning zero variation, and the rest of listed profiles must be highly similar, meaning meeting the tier testing limits. While the data presentation will be determined by the type of tier selection, Figure 9.2 shows an overall approach that is required to provide a meaningful presentation to the FDA.

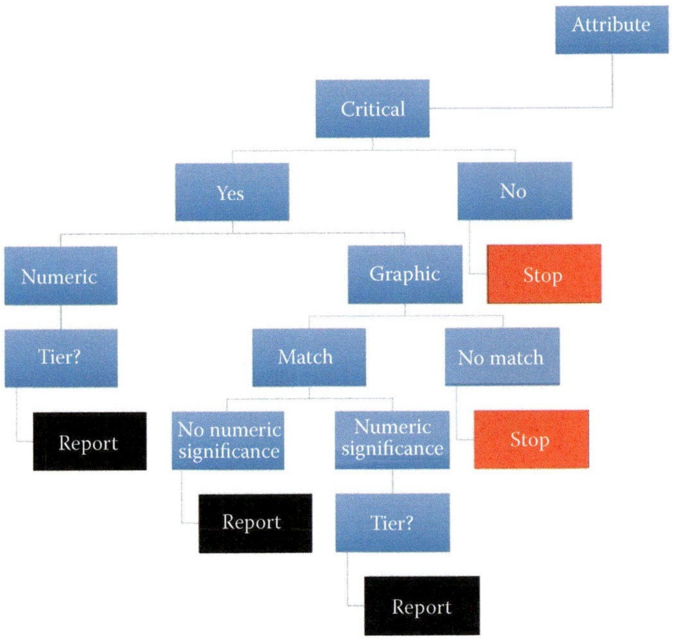

Figure 9.2 Tier testing plan.

9.4.1 Tier determination

The variability in biological products comes two sources: one is during the expression stage and the other at the post-expression processing level inside the cell—posttranslational modifications. Posttranslational modifications appear only in the mammalian cell and do not apply to such products as filgrastim, HGH, or insulins expressed in bacteria or yeast. Regardless of the mechanism involved, the primary structure must be identical such as the total mass, amino acid sequence, the position of disulfide bonds, immunoblotting and pI values, etc. For molecules undergoing post translational modifications (PTM), there can be variability at the primary structure level as well, and these may be tested in a tier that best describes the relative importance of the PTMs. Recently, the FDA approved its first biosimilar cancer drug, bevacizumab (MVASI, Amgen), and while there were significant variations in the glycosylation pattern, these were construed acceptable since these differences did not produce any impact on the safety and efficacy of the product—essentially calling them clinically not meaningful. However, there may be other drugs where the PTMs can be critical, so one must realize that there is no clear definition of tiers and how they are applied.

However, one should be aware that any statistical test result is subject to its suitability evaluation. For example, a Tier 1 test for the recently approved first anticancer drug bevacizumab shows that the biosimilar

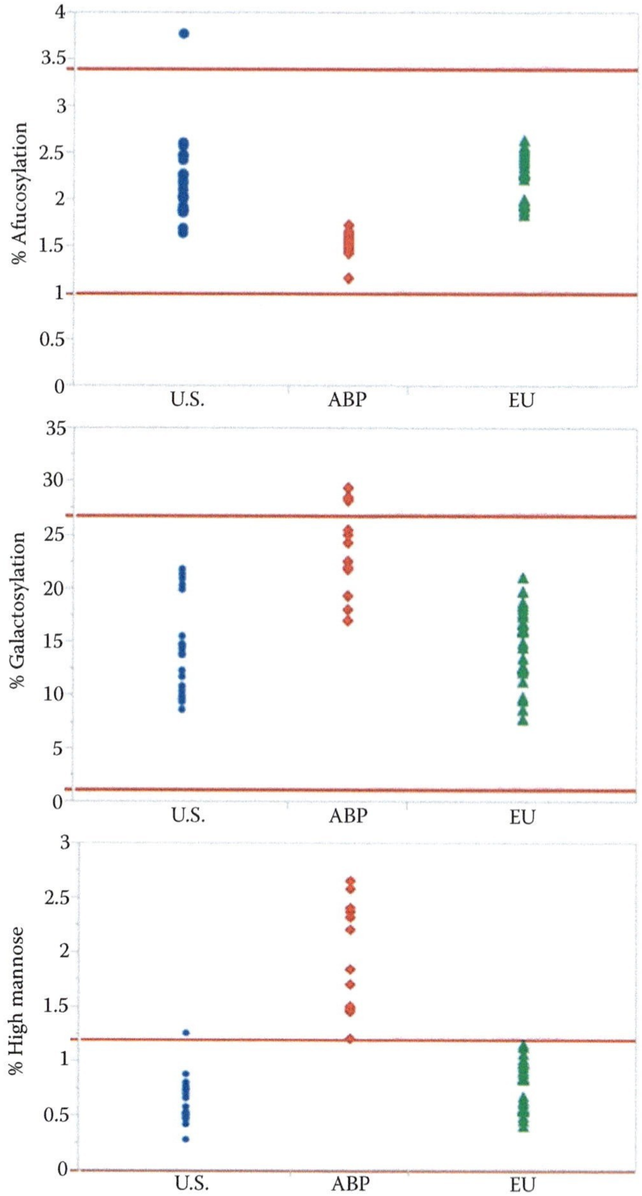

Figure 9.3 Comparison of glycan profile for ABP215, U.S.-licensed Avastin, and EU-approved bevacizumab. (From https://www.fda.gov/downloads/AdvisoryCommittees/CommitteesMeetingMaterials/Drugs/OncologicDrugsAdvisoryCommittee/UCM566365.pdf)

product did not have highly similar glycan profile, yet the FDA concluded that this is not clinically meaningful (Figure 9.3).

The primary structure attributes are mostly well established in legacy values, such as the reported total mass or amino acid sequence; the

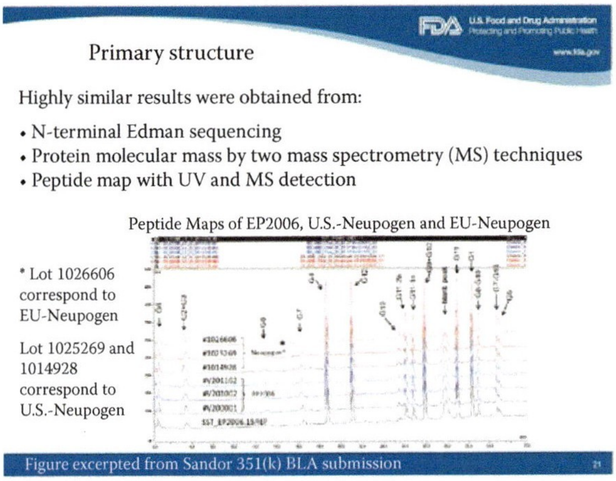

Figure 9.4 Retention time for mass spectrometry of two filgrastim product; multiple lots of each are presented overlapping. (From http://www.fda.gov/downloads/AdvisoryCommittees/CommitteesMeetingMaterials/Drugs/OncologicDrugsAdvisoryCommittee/UCM428780.pdf)

biosimilar product must conform to these fixed attributes, regardless of the appearance of these attributes in the reference product. Therefore, the absolute value of CQAs may come from side-by-side testing with the reference product or from legacy values. Further measure of being identical is established by the retention time and a deconvolution of the mass spectra; this is generally required by the FDA as a measure of demonstration of the identical attribute. It is noteworthy that while the primary structure has to be identical, the methods of determining its attributes, like peptide map, can vary to some extent as shown in Figure 9.4.

Tier 1 testing is intended for those CQAs that have high significance to clinical effects, effectiveness, and safety. One such attribute is the protein content, especially for low-dose products, such as cytokines. Obviously, the basis for this comes from a proportionality between dose and effect. While a good scientific argument can be made for not including protein content as a Tier 1 attribute, such challenges are not likely to meet success, and I am recommending listing this attribute as Tier 1. How far this debate of protein content goes can be appreciated from Table 9.1 that shows filgrastim content in various EP2006 lots as tested against U.S. and EU Neupogen.

The FDA first tested six lots of EP2006 Commercial against 12 U.S. Neupogen lots; the test failed (light gray) even at 81.4% CI and the FDA suggested that this deficiency can be addressed in manufacturing steps. Later the developer added one more lot, but the test still failed against both the 12 lots of U.S. Neupogen and 49 lots of EU Neupogen even though the CI was reduced to 85.2%. (It is not sure why the FDA chose a different CI instead of 81.4% that was first used.) At this stage, the FDA allowed consolidation of clinical lots with commercial lots, and with this, the equivalence test passed. The argument for this allowance was

Table 9.1 Equivalence Interval Analysis of EP2006 by the FDA

Test (# Lots)	Reference (# Lots)	Confidence Level, % (1–2α)*100	CI, %	Acceptance, %, 1.5*σ_R	Result	*R/T* Ratio
EP2006 clinical (11)	U.S. Neupogen (12)	90	–1,75, +0.70	±2.26	Pass	1.09
EP2006 commercial (6)	U.S. Neupogen (12)	81.4	–3.87, –1.13	±2.08	Fail	2
EP2006 clinical (11)	EU Neupogen (11)	90	–2.32, +0.52	±3.23	Pass	1
EU Neupogen (49)	U.S. Neupogen (12)	90	+0.27, +2.09	±2.26	Pass	0.24
EP2006 clinical + commercial (20)	U.S. Neupogen (12)	90	–1,87, +0.15	±2.26	Pass	0.6
EP2005 clinical + commercial (20)	EU Neupogen (49)	90	–2.98, –0.85	±3.23	Pass	2.45
EU Neupogen (49)	U.S. Neupogen (12)	90	+0.27, +2.09	±2.26	Pass	0.24
EP2006 clinical (13)	U.S. Neupogen (12)	90	–1.78, +0.43	±2.26	Pass	0.92
EP2006 clinical (13)	EU Neupogen (49)	90	–3.13, –0.53	±3.26	Pass	3.7
EP2006 commercial (7)	U.S. Neupogen (12)	85.2	–2.33, +0.67	±2.28	Fail	1.7
EP2006 commercial (7)	EU Neupogen (49)	85.2	–3.71, -0.20	±3.23	Fail	7

Last column was added by the author.

Source: http://www.fda.gov/downloads/AdvisoryCommittees/CommitteesMeetingMaterials/Drugs/OncologicDrugsAdvisoryCommittee/UCM428780.pdf)

that the clinical lots meet the U.S. and EU Neupogen. When the U.S. and EU Neupogen meet together, the clinical and commercial lots meet, and therefore they can be combined (dark gray shaded rows).
A good example is the comparison of the total protein content of filgrastim between two products (Figure 9.5).

Since protein content is also a release attribute, a dilemma arises for the developers, where the release criteria are established independently of the comparison with the reference product. It would be suitable for a release specification to list the acceptance criteria as ±5%, yet the product, at the evaluation stage, must not have higher variability than the reference product. What if the reference product has an extremely low standard deviation? Multiplying it by 1.5 still provides a very narrow range for the biosimilar candidate to fit the similarity. An extreme example, not out of possibility, comes when say 10 out of 10 lots of the reference product have exactly the same protein content; with a SD of zero, every biosimilar candidate will fail. The reason why this observation

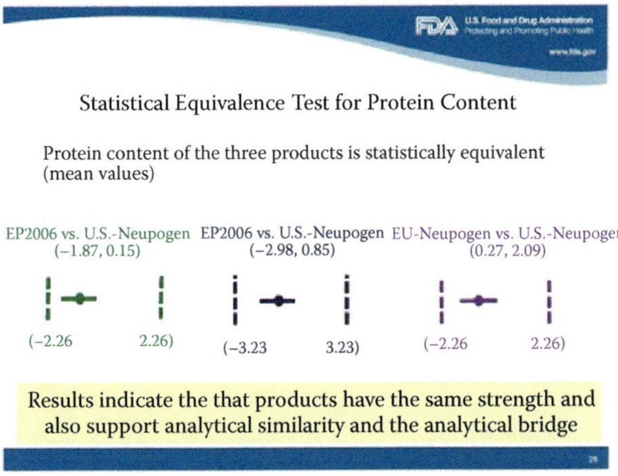

Figure 9.5 Tier 1 testing method for protein content of filgrastim; all three comparisons meet the test requirement. (From http://www.fda.gov/downloads/AdvisoryCommittees/CommitteesMeetingMaterials/Drugs/OncologicDrugsAdvisoryCommittee/UCM428780.pdf)

is not out of reality comes from the long experience of the originator company in compensating for manufacturing losses at all stages, more particularly, the filling stage.

Next to the protein content comes the bioassay or activity of the product. Primary biological activity falls under Tier 1 testing; however, given that all biological testing results have a variability that may not be proportional to protein content, as suggested above, the difficulties in passing this test are small, of course, if the product is the same (Figures 9.6 and 9.7).

Some biological or structural responses are tested as Tier 2, as shown in Figure 9.8.

The Tier 3 testing involves an approach that uses raw data/graphical comparisons for quality attributes with the lowest risk ranking. For CQAs in Tier 3 with lowest risk ranking, the FDA recommends an approach that uses raw data/graphical comparisons. The examination of similarity for CQAs in Tier 3 by no means is less stringent, which is acceptable because they have the least impact on clinical outcomes in the sense that a notable dissimilarity will not affect clinical outcomes. Depending on the nature of testing output, if a numerical output is a result of a graphical output, a Tier 3 analysis of the graphical output must always be made; a fluorescence spectrum is tested on a Tier 3 level, and the maximum emission wavelength or its ratio with 310 nm can be subjected to a Tier 2 level testing.

Figure 9.9 shows a typical example of data presented graphically to demonstrate similarity.

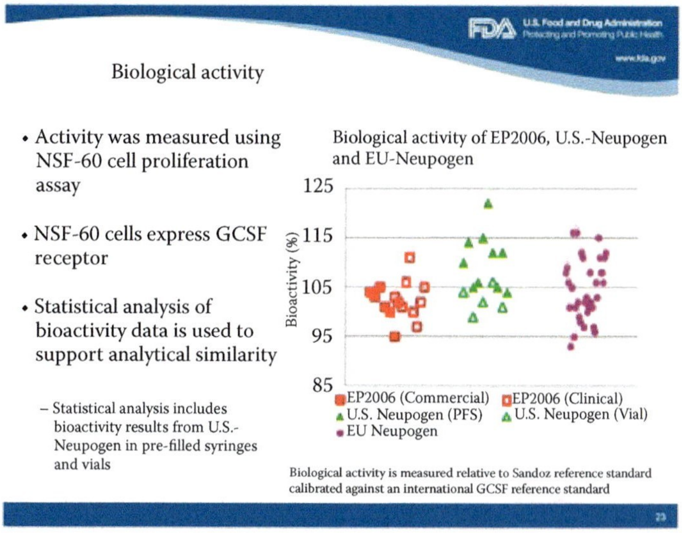

Figure 9.6 Statistical tier testing of biological activity of filgrastim. (From http://www.fda.gov/downloads/AdvisoryCommittees/CommitteesMeetingMaterials/Drugs/OncologicDrugsAdvisoryCommittee/UCM428780.pdf)

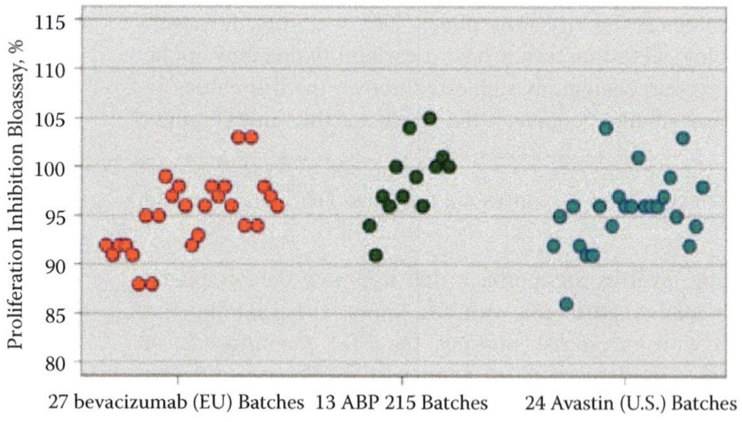

Figure 9.7 Scatter plots of proliferation bioassay for U.S.-licensed Avastin, ABP215, and EU-approved bevacizumab. (From https://www.fda.gov/downloads/AdvisoryCommittees/CommitteesMeetingMaterials/Drugs/OncologicDrugsAdvisoryCommittee/UCM566365.pdf)

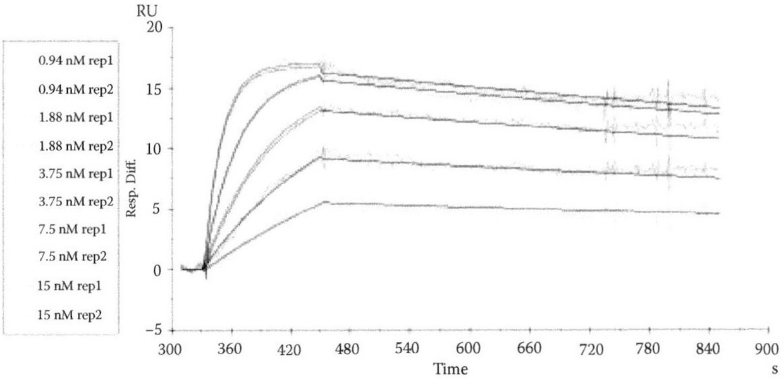

Figure 9.8 Receptor binding (surface plasmon resonance) that showed that the test product values for a filgrastim product were within 2*SD of the reference product as the quality range or Tier 2 testing. (From http://www.fda.gov/downloads/AdvisoryCommittees/CommitteesMeetingMaterials/Drugs/OncologicDrugsAdvisoryCommittee/UCM428780.pdf))

9.4.1.1 Examples of analytical similarity test protocols

Given below are three listings of the analytical similarity testing plans for cytokines like filgrastim and insulin and monoclonal antibodies like bevacizumab. There is enough information here to allow creating analytical similarity criteria for any biosimilar product. For summary purposes:

- Tier 1 means $-1.5\ \sigma R < 90\%$ C.I. of $(\mu T - \mu R) < 1.5\ \sigma_R$
- Tier 2 means % of the test results within $\hat{\mu}_R \pm 3.0\ \hat{\sigma}_R$
- Tier 3 means similar by visual comparison

9.5 How similar is similar?

Prior to conducting a formal analytical similarity study, the biosimilar product developer will set acceptance criteria for the study; every CQA will be assigned a criticality, a tier level, and the limits of acceptance, whether equivalence interval or quality range. The visual analysis of graphical presentation will be universal that there are no new or missing peaks or attributes. A keen understanding of statistical modeling is required to make sure the study does not fail for mathematical reasons. For example, the FDA may allow the protein content to be evaluated at 85.2% CI if measures can be placed to reduce the variation in protein

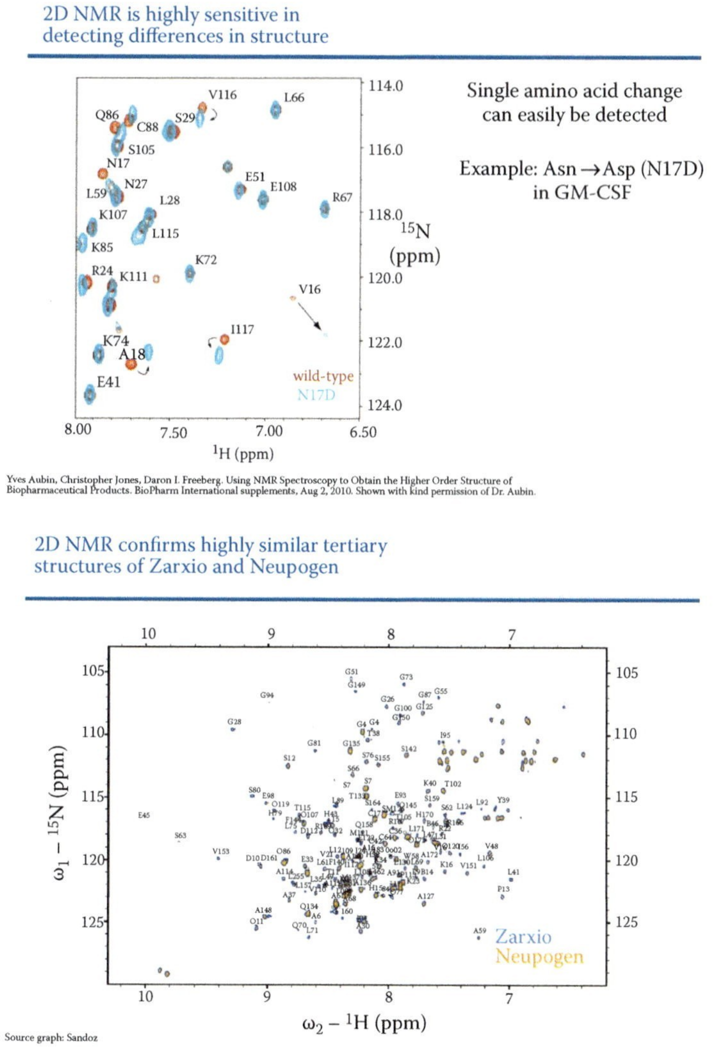

Figure 9.9 2D NMR spectra of test and reference product are showing graphical similarity. (From http://www.fda.gov/downloads/AdvisoryCommittees/CommitteesMeetingMaterials/Drugs/OncologicDrugsAdvisoryCommittee/UCM428780.pdf)

content; however, this equivalence testing interval modification may not apply to bioactivity that is more related to the cell line character rather than the process; however, in the case of products undergoing PTM, the bioactivity may also be managed in the manufacturing process, and therefore, the developer may test several Tier 1 attributes at a lower alpha value. How similar is similar is determined by the totality of evidence—taking into account both critical as well as noncritical attributes.

Table 9.2 Analytical Similarity Assessment Criteria and Tier Assignments for Filgrastim

Quality Attribute	Acceptance Criteria	Methodology	Statistical Tier Model
Identity: primary structure, total mass compared to theoretical mass 18,799 Da	100% of the mass values are within 18,799–18,800 Da.	Determination of filgrastim intact mass by LC-MS	No variation
Identity: primary structure, specific binding to antibody	The graphical representation shows positive identification of filgrastim.	Analysis of filgrastim by Western blotting	3
Identity: primary structure, position of disulfide bond	The graphical display identifies the correct location of two disulfide bonds.	Filgrastim disulfide linkages using peptide mapping with LC-MS[#]	No variation
Identity: primary structure; total amino acid sequence	Amino acid sequence completely matches theoretical sequence.	Mass spectrometry	No variation
Identity: primary structure (G2+G3, G4, G5)	90% of the total mass values are within the range $\mu_R \pm 3\sigma_R$.	Peptide mapping of filgrastim using RP-HPLC-MS	3
Identity: isoelectric point	$-1.5\sigma_R \leq$90% CI of $[\mu_T - \mu_R] \leq 1.5\sigma_R$	Analysis of filgrastim by cIEF	1
Identity and purity: reduced and nonreduced SDS-PAGE	The gels show similar migration patterns and intensity of all bands.	Analysis of filgrastim by using SDS-PAGE	3
Receptor binding (EC_{50})	90% of the EC_{50} values are within the range $\mu_R \pm 3\sigma_R$.	Enzyme-linked immunosorbent assay (ELISA) to determine receptor binding activity of filgrastim	2
Receptor binding (binding constants)	90% of the binding parameters are within the range of $\mu_R \pm 3\sigma_R$.	Characterization of the interaction of filgrastim with its receptor using the Biacore X100	2
Bioactivity	$-1.5\sigma_R \leq$ 90% CI of $[\mu_T - \mu_R] \leq 1.5\sigma_R$.	Filgrastim potency determination with rh-GCSF adapted M-NFS-60 cells	1
Content: filgrastim concentration	$-1.5\sigma_R \leq$ 90% CI of $[\mu_T - \mu_R] \leq 1.5\sigma_R$.	Determination of filgrastim concentration by UV absorbance spectroscopy	1
Content: filgrastim concentration	$-1.5\sigma_R \leq$90% CI of $[\mu_T - \mu_R] \leq 1.5\sigma_R$.	Protein concentration determination by RP-HPLC for filgrastim	1
Identity: tertiary structure	90% of the signal parameters are within the range $\mu_R \pm 3\sigma_R$.	Characterization of filgrastim solutions by one-dimensional proton nuclear magnetic resonance spectroscopy	2
Identity, tertiary structure: $310/\lambda_{max}$	Spectra are superimposable in shape with similar emission maxima.	Evaluation of filgrastim fluorescence spectrum	3

(*Continued*)

Table 9.2 (Continued) Analytical Similarity Assessment Criteria and Tier Assignments for Filgrastim

Quality Attribute	Acceptance Criteria	Methodology	Statistical Tier Model
Identity, higher order structure: melting temperature	90% of the melting point values are within the range $\mu_R \pm 3\sigma_R$.	Evaluation of filgrastim melting temperature using DSC differential scanning calorimetric system	2
Identity, secondary structure: P1/P2 helical content	90% of the helical content values are within the range $\mu_R \pm 3\sigma_R$.	Evaluation of the secondary structure of filgrastim using the Jasco J-815 circular dichroism spectropolarimeter	2
Identity, tertiary structure	The graphical representation shows highly similar spectral characteristics.	Evaluation of the tertiary structure of filgrastim using circular dichroism spectropolarimeter	3
Purity: total and single largest impurity	90% of impurities are $\leq \mu_R + 3\sigma_R$.	Determination of filgrastim purity by RP-HPLC	2
Purity: variants, acidic and basic	90% of the variants are within the range $\mu_R \pm 3\sigma_R$.	Determination of filgrastim related protein impurities by cation exchange chromatography	2
Safety: host cell proteins	90% of the host cell protein values are $\leq \mu_R + 3\sigma_R$.	Enzyme-linked immunosorbent assay (ELISA) for the determination of residual *E. coli* proteins in filgrastim	2
Safety: host cell DNA	90% of the host cell DNA values are $\leq \mu_R + 3\sigma_R$.	Residual DNA testing	2
Purity: aggregate and total high molecular weight impurities and largest single impurity	90% CI of $[\mu_T - \mu_R] \leq 1.5\sigma_R$.	Determination of filgrastim purity by SE chromatography	1

Source: From http://www.fda.gov/downloads/AdvisoryCommittees/CommitteesMeetingMaterials/Drugs/OncologicDrugsAdvisoryCommittee/UCM428780.pdf.

9.5.1 Fingerprint-like similarity

The FDA has yet to articulate fully its expectations of the level of fingerprint-like similarity. And none should be expected either since this will always be a case-by-case evaluation. Generally, the fingerprint-like similarity should be considered a continuous process, a step-by-step process to demonstrate similarity. For some cytokines where posttranslational modifications are not involved, it will be possible to demonstrate that all CQAs are entirely within the range of variation of the reference product and, therefore, the biosimilar product is fingerprint-like similar. The reward for this level of similarity demonstration is a reduced burden to demonstrate effectiveness, safety, and immunogenicity in patients. The minimum entry level is "highly similar," and in some instances, a "fingerprint-like similar" may reduce the cost and time of product development. In deciding what is critical, the FDA insists on establishing that the attributes that differ have no clinically meaningful difference—that may be challenging in some situations, and the path to modifying the process to bring the product

Table 9.3 Analytical Similarity Assessment Criteria and Tier Assignments for Insulin Products

Quality Attributes	Methodology	Similarity Acceptance Criteria	Tier
Assay	Protein concentration by RP-HPLC, USP method	$-1.5\ \sigma_R < 90\%$ C.I. of $(\mu_T - \mu_R) < 1.5\ \sigma_R$	1
Bioactivity	Bioactivity by USP Method	$-1.5\ \sigma_R < 90\%$ C.I. of $(\mu_T - \mu_R) < 1.5\ \sigma_R$	1
Receptor binding	Receptor binding by ELISA insulin receptor	90% of the test results within $\hat{\mu}_R \pm 3.0\,\hat{\sigma}_R$	2
	Receptor binding affinity IR-A, IR-B, and IGF1R)	90% of the test results of kinetic constants within $\hat{\mu}_R \pm 3.0\,\hat{\sigma}_R$	2
	Receptor activation (autophosphorylation)	90% of the test results of kinetic constants within $\hat{\mu}_R \pm 3.0\,\hat{\sigma}_R$	2
	Receptor binding by SPR with Biacore X100	90% of the test results of kinetic constants within $\hat{\mu}_R \pm 3.0\,\hat{\sigma}_R$	2
Metabolic activity	Metabolic activity (lipogenesis assay/ glucose incorporation assay)	90% of the test results of kinetic constants within $\hat{\mu}_R \pm 3.0\,\hat{\sigma}_R$	2
Bioactivity	Proliferative activity in IGF1R deficient and overexpressed cell lines.	90% of the test results of kinetic constants within $\hat{\mu}_R \pm 3.0\,\hat{\sigma}_R$	2
Size variants	SE-HPLC	90% of the test results within $\hat{\mu}_R \pm 3.0\,\hat{\sigma}_R$ for % total high molecular weight species (HMW)	2
Product-related impurities: charged species	CEX-HPLC	90% of the test results within $\hat{\mu}_R \pm 3.0\,\hat{\sigma}_R$ for % total charge variants	2
Ionization pattern	ESI-Q-TOF-MS	Comparison of three main ionization states: 1011 m/z (+6), 1213 m/z (+5), and 1516 m/z (+4)	2
Product-related impurities	RP-HPLC	90% of the test results within $\hat{\mu}_R \pm 3.0\,\hat{\sigma}_R$ for % total impurities. Presence of one peak; two degradation products upon thermal degradation	2
Secondary and higher order structure	Thermal unfolding melting point (DSC)	Thermograms similar by visual comparison, around 81°C	3
Secondary structure	Far-UV circular dichroism	Far-UV spectra similar by visual comparison.	3
Secondary structure	FTIR	Matching spectrum by visual comparison	3
Tertiary structure	Intrinsic fluorescence emission	Fluorescence emission spectrum similar by visual comparison	3
	Near-UV circular dichroism	Spectrum similar by visual comparison	3

(*Continued*)

Table 9.3 (Continued) Analytical Similarity Assessment Criteria and Tier Assignments for Insulin Products

Quality Attributes	Methodology	Similarity Acceptance Criteria	Tier
Primary structure: amino acid sequencing	Full sequence by peptide mapping with trypsin digestion and LC-MS/MS	Sequence matching at >95 % coverage. Detection of all the expected peptides according to the theoretical sequence*	3
	N-terminal sequencing by automated Edman degradation	N-terminal sequence matching based on published sequence 100%	3
	C-terminal sequencing by LC-MS/MS	C-terminal sequence matching based on published sequence 100%	3
	Intact mass by LC/MS	6,062.82 ±1 Da	3
	Amino acid composition	Matching composition 100%	3

Chain/Amino acids	Theoretical molecular weight (Da)	Amino acid sequence
A/1–21	2553.0644	GIVEQCCTSICSLYQLENYCG
B/1–23	2600.2628	FVNQHLCGSHLVEALYLVCGER
B/23–29	858.4276	GFFYTPK
B/1–30	6440.6798	FVNQHLCGSHLVEALYLVC GERGFFY TPKT

Quality Attributes	Methodology	Similarity Acceptance Criteria	Tier
Primary structure: disulfide bond integrity	Peptide mapping with LC-MS/MS of disulfide bonds in reduced and nonreduced condition	Matching location and number of disulfide bonds (two bands in reducing condition; one band in nonreducing condition)	3
Primary structure: free thiol	Reactivity with a fluorescent probe	Similar amount of free thiol (90–110% of reference)	3
Identity	SDS-PAGE with silver staining (nonreduced)	Matching principal band by visual comparison	3
	Western blot	Matching principal band and no new bands by visual comparison	3
	Isoelectric focusing point (pI=6.88)	Matching pI value (90–110% of reference)	3
Product-related impurities: deamidation	SDS-PAGE (Coomassie blue stain)	Matching principal band by visual comparison	3
UV exposure degradation (proprietary protocol)	RP-HPLC profile after exposure to 274 nm for 15, 30, and 60 min	Matching profile by visual comparison for all treatments	3
Subvisible particles	Light obscuration <787> USP method: subvisible particular matter in therapeutic proteins	Average number of particles ≥ 10 μm: NMT 6000 per container Average number of particles ≥25 μm: NMT 600 per container Subvisible particulates in the 2–10 μm range: report results	3

Table 9.4 Analytical Similarity Assessment Criteria and Tier Assignments for Bevacizumab, as an Example of Monoclonal Antibodies

Quality Attribute	Methods (Statistical Tier for testing analytical similarity with U.S.-Licensed Avastin)
Primary Structure	• Intact molecular mass by electrospray ionization time-of-flight mass spectrometry (ESI-TOF-MS) (Tier 3) • Reduced and deglycosylated molecular mass of heavy and light chains (ESI-TOF-MS) (Tier 3) • Amino acid analysis by reduced peptide mapping with ultraviolet (UV) and liquid chromatography (LC)-MS/MS (Tier 3) • Disulfide structure using nonreduced and reduced peptide mapping LC-MS (Tier 3)
Protein content	• Concentration by UV280 absorbance (Tier 1)
Higher order structure	• FTIR spectroscopy (Tier 3) • Near UV circular dichroism (Tier 3) • Differential scanning calorimetry (Tier 3)
Size variants/aggregates	• Size exclusion chromatography (SE-HPLC) (UV detection) (Tier 2) • SE-HPLC-static light scattering (SE-HPLC-SLS) (Tier 3) • Dynamic light scattering (DLS) (Tier 3) • Field flow fractionation (FFF) (Tier 3) • Analytical ultracentrifugation sedimentation velocity (AUC-SV) (Tier 3) • Capillary electrophoresis (CE)-SDS (reduced and nonreduced) (Tier 3)
Charge	• Capillary isoelectric focusing (cIEF) (Tier 3) • Cation exchange chromatography (CEX-HPLC) (Tier 3)
Glycosylation	• Afucosylation (Tier 3) • Galactosylation (Tier 3) • High mannose (Tier 3) • Sialic Acid (Tier 3)
Potency	• Inhibition of human umbilical vein endothelial cell (HUVEC) proliferation bioassay (Tier 1)
Binding assay VEGFA 165	• ELISA (Tier 3)
Binding assay and kinetics (VEGFA 111, 121, and 1651)	• Surface plasmon resonance (SPR) (Tier 3)
Binding assay-Fc	• FcRn (Alpha Screen) (Tier 3) • FcγRIa (AlphaLISA) (Tier 3) • FcγRIIa H type (SPR) (Tier 3) • FcγRIIb (SPR) (Tier 3) • FcγRIIIa V type and F type (AlphaLISA) (Tier 3) • FcγRIIIb (SPR) (Tier 3) • C1a (ELISA) (Tier 3)
Bioassay/specificity and cell-surface-associated VEGFA effects	• Specificity for VEGFA (VEGFR2 autophosphorylation in HUVEC) (Tier 3) • Absence of ADCC (cancer cell lines that secrete soluble V EGFA isoform with natural killer cell line) (Tier 3) • Absence of ADCC (cancer cell line that produces cell-surface-associated V EGFA isoform with peripheral mononuclear cells) (Tier 3) • Absence of CDC (cancer cell lines that secrete both soluble and cell-surface-associated VEGFA isoforms (Tier 3)

(*Continued*)

Table 9.4 (Continued) Analytical Similarity Assessment Criteria and Tier Assignments for Bevacizumab, as an Example of Monoclonal Antibodies

Quality Attribute	Methods (Statistical Tier for testing analytical similarity with U.S.-Licensed Avastin)
Subvisible particles	• Light obscuration (Tier 3) • Microfluid imaging (Tier 3)
Thermal degradation	• SE-HPLC (Tier 3) • rCE-SDS (Tier 3) • CEX-HPLC (Tier 3) • Potency (Tier 3)
General properties	• Deliverable volume (Tier 3) • Osmolality (Tier 3) • pH (Tier 3) • Appearance (Tier 3) • Color (Tier 3) • Clarity (Tier 3)

to the highest level of similarity may be a more practical approach. As an example, the ADCC values are relevant to the mode of action, but if these deviate significantly from the reference product, the FDA will be inclined to believe a difference in the process of manufacture that is significantly different; incidentally, the FDA requires the developers to match ADCC.

In establishing statistical testing limits, does the use of c=1.25 in Tier 1 make it more robust, or the use of X=2 makes a comparison more like a fingerprint? These questions can be addressed with the FDA, but generally demonstrating a closer value should augment the claim of fingerprint-like similarity. However, these choices should be made in a meaningful manner based on the various error levels and power calculations as described above. In all likelihood, meeting the similarity with narrower limits will be less significant than meeting across a larger number of orthogonal testing methods. The novelty of testing is an additional criterion to establish fingerprint-like similarity. Emerging trends in analytical methodologies may provide additional testing opportunities not generally involved in the release testing of biological products. For example, the author had established a fourth-dimensional thermodynamic testing (U.S. Patent Application 2014/0356968) that describes the behavior of protein molecules when stressed thermodynamically, and any blue or red shift in fluorescence or intensity of emission is related to the similarity of structure. This is an expanding trend to introduce newer testing methodologies to convince the regulatory agencies of the level of similarity.

9.6 Specific analytical topics

There are several specific testing issues that need to be well understood; these are not related to the statistical modeling but present a unique challenge in data analysis.

9.6.1 Stability profile

The FDA expects the biosimilar product to be tested side by side both qualitatively and quantitatively, for the type of degradants as well as their levels. Two questions arise. First, it is generally not possible to source lots of reference products with similar production dates as the biosimilar product. Second, how much deviation is allowable from theoretical degradation rates based on declared shelf life of the product?

The biosimilar developer is required to provide data on at least three lots that may include development lots; it is desirable to place at least three lots of reference product on stability testing; also these reference lots should represent a wider range of the remaining shelf life. The stability study should be conducted for six months and linear regression coefficients of degradation obtained with the expectation of high statistical significance (r^2). The slopes of degradation rates are then compared with theoretical rates. For example, if the product has a shelf life of 36 months and the stability limit is no more than 3% degradation, then the theoretical slope of the regression line can be calculated. The biosimilar product may not have a higher degradation rate than predicted theoretically, even if the reference product demonstrates a higher rate resulting in the reference product not meeting a projected expiration dating. Figure 9.10

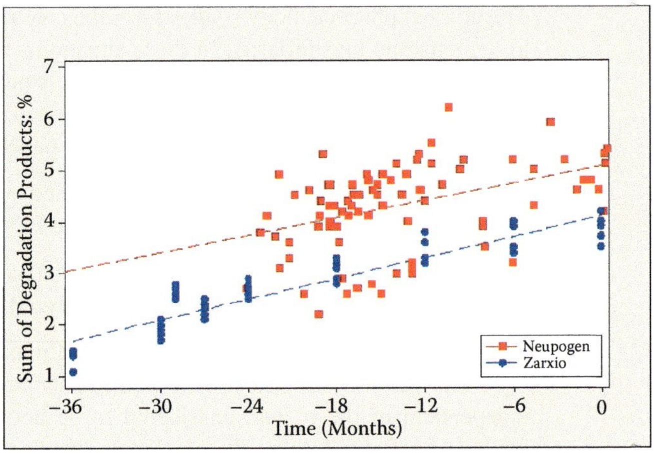

Figure 9.10 Display of stability data for test and reference products; the relative slope of the lines establishes similarity. Note that while full shelf-life data are presented for the test product, the reference product data will likely be limited by the inability to finder older lots from the market. (From http://www.fda.gov/downloads/AdvisoryCommittees/CommitteesMeetingMaterials/Drugs/OncologicDrugsAdvisoryCommittee/UCM428780.pdf)

shows what a typical stability data comparison will look like in a graphical representation.

9.6.2 HCP and residual DNA

When a new product is developed, the allowable limits of host cell proteins (HCP) and residual DNA are decided by demonstrating the feasibility of lowering this negative attribute, the relative safety risk of the specific products, and the measures in place to monitor these. Both HCP and residual DNA are organism strain dependent, so even if the biosimilar developer is using the same expression system, there is no possibility of matching the exact strain of the originator. Since the HCP and residual DNA are specific to the strain, a direct comparison of the relative safety of a biosimilar product is not possible, short of conducting complete safety studies evaluating these attributes. The FDA requires a critical analysis of HCP and residual DNA and accepts the fact that these may not be similar to the HCP and residual DNA in the originator product; a 2D SDS is also recommended to resolve these components for both the test and reference product. How does one then claim a similarity between the HCP and residual DNA between the test and the originator product?

While it is accurate that the HCP and residual DNA in the two products may not be the same, if the same expression system is used (e.g., *E. coli*), then there is a good likelihood that the safety will be proportional to the quantity of these components, notwithstanding any specific activity associated with any particular component. It is, therefore, possible for the test product to demonstrate a non-inferiority test evaluation using a Tier 2 approach.

The clinical pharmacology studies form the core of the required studies to demonstrate biosimilarity. In those situations, where a pharmacodynamic model exists in healthy subjects, these studies can be combined; for example, filgrastim has an excellent pharmacodynamic model that is better represented in healthy subjects than in patients.

When data are collected using a U.S.-licensed or EU-approved reference, a bridging study is recommended by the FDA (Figure 9.11).

To evaluate the bridging potential, a method that has recently come under FDA review as not necessary, the data are analyzed as shown in Table 9.5.

The statistical analysis of the total AUC and Cmax is conducted according to a Tier 1 basis wherein the equivalence acceptance criterion is independent of the σ_R and considered to be between 80% and 120% for log-transformed data. This applies to standard evaluation; in those instances where the coefficient of variation is very large, such as over 30–40%, the FDA allows the use of scaled average bioequivalence testing, wherein α_R is used to establish the EAC.

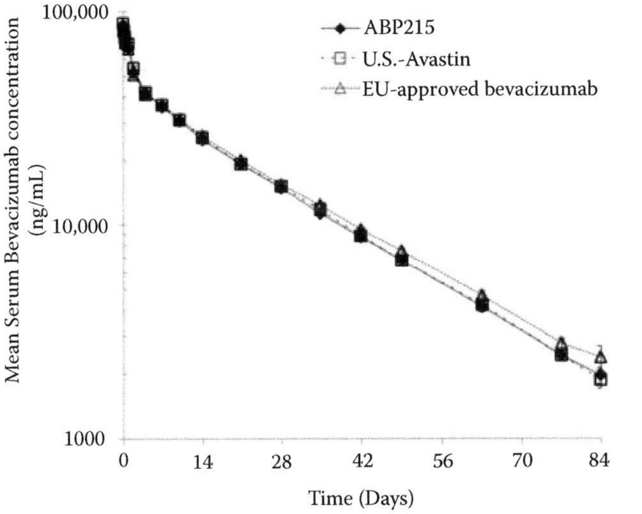

Figure 9.11 Pharmacokinetic profiles following 3 mg/kg single intravenous injection of bevacizumab in healthy subjects. (From https://www.fda.gov/downloads/AdvisoryCommittees/CommitteesMeetingMaterials/Drugs/OncologicDrugsAdvisoryCommittee/UCM566365.pdf)

Table 9.5 Pharmacokinetic Parameter Evaluation of Bevacizumab Biosimilar

	Geometric Mean Ratio (90% CI)		
Comparison	C_{Max}	AUC_{0-t}	AUC_{0-inf}
ABP215 vs U.S.-Avastin	98.1 (93.7–102.8)	98.3 (94.0–102.9)	98.3 (94.0–102.9)
ABP215 vs EU-bevacizumab	102.9 (98.2–107.8)	95.6 (91.3–100.0)	95.6 (91.3–100.0)
U.S.-Avastin vs EU-bevacizumab	104.9 (100.1–109.9)	97.2 (92.8–101.7)	97.2 (92.8–101.7)

Source: FDA analysis of data from the Applicant's 351(k) BLA submission https://www.fda.gov/downloads/AdvisoryCommittees/CommitteesMeetingMaterials/Drugs/OncologicDrugsAdvisoryCommittee/UCM566365.pdf

Where a pharmacodynamic model is available, a direct comparison of treatment emergent adverse events is made by calculating the 95% confidence interval for the difference in proportions:

$$P1 - P2 \pm Z_{\alpha/2} * SE,$$

where SE is the pooled standard error of P1–P2, which is given by

$$SE = \sqrt{\frac{P1(1-P1)}{N1} + \frac{P2(1-P2)}{N2}}.$$

For each AE, P1, P2, Diff =P1–P2, SE, and Lower CI bound and Upper CI bound are calculated and graphically presented as the difference between P1 and P2.

9.7 Concluding remarks

Presenting analytical similarity data to the FDA requires a clear understanding of the relative importance of each test, how it is conducted, and a discussion of any variability. Note the differences observed and how they are overcome by other attributes leading to the conclusion that there is no clinically meaningful difference.

9.8 Glossary of terms and concepts

The FDA provides details of several statistical approaches; the glossary given here provides a clarity of definition of these terms.

9.8.1 Significance level (also called size of a test) and error types

The size of a test, often called the significance level, is the probability of committing a Type I error (Table 9.6). A Type I error occurs when a null hypothesis is rejected when it is true. This test size is denoted by α (alpha). The $1-\alpha$ is called the confidence level, which is used in the form of the $(1-\alpha)*100$ percent confidence interval of a parameter.
The risk evaluation is based on a trade-off between the FDA risk and the developer's risk based on error types (Table 9.6).

9.8.2 Confidence level

Confidence level refers to the percentage of all possible samples that can be expected to include the true population parameter. For example, suppose all possible samples were selected from the same population, and a confidence interval was computed for each sample. A 90% confidence level implies that 90% of the confidence intervals would include the true population parameter. The confidence level can be lowered in

Table 9.6 Risks in Equivalence Demonstration

Reality of Attribute	Conclusions about Attribute	Description
Not similar	Similar	Type I error: patient (or FDA) risk (α)
Similar	Not similar	Type II error: developer's risk (β)
Similar	Similar	Power ($1-\beta$)

some instances, and in the literature reports, the lowest confidence level that the FDA had used to evaluate analytical similarity was 81.4%; the FDA also used 85.2% level. There are specific circumstances for these choices as will be discussed later in this chapter.

The FDA suggests using a 90% confidence interval of the difference between the means of the test and reference products to lie within the equivalence interval limits based on $1.5^*\sigma_R$ in a Tier 1 testing; what happens if the product does not meet this test? If the CQA fails, the test is related to process parameters, not the product parameters; for example, the protein content will be a process parameter since this can be adjusted in a process that is better controlled, but the potency, which is calculated on the basis of quantity, is a product-related CQA that cannot be adjusted without making a significant alteration in the expression of proteins—the latter cannot be a subject of consideration. For process-related CQAs, the testing limits can be adjusted to bring it within the limits to be made part of controls in the manufacturing of the product. What should be the smaller confidence level used to establish equivalence?

Very clearly, the choice of confidence level will have to be justified on the basis of the criticality of the attribute and a detailed plan for controlling the attribute to bring it to 90% level through manufacturing process controls.

9.8.2.1 Confidence interval

Confidence interval expresses the degree of uncertainty associated with a sample statistic. A confidence interval is an interval estimate combined with a probability statement. For example, suppose an analysis allows computation of an interval estimate; a confidence level will be used to describe uncertainty associated with the interval estimate. One may describe the interval estimate as a "90% confidence interval." This means that if we used the same sampling method to select different samples and computed an interval estimate for each sample, we would expect the true population parameter to fall within the interval estimates 90% of the time.

9.8.3 Statistical power

The statistical power is a function of the sample size, the effect size, and the probability level chosen (Figure 9.12).

9.8.4 Population vs. sample

The size (n) of a statistical sample affects the standard error for that sample. Because n is in the denominator of the standard error formula, the standard error decreases as n increases. The FDA requires developers to select a specific number based on variability to establish a reasonable standard deviation.

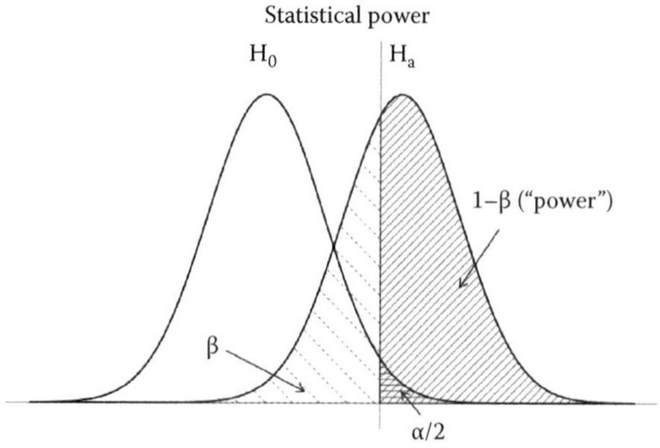

Figure 9.12 Statistical power of test.

9.8.5 Equivalence interval

This is an interval established based on the variability of the reference product, such as $1.5^*\sigma_R$; the σ value is derived from an independent set of reference lots. The 90% CI for the difference of means of the test and reference product (separate lots tested side by side) should reside within the equivalence interval.

9.8.6 Quality range

This is a range established based on the standard deviation of the reference product, $X^*\sigma_R$ side by side; the majority of values of the test product are expected to fall within this range; this will likely be 90% of values, and the X value will be 3, but the developer will have to justify this range.

9.8.7 One sample

Each lot contributes one value for each attribute being assessed. This condition, in essence, ignores any lot-to-lot variability of both the reference product and the proposed biosimilar product; the difference between means; and the inflation/deflation in variability between the reference product and the proposed biosimilar product. However, this is allowed by intention. Some researchers have criticized it mainly because of their lack of understanding of GMP considerations. In Tier 1 and Tier 2 testing, the standard deviation of the reference product is obtained from one lot contributing one value and not multiple samples from the same lot because if the lot is released, it is expected to have statistical compliance with within-lot variability; a similar assumption is made for the test product. This fine point is missed by commentators who are not fully familiar with GMP manufacturing aspects, and several suggestions have been made including testing multiple samples from each lot; using the lower of the 95% confidence limit of standard deviations; or using a Bayesian approach with appropriate choices of priors for the mean and standard deviation of the reference product in order to take into consideration the heterogeneity of mean and variability. The Bayesian approach is to obtain a Bayesian creditable interval, which will consider EAC for the assessment of analytical similarity. None of these are required by the FDA and unless the FDA changes its stance, none of these considerations are needed.

9.8.8 Orthogonal testing

At times, the developer will use two different tests to confirm an attribute; a good example is the protein content where it is measured by UVAS and RPHPLC methods. The question arises, what if the test fails in one and meets in the other? The FDA has not provided any clear guidance. However, generally, the protein content issue can be resolved, as the FDA suggested in its review of EP2006, through manufacturing controls, so the developer may want to test if the attribute passes at a lower confidence interval, say 81.4%. If that is true, then the test may be considered as passing since an orthogonal method is supporting similarity.

9.8.9 Replicates

It is recommended that the same number of replicates be performed within each proposed biosimilar lot as within each reference product lot and that the same lots be used for equivalence testing, quality range testing, and visual assessment of graphical displays.

9.8.10 Equal number side by side

There should be an equal number of lots when tested side by side; so if there are more lots available for reference, an unbiased selection should be made to select the equal number, and the rest can be used separately to develop the range acceptance criteria. This recommendation is challengeable once we demonstrate sufficient power of the test. If the number of samples of reference product is higher, this will lead to a smaller standard deviation and thus a larger difference range that may cause the test to fail because of β error. The critical minimum number of lots tested side by side is approximately 8; however, if there is an unbalanced selection between test and reference, a higher number may be required.

9.8.11 Side-by-side testing

The FDA recommends a side-by-side testing of the test and reference product in an equal number of lots and makes the Tier 1 and Tier 2 analysis by using the standard deviation derived from different lots of the reference product. Several questions arise. For those tests where the output is not numerical, and the comparison is made on the basis of overall similarity between the graphical output, should these comparisons be made with the reference product tested side by side or the different set of reference product? What if the reference product tested side by side does not match the reference product graphic output from a different set of lots tested earlier or with the lots tested side by side?

For comparison of graphical output where no numerical comparisons are made, it is preferred to use the reference product tested side by side; the data collected from the separate sets of lots are preferred over those tests that yield numerical data that have clinical relevance. However, if there are any testing-related anomalies found in the side-by-side testing, due to variability in testing, the developer should increase the number of lots and present the data on the basis of overall similarity.

9.8.12 Unbalanced samples

Samples of reference and test products are blinded prior to the testing of analytical similarity; if the reference samples to be tested are out of specification, these are to be removed from the statistical calculation, creating an unbalanced design since the FDA requires an equal number of samples of test and reference products to be tested side by side. How can this be resolved?

The developer should remove an equivalent number of test samples through a randomization process; this process must be presented in the analytical testing SOP and properly documented. It is important that if the reference product fails one attribute and is declared out of specification, other values drawn from that samples cannot be used, even if they are not affected by the out of specification reading for one attribute. This exercise will create a situation where the power of the test is reduced; to overcome this possibility, the biosimilar developer should try to start with a larger number of samples, such as 11 instead of 10, if the target is 10 samples. The developer may also adopt a procedure wherein the reference samples are tested prior to being blinded to avoid this situation. However, the selection and blinding of reference products must still be made on a random basis. A significant finding is that the briefing document released by the FDA on the approval of EP2006 shows that the test and reference samples were different in number and not all lots tested across for all attributes in the analytical similarity demonstration. The count of test samples and reference samples need not be the same as shown in where Tier 1 comparisons were made using ratios of reference/test ranging from 0.6 to 7. However, the agency discourages the use of unbalanced design in analytical similarity demonstration. One impact of the unbalanced design is a significant change in the statistical power of the test.

9.8.13 Different lots for EAC

The FDA suggests using a different set of lots to establish equivalence acceptance criteria (EAC), choosing a suitable number of lots based on the statistical acceptance criteria of the confidence interval for Tier 1 and Tier 2 testing. A valid hypothesis is not based on the sample to be used to test the hypothesis. Using the same lots tested to generate the EAC is a tautological logic that does not generate any productive information. This behavior is called "data fishing," which just hunts the model that best fits the sample, not the population. It is for this reason that the FDA recommends that the acceptance criteria be established using the separate lots of the reference product. However, where a numerical null hypothesis is not possible to establish a priori, this testing of separate lots can be omitted; the same argument will apply to those numerical data where legacy values or a published values (e.g., Briefing Documents [FDA] or EPARs [EMA]) are used as acceptance criteria such as molecular mass (non-PTM), amino acid sequence, disulfide bonds, and Western blot, where these attributes must be identical, not similar. It is highly recommended that the developer present to the FDA a comprehensive plan, in a Type II meeting, to determine and control the reference variability, σ_R. This may be a challenge when there are a limited number of lots available.

9.8.14 Declared attributes

For Tier 1 testing, if an attribute is declared on the label such as protein content, then a more robust approach is to use the mean value of the reference tested side by side and should be 100%, not the actual percentage of the reference lots.

9.8.15 Reference product variability

Whereas some primary structure attributes are well defined, how would the developer treat a sample of the reference product that does not meet the legacy attributes such as amino acid sequence (e.g., 1 out of 10 samples is not compliant) or the total degradants in the reference lots are above the release limits of the biosimilar product?

Since the primary structure attributes must be identical, not similar or highly similar, there is no variance allowed in the comparison exercise; if the reference product does not meet these attributes, then that specific lot would be labeled as out of specification and excluded from similarity demonstration exercise. The same principle applies to attributes for which a release criterion exists (those not requiring to be identical); the reference lots, in this case, will be excluded if they do not meet predetermined release criteria of the biosimilar product. Examples may include an out of specification impurity level or the formulation attributes.

9.8.16 Assay variability

Other aspects of the FDA understanding is that the high assay variability would not justify a large σ_R. In such a situation, the assay would need to be optimized, and/or the number of replicates increased to reduce variability. Also, in cases where the equivalence margins or quality ranges are too wide, it may be scientifically justified and appropriate to narrow the margins or range. In those cases where data do not follow a normal distribution, the developer may use nonparametric tolerance interval, but the large sample size is generally required.

The high assay variability would not justify a large σ_R. In such a situation, the assay would need to be optimized, and/or the number of replicates increased to reduce variability. What is considered a high variability that is acceptable is a difficult question to answer, but there are several guiding principles that can be applied. First, it involves instrumentation variability—can we use a better equipment? Second, it requires understanding what limit of the variability of CQA is acceptable—for example, many pharmacodynamic responses are highly variable by nature involving biological testing systems—the same applies to bioassays (Tier 1 testing) or binding assays (which will likely be Tier 2 tested). For example, if literature confirms, especially the reports from the originator data that the variability is ±30%, then that could be taken as the limit to achieve. The developers may also want to adopt tests other than those prescribed in the compendia (if so) or other routine methods of testing, and also adopt higher sensitivity and repeatability testing. There is no particular method that the FDA requires one to use, as long as it can be justified and demonstrated to be appropriate and suitable—later it can be validated if it is used for release purpose. (Note: Even though the guidance suggests that for analytical similarity demonstration, the methods must be suitable, the FDA may require validation, so be prepared and always remember that the FDA is never bound by its own guidance—this disclaimer is provided in every guidance document—read it and understand it.)

9.8.17 Margins and ranges

In cases where the equivalence margins or quality ranges are too wide, it may be scientifically justified and appropriate to narrow the margins or range. This position of the FDA creates a scientific challenge for the developer; this applies to both Tier 1 and Tier 2 testing. The scientific basis first comes from the lot release specification. For example, if the release specification calls for a smaller EAC, this should override a higher limit drawn from the testing of the reference product—this can happen, for example, if a few lots of the reference products have out of range values—whether these reference lots should be excluded is another consideration discussed below. The biosimilar developer should examine the legacy values, the known and accepted standards of variability, in determining the interval or range of a critical quality attribute.

9.8.18 Nonparametric

A nonparametric tolerance interval is available if data do *not* follow the normal distribution, but the large sample size is generally required.

9.8.19 Random lots

The FDA suggests that one sample is selected randomly from each lot for both the reference and the test. The fact is that the developer may not have the luxury of securing a sufficient number of originator lots to randomize the selection; the same may hold true for the test lots. Several publications have criticized that the differences between lots and heterogeneity among lots are major challenges to the validity of the FDA's proposed approaches for both equivalence testing for CQAs in Tier 1 and the concept of quality range CQAs from Tier 2. This is not entirely correct since released lots are supposed to have homogeneity, a concept that may be alien to many researchers who have criticized this approach. The FDA expects the lots of reference product used for establishing the acceptance criteria be selected on a random basis. Given the limited number of reference lots available to the developer, how does one assure this randomness? Also, how is the selection of the number of samples tested related to the confidence level used in a Tier 1 test?

In practice, it may be a challenge when there are a limited number of lots available. Thus, the FDA suggests the sponsor providing a plan for how the reference variability σ_R will be estimated with a justification. The developer may start with a larger number of lots of reference product and randomly select the desired number that will have to be justified on the basis of the power (probability of confidence interval within the limits).

9.8.20 Number of lots

The number of selected lots tested side by side will depend on three factors:

- *The power of testing accepted*; Figure 9.13 provides a correlation curve between power, confidence level, and the number of lots. Generally, like the bioequivalence testing, an 80% (0.80) power will be accepted.
- *Confidence level*; generally it is taken to be 5% giving a CL of 0.90, but the FDA has allowed testing at 0.814 and 0.852.
- *Standard deviation*; large standard deviations can be reduced either by increasing the number of lots or adjusting the analytical methods that are less variable.

With sample size ranging from 3 to 12 and with confidence level (CL) set to 0.814, 0.852, and 0.9, the probability (confidence interval within limits) (Power) will be ranging from 0.10596 to 0.97097 when testing

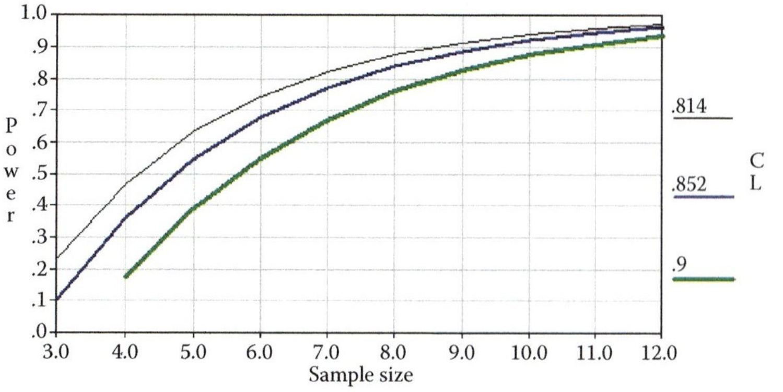

Figure 9.13 Power and sample size dependence at different alpha values.

the null hypothesis H_0: nonequivalence, with left equivalence limit = −1.5 and right equivalence limit = 1.5, against the alternative hypothesis H_1: mean 2 – mean 1 = 0.125 (equivalence). The test used is an equivalence test (confidence interval, a difference of means; *t*-distribution, two-sided CI). The calculation is based on the assumptions that the standard deviation is 1, and the sample size 2 / sample size 1 is 1. Note that confidence level is $(1\text{-}2\sigma) \times 100$. Generally 80% or a higher power will be sufficient to convince the FDA of the suitability of the number of lots selected. The choice of 0.814 and 0.852 confidence level was chosen in light of the FDA analysis of EP2006 using these confidence levels.

For all those attributes that must be tested using a Tier 1 approach, the developer needs to demonstrate equivalence at 90% confidence level to begin with; however, if the testing fails, the developer needs to demonstrate a reasonable confidence interval at which it would pass and then suggest a plan of controlling this variability during manufacturing operations, if it happens to be an attribute that can be controlled.

In practice, one of the major problems to a biosimilar sponsor is the availability of reference lots for analytical similarity testing. The FDA suggests that an appropriate sample size (the number of lots from the reference product and from the test product) be used for achieving the desired power (say 80%) to establish similarity based on a two-sided test at the 5% level of significance assuming that the mean response of the test product differs from that of the reference product by $\sigma_R/8$. Furthermore, because sample size is a function of α (type I error), β (type II error or 1 minus power), δ (treatment effect), and σ_2 (variability), it is a concern that we may have inflated the Type I error rate for achieving the desired power to detect a clinically meaningful effect size (adjusted for variability) with a preselected small sample size (i.e., a small number of lots).

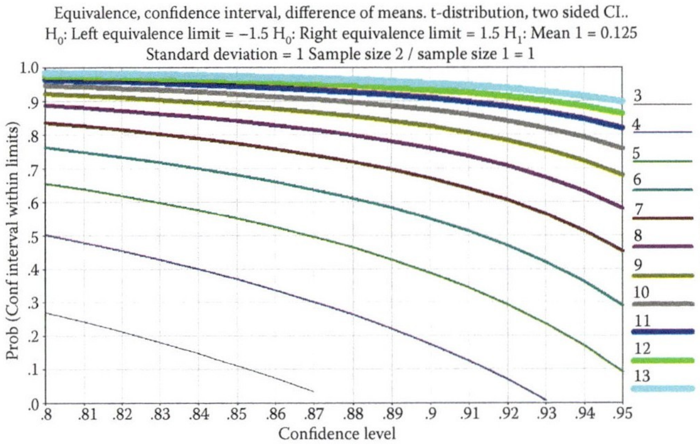

Figure 9.14 Probability that confidence interval is within limits as a function of confidence level and number of lots selected for side-by-side testing.

Figure 9.14 shows the power (probability of confidence interval within limits) as a function of sample size and the study size or the α value expressed as (1–2σ) × 100.

When seven lots are used side by side, the power drops to 67%. Generally, 80% or a higher power will be sufficient to convince the FDA of the suitability of the number of lots selected. The number of samples tested is also justified based on the confidence level used; for example, in the case if 81.4% or 85.2% is used, the number of samples required will change, as a minimum.

A significant concern arises when testing Tier 0 and Tier 3 attributes where no numerical calculations are required; in the case of Tier 0, all tested samples must either be identical to the reference product or meet the legacy value (e.g., total mass); for Tier 3, it is simply a display of numbers (where available) and an overall comparison of the shape and details of the graphical output. While one can argue that a smaller number of lots will be sufficient for this exercise, this concern becomes moot due to the fact that the FDA wants you to conduct all tests for the chosen test lots. The developer must present data for Tier 0 and Tier 3 testing for the same lots used for Tier 1 and Tier 2 testing.

9.8.21 Blinding

Prior to conducting the side-by-side analytical similarity testing, the biosimilar developer would create a protocol that will include all acceptance criteria as well as blind the test and reference samples; where a larger number of samples are available, this will be preceded by a random selection of lots. However, when establishing EAC or other acceptance attributes using a separate set of lots, there is no need for blinding the reference samples.

9.8.22 Degree of similarity

How similar is similar? Does being highly similar mean that all Tier 1 tests must meet? Does it mean that the α value can be lowered and the manufacturing process controlled to reduce the risk to patients (this is called the FDA risk)? Is there a degree of similarity in Tier 3 evaluations? How close is close? These are some of the key aspects that the developer would need to address in presenting the data. Know that the guidance by the FDA is merely a guidance, not an obligation by the FDA to follow this.

9.8.23 Legacy values

The CQAs that are the subject of analytical similarity can be classified into two categories: inherent and legacy attributes. Inherent attributes are those variable properties that are inherent in the manufacturing of the product that result in the lot-to-lot variability. This classification of attributes includes both process- and product-related factors. A good example will be all types of posttranslational modifications for both cytokines as well as antibodies. Legacy attributes are those characteristics that are not subject to a lot-to-lot variation and must be met essentially in their entirety. A good example of a legacy attribute is the total mass of a protein, its amino acid sequence, and other declared properties such as disulfide bonds, etc., that we widely and completely reported in several protein databanks, patents, and publications, as well as the pharmacopeia. Another category of legacy attributes is the labeled specification of inactive ingredients, the product characteristics such as pH, etc. Historically, we have established rational variance of these attributes, such as a range of content, a range of physical attributes, as well as the expected stability profiles.

Legacy attributes can be tested without reference to the originator product; the inherent attributes require a detailed evaluation of the originator product. Whereas the primary structural attributes must conform to established legacy values, a side-by-side testing of the test and reference product is required to assure that the test methods used are suitable for detecting any differences in these attributes. However, for these attributes the developer need not to develop acceptance criteria using a separate set of lots of the reference product.

9.8.24 Compendia specifications

Drug substance monographs of several biological products are provided in official compendia like EP, BP, and USP; compendia also provide acceptance criteria for attributes such as glycan distribution, isomers, and other structural variants. How much can the biosimilar product developer rely on compendia limits to develop release criteria and also use these values as legacy limits to demonstrate analytical and functional similarity?

The FDA has two concerns regarding the variability: first, the inherent variability in protein structures, and second, the variability introduced by the manufacturing process used by the biosimilar product developer. Whereas the compendial specifications for drug substance may be useful in extrapolating the specification for the drug product with regard to primary and higher-order attributes, the goal of demonstrating that the variability between the biosimilar product and the originator product is comparable can only be reached in a side-by-side testing. A good example is the level of protein content, which may be allowed a range of establishing ±5% for the release purpose, but for the analytical similarity demonstration, the difference in the mean of the test and originator product will be based on $1.5^*\sigma_R$. In the case of EP2006, the FDA reported the acceptance intervals to be 2.08–2.26%. The same applies to Tier 2 range testing, where the goal is to demonstrate a similar variability. As a result, it is entirely possible for the lots of the biosimilar product to meet all release specifications, yet fail in the analytical similarity demonstration. For example, the biosimilar product may use release criteria where total impurities are not more than 2% and no single impurity is more than 1%; however, if minor impurities are found in the biosimilar product, but not in the originator product, this may be a reason for failing similarity.

9.8.25 Mixed graphic and numerical data

Some testing provides a graphical output, but the values such as peak height and area under the peak curve can be quantitated. Should these data output be treated as numerical or graphical?

Whenever there is a graphical output, it should demonstrate no extraordinary peak, no extraordinary heights of the peaks, and no extraordinary baseline—this is an overall evaluation of the graphical output and applies to all tiers (1–3). However, peaks have known significance relating to potency, purity, and safety, and as a result, the quantifiable graphical attributes have clinical meaningfulness; these can be compared for Tier 1 and Tier 2 analysis. For Tier 3 testing, there is no further need to perform any quantitative evaluation. In this situation, the data analysis will be presented both as highly similar graphical presentation as well as a tier-sensitive equivalent interval or range. However, if the numerical comparisons do not have any clinical relevance, a graphical representation alone would be sufficient, regardless of the attribute.

9.8.26 Non-inferiority testing

There can be several situations where the attribute tested less desirable in Tier 1 and Tier 2 testing; the comparison test may fail if the TOST approach is used instead of one-sided testing or non-inferiority testing. How should these data be analyzed and interpreted?

The developer should define the attributes that are characterized in this category, such as level of aggregates, impurities adversely affecting activity or safety, degradation rate, HCP, residual DNA, etc., for which the acceptance criteria should be established to show non-inferiority. In the case of Tier 1, testing should be done with this model = $1.5*\sigma_R \leq 90\%$ CI $(\mu_T - \mu_R)$, and in Tier 2 testing, values outside the lower limits of $X*\sigma_R$ are excluded. The statistical power will increase in one-sided testing.

To make sure that the similarity testing does not fail where it is supposed to be not within the interval or range, but desirably higher or lower, the acceptance criteria can be developed accordingly. For some attributes, the test should be a non-inferiority testing and not a testing of equivalence. Examples of these tests would include the level of aggregates, potentially toxic or undesirable impurities, process-related impurities that impact negatively (e.g., tungsten level), and all other attributes where a lower level is preferred. These should be tested as $(\mu_T - \mu_R) \leq - c*\sigma_R$, where μ_T is the test product sample mean, μ_R is the reference product sample mean, and σ_R is the standard deviation of the reference product.

9.8.27 Use of public domain values

There may be situations where detailed information on reference product may be available in regulatory documents that are made public, in research publications, or in patent documents that will qualify as the population values of variation (σ_R). A good example is the EAC reported by the FDA for a filgrastim product in its ODAC Committee Meetings. Based on samples ranging from 12 to 39, this range represents in all likelihood the narrowest range; for protein content it was ±2.26% and ±2.08% for U.S. Neupogen; for bioassay, the EAC was ±9.26% in Tier 1 testing for the 90% CI for the difference in the mean.

A justification for using this approach can be that the reported data on the reference product are based on a larger number of lots with different expiry dates and thus provide a better sampling of the population standard deviation, increasing the reliability of the ranges established. This is more applicable to bioassays where the variation is likely going to be higher, and thus a larger number of samples are required to narrow down the standard deviation. However, the developer must also demonstrate that the test methods used are not providing any testing bias. One way to demonstrate this is to compare the 90% CI of the reference products tested side by side with the acceptance criteria established above; if that test passes, then there is strong justification for using this approach. This is a bridging study. However, for some tests where sample handling may contribute to variation such as stability testing, etc., publicly available data may not be used.

9.8.28 Testing across

The FDA recommends that all lots of the test products be tested for all attributes. Are there any situations where not all lots are tested for specific tests?

In reporting other attributes like bioassay as Tier 1, a different number of lots were used as reported in the Briefing Document, to analyze protein content, indicating that not all tests were conducted on the same lots. This is against the suggestions by the FDA that all similarity testing be done on all lots. This may be a subject of discussion with the FDA. One reason why a different number of lots for different tests may be admissible may have to do with the degree of variability in the test method and assays used. Generally, the FDA will want you to increase the number of test lots or improve the method of analysis where variation is high.

9.8.29 Combining lots

Biosimilar developer conducts several biosimilarity studies at different stages and accordingly conducts analytical and functional similarity testing. Can these lots be combined to provide a composite description instead of one study?

As reported by the FDA in its Briefing Report, data from different studies can be combined to produce the acceptance criteria and for testing as long as there is a bridging evidence between the sets of lots that were tested separately. The argument provided by the FDA is based on philosophical syllogism and goes as follows. If A=B, and B=C, then C must be equal to A. The EP2006 commercial was similar to EP2006 clinical, which was similar to both U.S. and EU Neupogen. Therefore, EP2006 must be highly similar to U.S. and EU Neupogen. However, the FDA may be changing its mind on this. It is not sure if this is the current expectation of the FDA. However, the FDA may change its mind as more data become available, so, to improve the power of testing, the developer may offer data with combined study lots.

9.8.30 Release criteria

One question that resonates in the mind of biosimilar developers relates to the importance of release testing. It is likely that a developer would use a different set of testing to establish analytical similarity than that used for release purpose, though inevitably some tests will overlap. However, the release criteria may not be used to establish analytical similarity since these ranges may be based on generally analytical standards; for example, it would be admissible to have a 10% variability in the content of drug for release purpose, but for similarity purpose, the developer must demonstrate the similarity with the variability in the reference product, lot to lot. That number may be significantly lower than 10%, so while all lots of a biosimilar product may pass release criteria, they may fail in analytical similarity testing.

Bibliography

Aapro MS. What do prescribers think of biosimilars? *Target Oncol.* 2012 Mar;7 Suppl 1:S51–5.

Araújo F, Cordeiro I, Teixeira F, Gonçalves J, Fonseca JE. Pharmacology of biosimilar candidate drugs in rheumatology: A literature review. *Acta Reumatol Port.* 2014 Jan–Mar;39(1):19–26. Review.

Azevedo VF. Biosimilars require scientifically reliable comparative clinical data. *Rev Bras Reumatol.* 2013 Feb;53(1):129–31.

Bickel PJ, Doksum K. *Mathematical Statistics: Basic Concepts and Selected Ideas*, Vol. I; 2007.

Casadevall N, Edwards IR, Felix T, Graze PR, Litten JB, Strober BE, Warnock DG. Pharmacovigilance and biosimilars: Considerations, needs and challenges. *Expert Opin Biol Ther.* 2013 Jul;13(7):1039–47.

Challand R, Gorham H, Constant J. Biosimilars: Where we were and where we are. *J Biopharm Stat.* 2014;24(6):1154–64.

Chow SC. Assessing biosimilarity and interchangeability of biosimilar products. *Stat Med.* 2013 Feb 10; 32(3):361–3.

Chow SC. *Biosimilars: Design and Analysis of Follow-on Biologics*. New York: Chapman & Hall/CRC Press, Taylor & Francis; 2013.

Chow SC. On assessment of analytical similarity in biosimilar studies. *Drug Des.* 2014;3:119.

Chow SC, Endrenyi L, Lachenbruch PA. Comments on the FDA draft guidance on biosimilar products. *Stat Med.* 2013 Feb 10; 32(3):364–9.

Chow SC, Hsieh TC, Chi E, Yang J. A comparison of moment-based and probability-based criteria for assessment of follow-on biologics. *J Biopharm Stat.* 2010 Jan; 20(1):31–45.

Chow SC, Liu JP. *Design and Analysis of Bioavailability and Bioequivalence Studies*, 3rd ed. New York: Chapman & Hall/CRC Press, Taylor & Francis; 2008.

Chow SC, Liu JP. Statistical assessment of biosimilar products. *J Biopharm Stat.* 2010 Jan;20(1):10–30.

Chow SC, Lu Q, Tse SK, Chi E. Statistical methods for assessment of biosimilarity using biomarker data. *J Biopharm Stat.* 2010 Jan; 20(1):90–105.

Chow SC, Wang J, Endrenyi L, Lachenbruch PA. Scientific considerations for assessing biosimilar products. *Stat Med.* 2013 Feb 10; 32(3):370–81.

Chow SC, Yang LY, Starr A, Chiu ST. Statistical methods for assessing interchangeability of biosimilars. *Stat Med.* 2013 Feb 10; 32(3):442–8.

Christi L. Overview of the regulatory pathway and FDA's guidance for the development and approval of biosimilar products in the US. Presented at the Oncologic Drugs Advisory Committee meeting; January 7, 2015; Silver Spring, MD.

Combe C, Tredree RL, Schellekens H. Biosimilar epoetins: An analysis based on recently implemented European medicines evaluation agency guidelines on comparability of biopharmaceutical proteins. *Pharmacotherapy.* 2005 Jul;25(7):954–62.

Davis R, Batur P, Thacker HL. Risks and effectiveness of compounded bioidentical hormone therapy: A case series. *J Womens Health (Larchmt).* 2014 Aug;23(8):642–8. doi: 10.1016/j.jaad.2011.08.034.

Dong X, Tsong Y, Shen M, Zhong J. Using tolerance intervals for assessment of pharmaceutical quality. *J Biopharm Stat.* 2015; 25(2):317–27.

Dranitsaris G, Amir E, Dorward K. Biosimilars of biological drug therapies: Regulatory, clinical and commercial considerations. *Drugs.* 2011 Aug 20;71(12):1527–36.

Dranitsaris G, Dorward K, Hatzimichael E, Amir E. Clinical trial design in biosimilar drug development. *Invest New Drugs.* 2013 Apr;31(2):479–87.

Drouet L. Low molecular weight heparin biosimilars: How much similarity for how much clinical benefit? *Target Oncol.* 2012 Mar;7 Suppl 1:S35–42.

Ebbers HC, van Meer PJ, Moors EH, Mantel-Teeuwisse AK, Leufkens HG, Schellekens H. Measures of biosimilarity in monoclonal antibodies in oncology: The case of bevacizumab. *Drug Discov Today*. 2013 Sep;18(17–18):872–9.

EMA, 2013: EMA Concept Paper on the need for a reflection paper on the statistical methodology for the comparative assessment of quality attributes in drug development. Available at http://www.ema.europa.eu/docs/en_GB/document_library/Scientific_guideline/2013/06/WC500144945.pdf

FDA 2015: Quality Considerations in Demonstrating Biosimilarity of a Therapeutic Protein Product to a Reference Product. Available at https://www.fda.gov/downloads/Drugs/GuidanceComplianceRegulatoryInformation/Guidances/UCM291134.pdf

FDA: Briefing Information for the January 7, 2015 Meeting of the Oncologic Drugs Advisory Committee (ODAC). Available at http://www.fda.gov/AdvisoryCommittees/CommitteesMeetingMaterials/Drugs/OncologicDrugsAdvisoryCommittee/ucm428779.htm

FDA: Committee Roster for the January 7, 2014 Meeting of the Oncologic Drugs Committee Roster for the January 7, 2014 Meeting of the Oncologic Drugs Advisory Committee (PDF—28 kb). Available at http://www.fda.gov/downloads/AdvisoryCommittees/CommitteesMeetingMaterials/Drugs/OncologicDrugsAdvisoryCommittee/UCM428777.pdf)

FDA: Final Agenda for the January 7, 2015 Meeting of the Oncologic Drugs Advisory Committee (ODAC) (PDF—29 kb). Available at http://www.fda.gov/downloads/AdvisoryCommittees/CommitteesMeetingMaterials/Drugs/OncologicDrugsAdvisoryCommittee/UCM431113.pdf

FDA: Final Meeting Roster for the January 7, 2015 Meeting of the Oncologic Drugs Advisory Committee (ODAC) (PDF—27 kb). Available at http://www.fda.gov/downloads/AdvisoryCommittees/CommitteesMeetingMaterials/Drugs/OncologicDrugsAdvisoryCommittee/UCM431115.pdf

FDA: Final Questions for the January 7, 2015 Meeting of the Oncologic Drugs Advisory Committee (ODAC) (PDF—26 kb). Available at http://www.fda.gov/downloads/AdvisoryCommittees/CommitteesMeetingMaterials/Drugs/OncologicDrugsAdvisoryCommittee/UCM431114.pdf

FDA: Guidance Compliance. Available at https://www.fda.gov/Drugs/GuidanceComplianceRegulatoryInformation/Guidances/default.htm

FDA: January 7, 2015: Oncologic Drugs Advisory Committee Meeting Announcement. Available at http://www.fda.gov/AdvisoryCommittees/Calendar/ucm426350.htm

FDA: Minutes for the January 7, 2015 Meeting of the Oncologic Drugs Advisory Committee (ODAC) (PDF—41 kb). Available at http://www.fda.gov/downloads/AdvisoryCommittees/CommitteesMeetingMaterials/Drugs/OncologicDrugsAdvisoryCommittee/UCM436385.pdf

FDA: Slides for the January 7, 2015 Meeting of the Oncologic Drugs Advisory Committee (ODAC) Available at http://www.fda.gov/AdvisoryCommittees/CommitteesMeetingMaterials/Drugs/OncologicDrugsAdvisoryCommittee/ucm431116.htm

FDA: Transcript for the January 7, 2015 Meeting of the Oncologic Drugs Advisory Committee (ODAC) (PDF—736 kb). Available at http://www.fda.gov/downloads/AdvisoryCommittees/CommitteesMeetingMaterials/Drugs/OncologicDrugsAdvisoryCommittee/UCM436387.pdf.

FDA ODAC 2015: https://www.pbwt.com/content/uploads/2016/09/20150107-ODAC-B1-01-FDA_Backgrounder.pdf

FDA: Webcast Information for the January 7, 2014 Meeting of the Oncologic Drugs Advisory Committee (PDF—43 kb). Available at http://www.fda.gov/downloads/AdvisoryCommittees/CommitteesMeetingMaterials/Drugs/OncologicDrugsAdvisoryCommittee/UCM428778.pdf.

FDA. Guidance on Bioavailability and Bioequivalence Studies for Orally Administrated Drug Products—General Considerations. Rockville, MD: Center for Drug Evaluation and Research, the US Food and Drug Administration; 2003.

Feagan BG, Choquette D, Ghosh S, Gladman DD, Ho V, Meibohm B, Zou G, Xu Z, Shankar G, Sealey DC, Russell AS. The challenge of indication extrapolation for infliximab biosimilars. *Biologicals.* 2014 Jul;42(4):177–83.

Fox A. Biosimilar medicines—New challenges for a new class of medicine. *J Biopharm Stat.* 2010 Jan;20(1):3–9.

García-Arieta A, Blázquez A. Regulatory considerations for generic or biosimilar low molecular weight heparins. *Curr Drug Discov Technol.* 2012 Jun 1;9(2):137–42.

Gascon P. Presently available biosimilars in hematology–oncology: G-CSF. *Target Oncol.* 2012 Mar;7 Suppl 1:S29–34.

Gecse KB, Khanna R, van den Brink GR, Ponsioen CY, Löwenberg M, Jairath V, Travis SP, Sandborn WJ, Feagan BG, D'Haens GR. Biosimilars in IBD: Hope or expectation? *Gut.* 2013 Jun;62(6):803–7.

Genazzani AA, Biggio G, Caputi AP, Del Tacca M, Drago F, Fantozzi R, Canonico PL. Biosimilar drugs: Concerns and opportunities. *BioDrugs.* 2007;21(6):351–6.

Gomollón F. Biosimilars: Are they bioequivalent? *Dig Dis.* 2014;32 Suppl 1:82–7.

Haidar SH, Davit B, Chen ML et al. Bioequivalence approaches for highly variable drugs and drug products. *Pharm Res.* 2008;25:237–41.

Hsieh TC, Chow SC, Yang LY, Chi E. The evaluation of biosimilarity index based on reproducibility probability for assessing follow-on biologics. *Stat Med.* 2013 Feb 10;32(3):406–14.

Iyer V, Maddux N, Hu L, Cheng W, Youssef AK, Winter G, Joshi SB, Volkin DB, Middaugh CR. Comparative signature diagrams to evaluate biophysical data for differences in protein structure across various formulations. *J Pharm Sci.* 2013 Jan;102(1):43–51.

Jelkmann W. Biosimilar epoetins and other "follow-on" biologics: Update on the European experiences. *Am J Hematol.* 2010 Oct;85(10):771–80.

Jeske WP, Walenga JM, Hoppensteadt DA, Vandenberg C, Brubaker A, Adiguzel C, Bakhos M, Fareed J. Differentiating low-molecular-weight heparins based on chemical, biological, and pharmacologic properties: Implications for the development of generic versions of low-molecular-weight heparins. *Semin Thromb Hemost.* 2008 Feb;34(1):74–85.

Kálmán-Szekeres Z, Olajos M, Ganzler K. Analytical aspects of biosimilarity issues of protein drugs. *J Pharm Biomed Anal.* 2012 Oct;69:185–95.

Kang SH. Avoiding ambiguity with the Type I error rate in non-inferiority trials. *J Biopharm Stat.* 2015.

Kang SH, Chow SC. Statistical assessment of biosimilarity based on relative distance between follow-on biologics. *Stat Med.* 2013 Feb 10;32(3):382–92.

Kang SH, Kim Y. Sample size calculations for the development of biosimilar products. *J Biopharm Stat.* 2014;24(6):1215–24.

Karalis V, Macheras P. Current regulatory approaches of bioequivalence testing. *Expert Opin Drug Metab Toxicol.* 2012 Aug;8(8):929–42.

Kessler M, Goldsmith D, Schellekens H. Immunogenicity of biopharmaceuticals. *Nephrol Dial Transplant.* 2006 Oct;21 Suppl 5:v9–12.

Krämer I. Pharmacy and pharmacology of biosimilars. *J Endocrinol Invest.* 2008 May;31(5):479–88.

Kuhlmann M, Covic A. The protein science of biosimilars. *Nephrol Dial Transplant.* 2006 Oct;21 Suppl 5:v4–8.

Lee JF, Litten JB, Grampp G. Comparability and biosimilarity: Considerations for the healthcare provider. *Curr Med Res Opin.* 2012 Jun;28(6):1053–8.

Li Y, Liu Q, Wood P, Johri A. Statistical considerations in biosimilar clinical efficacy trials with asymmetrical margins. *Stat Med.* 2013 Feb 10;32(3):393–405.

Liao JJ, Darken PF. Comparability of critical quality attributes for establishing biosimilarity. *Stat Med.* 2013 Feb 10;32(3):462–9.

Lin JR, Chow SC, Chang CH, Lin YC, Liu JP. Application of the parallel line assay to assessment of biosimilar products based on binary endpoints. *Stat Med.* 2013 Feb 10;32(3):449–61.

Locatelli F, Roger S. Comparative testing and pharmacovigilance of biosimilars. *Nephrol Dial Transplant.* 2006 Oct;21 Suppl 5:v13–6.

Lu Y, Zhang ZZ, Chow SC. Frequency estimator for assessing of follow-on biologics. *J Biopharm Stat.* 2014;24(6):1280–97.

Mellstedt H, Niederwieser D, Ludwig H. The challenge of biosimilars. *Ann Oncol.* 2008 Mar;19(3):411–9. Epub 2007 Sep 14.

Mellstedt H. [Biosimilar products--cheaper version of biological drugs. New possibilities within several therapeutic fields]. *Lakartidningen.* 2009 Jun 3–9;106(23):1563–6. Swedish.

Mikhail A, Farouk M. Epoetin biosimilars in Europe: Five years on. *Adv Ther.* 2013 Jan;30(1):28–40.

Miller KL, Lanthier M. Regulatory watch: Innovation in biologic new molecular entities: 1986–2014. *Nat Rev Drug Discov.* 2015 Feb;14(2):83.

Nandurkar H, Chong B, Salem H, Gallus A, Ferro V, McKinnon R; Australian Low-Molecular-Weight Heparin Biosimilar Working Group (ALBW). Low-molecular-weight heparin biosimilars: Potential implications for clinical practice. Australian Low-Molecular-Weight Heparin Biosimilar Working Group (ALBW). *Intern Med J.* 2014 May;44(5):497–500.

Owens DR, Landgraf W, Schmidt A, Bretzel RG, Kuhlmann MK. The emergence of biosimilar insulin preparations—A cause for concern? *Diabetes Technol Ther.* 2012 Nov;14(11):989–96.

Papamichael K, Van Stappen T, Jairath V, Gecse K, Khanna R, D'Haens G, Vermeire S, Gils A, Feagan BG, Levesque BG, Vande Casteele N. Pharmacological aspects of anti-TNF biosimilars in inflammatory bowel diseases. *Aliment Pharmacol Ther.* 2015 Nov;42(10):1158–69.

Parnham MJ, Schindler-Horvat J, Kozlović M. Non-clinical safety studies on biosimilar recombinant human erythropoietin. *Basic Clin Pharmacol Toxicol.* 2007 Feb;100(2):73–83.

Poh J, Tam KT. Registration of similar biological products—Singapore's approach. *Biologicals.* 2011 Sep;39(5):343–5.

Prugnaud JL. [Similarity of biotechnology-derived drugs: Regulatory framework and specificity]. *Ann Pharm Fr.* 2008 Aug;66(4):206–11.

Radtke MA, Augustin M. Biosimilars in psoriasis: What can we expect? *J Dtsch Dermatol Ges.* 2014 Apr;12(4):306–12.

Ranjan N, Mahajan VK, Misra M. Biosimilars: The 'future' of biologic therapy? *J Dermatolog Treat.* 2011 Dec;22(6):319–22.

Roger SD, Mikhail A. Biosimilars: Opportunity or cause for concern? *J Pharm Pharm Sci.* 2007;10(3):405–10.

Schellekens H. Assessing the bioequivalence of biosimilars. The Retacrit case. *Drug Discov Today.* 2009 May;14(9–10):495–9.

Schellekens H. The first biosimilar epoetin: But how similar is it? *Clin J Am Soc Nephrol.* 2008 Jan;3(1):174–8. Epub 2007 Dec 5.

Scotté F, Launay-Vacher V, Rey JB. Colony stimulating factors (CSF) biosimilars. Progress? *Target Oncol.* 2012 Mar;7 Suppl 1:S17–24.

Sharma B. Immunogenicity of therapeutic proteins. Part 1: Impact of product handling. *Biotechnol Adv.* 2007 May–Jun;25(3):310–7. Epub 2007 Jan 30.

Strober BE, Armour K, Romiti R, Smith C, Tebbey PW, Menter A, Leonardi C. Biopharmaceuticals and biosimilars in psoriasis: What the dermatologist needs to know. *J Am Acad Dermatol.* 2012 Feb;66(2):317–22.

Subramanyam M. Clinical development of biosimilars: An evolving landscape. *Bioanalysis.* 2013 Mar;5(5):575–86.

Tamilvanan S, Raja NL, Sa B, Basu SK. Clinical concerns of immunogenicity produced at cellular levels by biopharmaceuticals following their parenteral administration into human body. *J Drug Target.* 2010 Aug;18(7):489–98.

Tothfalusi L, Endrenyi L, Garcia Areta A. Evaluation of bioequivalence for highly-variable drugs with scaled average bioequivalence. *Clin Pharmacokinet.* 2009;48:725–43.

Tsou HH, Chang WJ, Hwang WS, Lai YH. A consistency approach for evaluation of biosimilar products. *J Biopharm Stat.* 2013;23(5):1054–66.

Vulto AG, Crow SA. Risk management of biosimilars in oncology: Each medicine is a work in progress. *Target Oncol.* 2012 Mar;7 Suppl 1:S43–9.

Warren JB. Generics, chemisimilars and biosimilars: Is clinical testing fit for purpose? *Br J Clin Pharmacol.* 2013 Jan;75(1):7–14.

Weise M, Kurki P, Wolff-Holz E, Bielsky MC, Schneider CK. Biosimilars: The science of extrapolation. *Blood.* 2014 Nov 20;124(22):3191–6.

Wiatr C. US biosimilar pathway unlikely to be used: Developers will opt for a traditional BLA filing. *BioDrugs.* 2011 Feb 1;25(1):63–7.

Woroń J, Kocić I. [The story of biosimilars—Chance or threat?]. *Pol Merkur Lekarski.* 2014 Nov;37(221):311–5. Review. Polish. PubMed PMID: 25546996.

Xu S, Barker K, Menon S, D'Agostino RB. Covariate effect on constancy assumption in noninferiority clinical trials. *J Biopharm Stat.* 2014;24(6):1173–89.

Yang J, Zhang N, Chow SC, Chi E. An adapted F-test for homogeneity of variability in follow-on biological products. *Stat Med.* 2013 Feb 10;32(3):415–23.

Yang LY, Lai CH. Estimation and approximation approaches for biosimilar index based on reproducibility probability. *J Biopharm Stat.* 2014;24(6):1298–311.

Yu LX. Bioinequivalence: Concept and definition. Presented at Advisory Committee for Pharmaceutical Science of the Food and Drug Administration; April 13–14, 2004; Rockville, MD.

Zajdel J, Zajdel R. Brand-name drug, generic drug, orphan drug. Pharmacological therapy with biosimilar drugs—Provision of due diligence in the treatment process. *Contemp Oncol (Pozn).* 2013;17(6):477–83.

Zhang A, Tzeng JY, Chow SC. Statistical considerations in biosimilar assessment using biosimilarity index. *J Bioequiv Availab.* 2013 Sep 2;5(5):209–14.

Zhang N, Yang J, Chow SC, Chi E. Nonparametric tests for evaluation of biosimilarity in variability of follow-on biologics. *J Biopharm Stat.* 2014;24(6):1239–53.

Zhang N, Yang J, Chow SC, Endrenyi L, Chi E. Impact of variability on the choice of biosimilarity limits in assessing follow-on biologics. *Stat Med.* 2013 Feb 10;32(3):424–33.

Zuñiga L, Calvo B. Biosimilars: Pharmacovigilance and risk management. *Pharmacoepidemiol Drug Saf.* 2010 Jul;19(7):661–9.

Chapter 10 Biosimilarity

The final frontier

You never really understand a person until you consider things from his point of view.

Harper Lee

10.1 Leadership

The FDA has taken a leading role to a suggest novel analytical and objective approach to approving biosimilars pursuant to the BPCI Act of 2009. A historic snapshot points out that the Biologics Control Act was passed in 1902 to ensure purity and safety of serums, vaccines, and similar products used to prevent or treat diseases in humans, years before Congress passed the original Food and Drugs Act on June 30, 1906 (Figure 10.1). It is no wonder that the FDA has taken a major initiative over the past 107 years leading to providing a safe pathway for the approval of biological drugs coming off patent.

The term *biosimilarity* was coined after much debate, and more debates went on understanding the scope of the term. In describing it, the FDA has adopted a vocabulary that is just as interesting as it is instructional.

1. No one size fits all: The size refers to the scope of studies; the breadth and depth of studies, from the laboratory to patients, will always be molecule driven. So, do not expect the FDA to treat every application, even for the same molecule, similarly.
2. Totality of the evidence: The evidence pertains to identity, potency, safety, and purity (identity added by author). One would not do; all must conform.
3. No residual uncertainty: Residual is what is not clearly understood—there can be differences, but not those that could not be connected to potency, safety, and purity.
4. No clinically meaningful difference: *Clinically* refers to potency and safety; first correlate the CQAs to potency and safety and then justify differences.
5. Tier-based evaluation: Tiers range from not similar to fingerprint-like similar; the sponsor can maximally call its product similar. Also applies to the statistical evaluation of data, from Tier 1 to Tier 3.

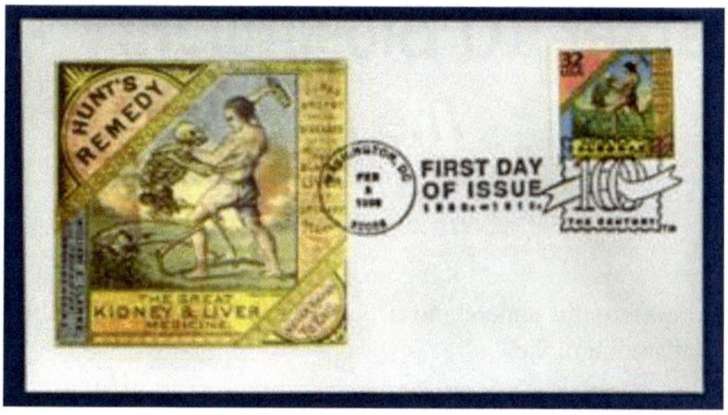

Figure 10.1 The U.S. Post Office recognized the 1906 Act as a landmark of the 20th century when it released this stamp, the design of which was based on a 19th-century patent medicine trading card.

10.2 Biosimilarity

This is the final judgmental call by the FDA, not by the sponsor, and it is based on the FDA, not the sponsor, to conclude that CQAs are highly similar. The sponsor can only label its submission as *similar*, and not claim it to be highly similar.

Biosimilarity is a description that a sponsor candidate product is indeed biosimilar. Note that *biosimilarity* means "biological response similarity," not "biological products that are similar." There is a fine defining line here. To assure that the biological response is similar, the sponsor has to demonstrate on a formal tier basis that starts with analytical and functional characterization of the biosimilar candidate, followed by any safety evaluations in nonclinical setting, where possible, and the required clinical pharmacology evaluation, at least at the level of PK and additionally, PD, where possible. For example, the FDA will require both PK and PD studies in healthy subjects for filgrastim, but only a PK study for adalimumab in healthy subjects, since the latter does not have a PD model in healthy subjects.

Clinical trials in patients are different from the trials conducted for new molecules. The focus in conducting patient trials of biosimilars is intended to demonstrate equivalent effectiveness (not efficacy) and safety. Figure 10.1 shows the interrelationship of these two attributes to the expectation of the FDA for new biologics. Note the subtle difference between effectiveness and efficacy. The efficacy of the products has already been established; the biosimilar sponsor is required to prove equal effectiveness if potency and content can be proven to be equivalent using analytical and functional similarity and, where a PD model does not exist, in limited trials in one sensitive indication.

The safety is proven in analytical and functional similarity testing and in clinical pharmacology studies or in the studies planned for demonstrating equivalent effectiveness (Figure 10.2).

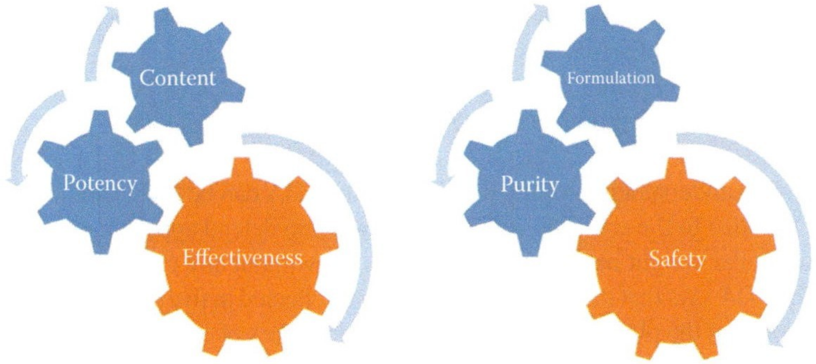

Figure 10.2 Dependency of effectiveness and safety of biosimilars.

10.3 No phase 3

Perhaps the most significant aspect of the FDA perspective on biosimilarity comes from a view that is diametrically opposed to what other regulatory agencies consider pivotal—the phase 3–type trials. Recently, agencies such as EMA have begun to take the same stance but with a lot of hesitation and without the FDA frankness in making decisions.

The biosimilar application for epoetin alfa was submitted by Hospira to the FDA on December 16, 2014. It was Hospira's first submission for a biosimilar in the United States and submitted as an abbreviated BLA. This product has been available in Europe since 2008 under the name *Retacrit* for the treatment of anemia associated with chronic renal failure. On its quarterly earnings call, Pfizer (now the owner of Hospira) revealed that the FDA has rejected Hospira's application. In securing approval in Europe, Hospira ran phase 3–type studies in thousands of patients and had a history of over 6 years of use in a large patient population, yet all of this was not enough to convince FDA; the lesson we learned is that phase 3 trials do not replace any residual uncertainty and a proof of clinical effectiveness does not overcome the tier-based biosimilarity assessment (http://www.bigmoleculewatch.com/2015/10/27/fda-rejects-hospiras-epogen-biosimilar/).

The reason why the FDA does not anticipate seeing any phase 3–type trials is based on several considerations:

- New drug approval requires demonstration of efficacy and adverse events for each indication, forming a basis for risk analysis; each indication requires a separate clinical trial.
- Biosimilar clinical testing will require NI testing against the reference, *not* the placebo, increasing the need for a larger population—the question, can one trial be sufficient to allow all other claims? arises.
- To allow all claims, the molecule must be highly similar to the reference molecule with no residual uncertainty, and that can

be readily established using analytical similarity studies and clinical pharmacology studies.

- A product that needs a trial in patients is likely a borderline biosimilar product, the Agency asserts.

A clear understanding of the mind-set of the FDA can be had from how it responded to the criticism as well as a lawsuit to defend approving a low–molecular weight heparin (LMWH) product without any clinical studies. The FDA says that this scientific approach is reflected in five criteria, which involve (a) the physical and chemical characteristics of enoxaparin, (b) the nature of the heparin material and the chemical process used to break up heparin chains into smaller pieces, (c) the nature and arrangement of components that constitute enoxaparin, (d) certain laboratory measurements of the product's anticoagulant activity, and (e) certain aspects of the drug's effect in humans. These five criteria ensure that a generic enoxaparin drug product will have the same effects as the brand name drug product when injected into a patient. Although the EMA guideline requires clinical studies to demonstrate comparable effectiveness to a similar LMWH, the FDA notes that its approach (i.e., the five criteria) is more sensitive to differences between two enoxaparin products than the clinical studies recommended in the EMA guideline are (http://www.fda.gov/Drugs/DrugSafety/Postmarketdrugsafetyinformationforpatientsandproviders/ucm220037.htm).

The most significant advice that I can offer to biosimilar sponsors is *not* to offer to do any phase 3–type studies unless specifically asked for by the FDA, in the review of data at the Type 3 meeting level. When the FDA tells you the design and scope of the study needs a review—you would know then that your application is weak.

If it takes a clinical study in patients to establish effectiveness, then it is not a good biosimilar product; clinical testing does not replace analytical similarity, the clinical pharmacology, and, where applicable, nonclinical evaluation.

10.4 Meeting the FDA

From the initial advisory meeting (which is free) to Type 4 meetings, the FDA has opened its doors for continued consultation with biosimilar developers; the sponsor must take advantage of these meetings regardless of how confident it feels about its product. There is no hearsay reliance on approvals given to others. Because of the stiff fee you will pay under BsUFA as shown in Table 10.1 for 2016, it pays to make use of these meetings. Know that if you fail to pay on a timely basis, you will have an automatic full clinical hold.

Notice the fee structure wherein a separate category of without clinical studies is provided, which simply asserts the mind-set of the FDA that

Table 10.1 The FDA BsUFA Fee Structure for 2016

Category	Stage/Type	Fee
BPD	Initial	$237,420
	Annual	$237,420
Application	With clinical studies	$2,374,200
	Without clinical studies	$1,187,100
Supplement	With clinical studies	$1,187,100
Product		$114,450
Establishment		$585,200
Reactivation		$474,840

Source: FDA, http://www.fda.gov/ForIndustry/UserFees/BiosimilarUserFeeActBsUFA/default.htm.

not all applications require a clinical trial—and that is one mind-set of the FDA that must be clear to all. Unfortunately, the biosimilar product industry is being populated with scientists and administrators from the big pharma, to whom the thought of getting a biological product approved without a massive clinical trial is unthinkable. If you take a look at ClinicalTrials.gov and figure out who is doing what, you will find that all deep-pocket sponsors still continue doing clinical trials; the argument in favor of clinical trials comes from the marketing teams, who still have to understand how to present their product to clinicians and other stakeholders without clinical trials.

The FDA has also released data on its workload in handling biosimilar applications (Table 10.2). It also provides its workload summary (Table 10.3). These data show us how the FDA sees the future of biosimilars approval, the competition in making, and how the FDA sees the workload to review these applications.

10.5 The future

In 2005, I wrote my first book on this subject and titled it *Handbook of Biogeneric Therapeutic Proteins*, hoping that *biogeneric* would stick—a subliminal message to regulatory agencies—it did not. Instead, we have the universally accepted *biosimilar*. However, only the FDA has created a category of interchangeable biosimilar products, which is quite akin to biogeneric, legal subtleties notwithstanding. A few years ago, "product by the process" was the mantra of the originator companies; that is blown away. A few years from today, all uncertainty about the safety and effectiveness of biosimilars will be gone, and the market for these products will take a more generic stance. However, given that the cost of regulatory filing with the FDA will remain high, there is not going to be a crowding of players in these markets. The FDA will continue to push the scientific envelope, and the sponsors of biosimilars who will

Table 10.2 Volume of Biosimilar Program Submissions and Applications

Category	FY13	FY14	FY15 (First 2 Quarters)	Total
Number of sponsors in the program (cumulative totals)	33	48	52	52
Biosimilar Application Review				
Original biosimilar product applications	0	2	3	5
Resubmitted original biosimilar product applications	0	0	0	0
Original supplements with clinical data	0	0	0	0
Resubmitted supplements with clinical data	0	0	0	0
Manufacturing supplements	0	0	0	0
Procedural Notifications				
Notification of issues identified during review	0	2	3	5
Notification of planned review timeline	0	2	3	5
Review of proprietary biosimilar product names (during BPD phase)	3	3	3	9
Review of proprietary biosimilar product names (with application)	0	1	4	5
Review of proprietary biosimilar product names (resubmitted or requests for reconsideration)	0	0	0	0
Procedural Responses				
Major dispute resolution	0	0	0	0
Responses to clinical holds	1	1	2	4
Special protocol assessments	0	2	1	3
Meeting Requests				
Biosimilar Initial Advisory	4	11	2	17
BPD Type 1	0	1	2	3
BPD Type 2	21	30	21	72
BPD Type 3	6	9	1	16
BPD Type 4	1	3	1	5
Scheduled Meetings				
Biosimilar Initial Advisory	3	9	2	14
BPD Type 1	0	1	2	3
BPD Type 2	20	25	19	64
BPD Type 3	6	9	1	16
BPD Type 4	1	3	1	5
Provided meeting minutes (all meeting types)	29	42	17	88

Source: FDA, http://www.fda.gov/downloads/forindustry/userfees/biosimilaruserfeeactbsufa/ucm459686.pdf.

Note: FY13: fiscal year 2013; FY14: fiscal year 2014; FY15: fiscal year 2015.

Table 10.3 Summary of Estimated Hours and Full-Time Equivalents (FTEs) by Cost Category and by Fiscal Year

Category	FY13	FY14	FY15 (First 2 Quarters Only)	Total
FTEs Estimated by Eastern Research Group, Inc. (ERG) for Biosimilar-Related Work				
IND, pre-IND, and BPD meetings	21.73	23.28	10.79	55.80
351(k) BLA review	0.00	0.95	11.79	12.75
Regular biosimilar-related meetings	3.56	2.90	2.15	8.62
Policy	8.96	8.42	6.31	23.69
Science and research	9.42	7.44	4.13	21.00
Outreach	0.00	0.00	1.29	1.29
CDER offices not covered by estimates above (provided by FDA)	10.95	11.02	21.40	43.37
FDA Office of the Commissioner[a]	12.98	13.43	11.41	37.82
Office of Regulatory Affairs (provided by FDA)	0.00	0.00	–	0.00
CBER (provided by FDA)	3.89	1.33	–	5.22
Total FTEs	70.99	68.90	70.93	210.83

Source: FDA, http://www.fda.gov/downloads/forindustry/userfees/biosimilaruserfeeactbsufa/ucm459686.pdf.

Note: FY13: fiscal year 2013; FY14: fiscal year 2014; FY15: fiscal year 2015.

[a] FTEs for fiscal years 2013 and 2014 for the FDA Office of the Commissioner were estimated based on the share of total FDA salary that the Office of the Commissioner represents. These percentages were 21.34% for fiscal year 2013 and 21.18% for fiscal year 2014. ERG used the fiscal year 2014 percentage for fiscal year 2015 since an estimate of the percentage for fiscal year 2015 is not yet available. These percentages were then applied to the sum of all CDER, CBER, and Office of Regulatory Affairs FTEs in this table.

emerge as winners will have sophisticated scientific abilities, more like the developers of new drugs.

The FDA perspective on biosimilarity will emerge with greater clarity as more complex molecules are approved as biosimilars; in all likelihood, the FDA will hold advisory meetings wherein much will be disclosed, and that will provide a more focused understanding that the biosimilar sponsors will find very useful.

So, stay tuned. The FDA has opened the doors to the most revolutionary modality of treatment of critical illnesses becoming affordable; the cost savings from these products will make the small-molecule generic industry a dwarf, The value to humankind will be immeasurable, if only we are able to pay attention to what the former Commissioner of the FDA, Dr. Margaret Hamburg, to whom this book is dedicated, said:

> Efforts to undermine trust in these [biosimilar] products are worrisome and represent a disservice to patients who could benefit from these lower-cost

treatments. (http://www.worldipreview.com/article/biosimilar-biologics-is-the-us-being-left-behind)

Bibliography

Bigmoleculewatch.com (2015, October 27) FDA rejects Hospira's epogen biosimilar. http://www.bigmoleculewatch.com/2015/10/27/fda-rejects-hospiras-epogen-biosimilar/.

Calvo, P. (2013, November 1). Biosimilar biologics: Is the US being left behind? *World IP Review*. http://www.worldipreview.com/article/biosimilar-biologics-is-the-us-being-left-behind.

FDA—Review of Biosimilar Biologic Product Applications. http://www.fda.gov/downloads/forindustry/userfees/biosimilaruserfeeactbsufa/ucm459686.pdf, 2015.

FDA—Postmarket Drug Safety Information for Patients and Providers. http://www.fda.gov/Drugs/DrugSafety/Postmarketdrugsafetyinformationforpatientsandproviders/ucm220037.htm, 2011.

FDA—Biosimilar User Fee Act (BsUFA). http://www.fda.gov/ForIndustry/UserFees/BiosimilarUserFeeActBsUFA/default.htm, 2015.

Index

Page numbers followed by f and t indicate figures and tables, respectively.

G

H

I

J

K

L

M

S

T

U

V